Recovery After Traumatic Brain Injury

Edited by

B. P. Uzzell
Memorial Neurological Association

and

Henry H. Stonnington
Memorial Medical Center

LEA

LAWRENCE ERLBAUM ASSOCIATES, PUBLISHERS
1996   Mahwah, New Jersey

Lawrence Erlbaum Associates, Inc., Publishers
10 Industrial Avenue
Mahwah, NJ 07430

Cover design by Semadar Megged

Library of Congress Cataloging-in-Publication Data

Recovery after traumatic brain injury / B. P. Uzzell and Henry H.
   Stonnington, editors.
       p.   cm.
   Includes bibliographical references and index.
   ISBN 0-8058-1823-5 (cloth : alk paper). — ISBN 0-8058-1824-3
(pbk. : alk. paper).
   1. Brain damage.   2. Brain damage—Patients—Rehabilitation.
I. Uzzell, Barbara P.   II. Stonnington, Henry H.
   [DNLM: 1. Brain Injuries—rehabilitation.   2. Brain Injuries
—complications.   3. Brain Injuries—physiopathology.   WL 354R3101
1996]
RC387.5.R37   1996
617.4'81044—dc20
DNLM/DLC
for Library of Congress   95-53004
                                                                    CIP

Books published by Lawrence Erlbaum Associates are printed on acid-free paper, and
their bindings are chosen for strength and durability.

Printed in the United States of America
10 9 8 7 6 5 4 3 2 1

Contents

Contributors

Carla Caetano, PhD
Neuropsychologist Center
  for the Rehabilitation
  of Brain Injury
University of Copenhagen
88 Njalsgade, DK 2300
Copenhagen, Denmark

Susanna Chang, MS
Department of Radiology (114M)
VAMC
2100 Ridgecrest Drive, SE
Albuquerque, NM 87108, USA

Anne-Lise Christensen, PhD
Professor and Director
Center for Rehabilitation
  of Brain Injury
University of Copenhagen
88 Njalsgade, DK 2300
Copenhagen, Denmark

D. Nathan Cope, MD
Senior Vice President,
  Medical Affairs
Paradigm Health Corporation
1001 Galaxy Way, Suite 412
Concord, CA 94520, USA

John D. Corrigan, PhD
Associate Professor
Department of Physical Medicine
  and Rehabilitation
The Ohio State University
480 West Ninth Avenue
Columbus, OH 43210, USA

Carolyn Curran, BBSc
Bethesda Hospital
30 Erin Street
Richmond, Victoria
Australia 3121

Ralph G. Dacey Jr., MD
Professor and Chair
Department of Neurosurgery
Washington University School of
  Medicine
Campus Box 8057
660 South Euclid Avenue
St. Louis, MO 63110-1093, USA

John T. Davis, PhD
Department of Radiology (114M)
VAMC
2100 Ridgecrest Drive, SE
Albuquerque, NM 87108, USA

W. Dalton Dietrich, PhD
Department of Neurology (D4-5)
University of Miami School
of Medicine
P.O. Box 016960
Miami, FL 33101, USA

Joshua L. Dowling, MD
Department of Neurosurgery
Washington University School of
Medicine
Campus Box 8057660
South Euclid Avenue
St. Louis, MO 63110-1093, USA

Chris Edgar, BA
Department of Radiology (114M)
VAMC
2100 Ridgecrest Drive, SE
Albuquerque, NM 87108, USA

Janet E. Farmer, PhD
Assistant Professor
Physical Medicine
and Rehabilitation
University of Missouri—
Columbia School
of Medicine
2R01 Rusk Rehabilitation Center
One Hospital Drive
Columbia, MO 65212, USA

Marcus J. Fuhrer, PhD
Director, National Center
for Medical Rehabilitation and
Research
National Institute of Child Health
and Human Development
Executive Building / Room 2A03
6100 Executive Boulevard MSC
7510
Bethesda, MD 20892-7510, USA

D. M. Hadley, MB, PhD
MRI Unit
Institute of Neurological Sciences
Southern General Hospital
Glasgow, Scotland

A. Harper, BA
Institute of Neurological Sciences
Southern General Hospital
Glasgow, Scotland

Blaine Hart, MD
Department of Radiology (114M)
VAMC
2100 Ridgecrest Drive, SE
Albuquerque, NM 87108, USA

Dina Hill, BA
Department of Radiology (114M)
VAMC
2100 Ridgecrest Drive, SE
Albuquerque, NM 87108, USA

Brick Johnstone, PhD
Director, Division of Health
Psychology and
Neuropsychology
Department of Physical Medicine
and Rehabilitation
University of Missouri—
Columbia
2R01 Rusk Rehabilitation Center
Columbia, MO 65212, USA

Zvi Kalisky, MD
Del Oro Institute
for Rehabilitation
Spring Branch Medical Center
and Baylor College
of Medicine
1501 Pech
Houston, TX 77054

Yoichi Katayama, MD, PhD
Professor and Head
Department of Neurological
Surgery
Nihon University School
of Medicine
30 Oyaguchi Kamimachi
Itabashi-Ku, Tokyo 173, Japan

Tatsuro Kawamata, MD, PhD
Assistant Professor
Department of Neurological
Surgery
Nihon University School
of Medicine
30 Oyaguchi Kamimachi
Itabashi-Ku, Tokyo 173, Japan

P. W. Kodituwakku, PhD
Department of Radiology (114M)
VAMC
2100 Ridgecrest Drive, SE
Albuquerque, NM 87108, USA

Bryan Kolb, PhD
Professor
Department of Psychology
The University of Letbridge
4401 University Drive
Lethbridge, AB, Canada T1K 3M4

Fred Krause, PhD
International Brain Injury
Association, Inc.
P.O. Box 18667
Washington, DC 20036-8667, USA

Jeffrey David Lewine, PhD
Scientific Director, Magnetic
Source Imaging Facility
Department of Radiology (114M)
VAMC
2100 Ridgecrest Drive, SE
Albuquerque, NM 87108, USA

Warren E. Lux, MD
Associate Professor
of Neurology
Washington University School of
Medicine
216 South Kingshighway
St. Louis, MO 63110, USA

Bruce E. Murdoch, PhD
Director, Motor Speech Research
Unit
The University of Queensland
Brisbane, Queensland 4072,
Australia

John H. Olver, MBBS
Bethesda Hospital
30 Erin Street
Richmond, Victoria
Australia 3121

William W. Orrison, MD
Department of Radiology (114M)
VAMC
2100 Ridgecrest Drive, SE
Albuquerque, NM 87108, USA

Jennie L. Ponsford, PhD
Chief Psychologist
Bethesda Hospital
30 Erin Street
Richmond, Victoria
Australia 3121

Gitte Rasmussen, MS
Registered Physical Therapist
Center for the Rehabilitation of
Brain Injury
University of Copenhagen
88 Njalsgade DK 2300
Copenhagen, Denmark

J. Scott Richards, PhD
National Center for Medical
  Rehabilitation Research
National Institute of Child Health
  and Human Development
Executive Building / Room 2A03
6100 Executive Boulevard MSC
  7510
Bethesda, MD 20892-7510

L. C. Scott, BA
Department of Psychological
  Medicine
University of Wales College
  of Medicine
Heath Park
Cardiff CF4 4XN, United
  Kingdom

Pat Shaw, BA, RN
Department of Radiology (114M)
VAMC
2100 Ridgecrest Drive, SE
Albuquerque, NM 87108, USA

John Henry Sloan, MD
Department of Radiology (114M)
VAMC
2100 Ridgecrest Drive, SE
Albuquerque, NM 87108, USA

Jon Spar, MD
Department of Radiology (114M)
VAMC
2100 Ridgecrest Drive, SE
Albuquerque, NM 87108, USA

**Henry H. Stonnington, MBBS,
  FRCP(E)**
Medical Director
Memorial Rehabilitation Center
Provident Office Bldg.
4750 Waters Avenue, Suite 307
Savannah, GA 31404, USA

Renée Stucky-Ropp, MA
Department of Psychology
University of Missouri-Columbia
Columbia, MO 65211, USA

J. Sherrod Taylor, JD
Law Offices of Taylor, Harp and
  Callier
P.O. Box 2645
Columbus, GA 31902-2645, USA

Robert Thoma, BA
Department of Radiology (114M)
VAMC
2100 Ridgecrest Drive, SE
Albuquerque, NM 87108, USA

Takashi Tsubokawa, MD, MDSc
Professor
Department of Neurologial
  Surgery
Nihon University School
  of Medicine
30 Oyaguchi Kamimachi
Itabashi-Ku, Tokyo 173, Japan

B. P. Uzzell, PhD
Associate Professor
Baylor College of Medicine
University of Texas Health
  Science Center
Memorial Neurological
  Association
7777 Southwest Freeway, Suite
  900
Houston, TX 77074, USA

V. Ann Waldorf, MS
Department of Radiology (114M)
VAMC
2100 Ridgecrest Drive, SE
Albuquerque, NM 87108, USA

Paul Wehman, PhD
Professor of Physical Medicine &
  Rehabilitation
Rehabilitation Research
  and Training Center
Virginia Commonwealth
  University
1314 West Main Street
Box 842011
Richmond, VA 23284-2011 USA

J. T. Lindsay Wilson, PhD
Department of Psychology
University of Stirling
Stirling FK9 4LA, Scotland

Atsuo Yoshino, MD, PhD
Assistant Professor
Department of Neurological
  Surgery
Nihon University School
  of Medicine
30 Oyaguchi Kaminachi
Itabashi-Ku, Tokyo 173, Japan

Nathan D. Zasler, MD
Executive Medical Director
National NeuroRehabilitation
  Consortium, Inc.
4198 Innslake Drive
Glen Allen, VA 23060, USA

Introduction

B. P. Uzzell
Henry H. Stonnington

Emotions, behaviors, thoughts, creations, planning, daily physical activities and routines are programmed within our brains. To acquire these capacities, the brain takes time to fully develop. This development goes far beyond the in utero stages, and may take the first 20 years of life. Disruptions of the brain involving neurons, axons, dendrites, synapses, neurotransmitters, or brain infrastructure (such as glial cells, trophic chemicals, circulation, and CSF) produce profound changes in development and functions of the one organ that makes us unique—the organ that gives us our personality and intelligence. Trauma to this organ can and does change us. To understand the functions and development of the brain is difficult enough, but to reverse the consequences of trauma and repair the damage is even more challenging. To meet this challenge and increase understanding, a host of disciplines working and communicating together is required.

Opportunities for transdisciplinary communications among individuals concerned with the brain are sometimes limited. The International Association for the Study of Traumatic Brain Injury (IASTBI) tried to correct this limitation during its meetings of international clinicians, researchers, and scientists from many fields. The most recent IASTBI conference, in St. Louis in September 1994, was no exception to this goal. Our friend, John Doronzo, PhD, was one of the organizers of this conference. Unfortunately, he was unable to attend due to his untimely death. He was enthusiastic, knowledgeable, and dedicated, and we miss him. We would also like to acknowledge the assistance of the Health South Corporation in making possible the conference, where ideas about brain injury could be freely exchanged.

It was felt that many of the outstanding ideas and thoughts from that meeting and from others working in the field of traumatic brain injury

1

(TBI) should be shared in written communication. Hence, this book was conceived not as proceedings of the conference—because several chapters of this book were written by individuals who were not speakers at the conference—but as a collection of knowledge for those working in the acute and chronic recovery aspects of head injury. Although the contents of this book do not attempt to be all encompassing, important aspects are addressed with current knowledge.

Part I of this book begins with methods used to improve diagnosis and management of head injury. Jeffrey David Lewine and associates (chap. 1) describe a methodology, namely the neuromagnetic evaluation of head-injured patients. Modern radiology has made significant advances in defining how to treat and prognosticate various types of brain injuries. J. T. Lindsay Wilson and colleagues (chap. 2) remind us of this methodology in correlating neuropsychological data in mild head injury with magnetic resonance imaging (MRI) findings. Joshua L. Dowling and Ralph G. Dacey Jr. (chap. 3) select an aspect of neurosurgery dealing with subarachnoid hemorrhage.

Intervention and prevention of complications are approached both from a basic science point of view with Yoichi Katayama and associates' (chap. 4) explanation of the role of excitatory amino acids and W. Dalton Dietrich's (chap. 5) reduction in morbidity in hypothermic rats. Takashi Tsubokawa (chap. 6) discusses his extensive experience in awakening patients who have been in persistent vegetative states using deep electrical brain stimulation. An area used more and more by rehabilitation practitioners to improve behavior, cognition, and neurological recovery of awake patients is neuropharmacology. Warren E. Lux (chap. 7) reviews the many ways to manipulate neurotransmitters, and shows the evidence for and against various pharmacological agents.

Part II of this book addresses clinical states after head injury. Brick Johnstone and Ty S. Callahan (chap. 8) provocatively discuss neuropsychological measurements in relation to rehabilitation in the United States. John D. Corrigan (chaps. 9 and 10) deals with problems of agitation and substance abuse after head injuries. He demonstrates how to accurately measure and manage agitation. Zvi Kalisky and B. P. Uzzell (chap. 11) provide fascinating examples of patients with florid confabulations. Bruce E. Murdoch (chap. 12) describes in detail outstanding research and its application to clinical aspects of motoric speech disorders. Nathan D. Zasler (chap. 13) reviews ethics, controversies, and definitions associated with persistent vegetative states, providing a point of view endorsed by many.

No book devoted to head injury would be complete without timing and outcome measurements, which are discussed in Part III. Rehabilitation depends on plasticity of the nervous system, and timing is important in integrating rehabilitation procedures with evolving plasticity. Early intervention is vital. Bryan Kolb (chap. 14) shows how plasticity works, as well as its limitations and developmental aspects. Outcome measurements are internationally presented from Australia and Denmark, respectively, by Jennie L. Ponsford (chap. 15) and Anne-Lise Christensen (chap. 16) and their respective colleagues. These chapters contain measures of social behavioral and community reintegration, as well as other aspects of life. Marcus J. Fuhrer and J. Scott Richards (chap. 17) review the past and provide direction for medical rehabilitation outcomes in the future. Work return is most important for the head-injured survivor; many professionals and family members view it as the ultimate successful outcome. Work reentry with supportive employment is described by Paul Wehman (chap. 18).

Part IV of this book is broad, including both family and community (which can be thought of as extended family) concerns. TBI has consequences far beyond the individual. How families are affected and how school reentry is accomplished are described by Janet E. Farmer and Renée Stucky-Ropp (chap. 19). As documented by Fred Krause (chap. 20), organizations such as the National Head Injury Foundation (NHIF), developed in the United States by families, demonstrate their strength in information dissemination and assistance in creating resources devoted to the care of their head-injured relatives. With managed health care both in the United States and elsewhere, there is a need to understand it better. D. Nathan Cope (chap. 21) describes an innovative type of managed care. On occasion, head injury is followed by litigation. J. Sherrod Taylor (chap. 22) describes the medicolegal aspects, as well as the importance of making an attorney a member of the rehabilitation team. A concluding chapter (chap. 23) focuses on summarizing and speculating about various points of view.

This book contains a wide variety of subjects, some of which are controversial and innovative. It is designed to be thought provoking. Chapters are of interest not only to professionals such as neurosurgeons; neurologists; case managers; psychologists; physiatrists, physical, occupational, speech, and recreational therapists; nurses; and educators but also for those who care for head-injured survivors changed by brain damage, family members who are significantly affected by those changes, and community members who are involved, including attorneys. We hope this book will help readers to rethink their ideas and stimulate them to come up with their own innovative methodologies and activities, advancing the future case of survivors and their families.

I

Diagnoses and Management

1

Neuromagnetic Evaluation of Brain Dysfunction in Postconcussive Syndromes Associated with Mild Head Trauma

Jeffrey David Lewine
William W. Orrison, Jr.
John T. Davis
Blaine Hart
Jon Spar
P. W. Kodituwakku
Dina Hill
Susanna Chang
V. Ann Waldorf
Pat Shaw
Chris Edgar
John Henry Sloan

In the United States alone, more than 2 million people suffer head traumas each year. Twenty-five percent of these cases require hospitalization, with 70,000–90,000 of the survivors demonstrating many of the chronic sequalae of traumatic brain injury (TBI; Department of Health and Human Services, 1989). The annual economic cost in the United States for the treatment of head trauma victims exceeds $25 billion, yet relatively little funding is available for the development of better diagnostic tools and efficient rehabilitation programs. Nevertheless, the "decade of the brain" has witnessed several advances in the diagnosis and treatment of trauma victims. Following a brief discussion of the uses of traditional brain imaging techniques in the evaluation of trauma, this chapter focuses on recent advances in the neuromagnetic evaluation of TBI.

STRUCTURAL BRAIN IMAGING

In the acute clinical evaluation of head trauma, rapid application of structural neuroimaging methods such as magnetic resonance imaging (MRI) or computed tomography (CT) is imperative for assessment of life-threatening situations. These methods provide detailed structural data on the skull and soft tissues of the brain. Acute neuroanatomical sequalae of significant head trauma may include skull fractures, extra-axial and intra-parenchymal hemorrhages, brain contusions, edema, ventricular dilation, and shearing injuries of the white matter (Fong, Teal, & Hieshima, 1984; Gentry, Godersky, Thompson, & Dunn, 1988). Head trauma may also cause gradual cell death, which can manifest as focal regions of encephalomalacia or diffuse brain atrophy (Fong et al., 1984; Gentry et al., 1988; Reider-Groswasser, Cohen, Costeff, & Groswasser, 1993).

For patients who survive TBIs, the long-term behavioral sequalae of head trauma may include pain, fatigue, attentional deficits, erratic mood swings, and mnemonic difficulties (Levin, Benton, & Grossman, 1982). In patients who have suffered severe head trauma, these behavioral symptoms can often be traced to specific structural changes. However, many individuals suffer significant postconcussive syndromes following mild head injuries that do not cause gross changes in brain structure. In cases with positive neuropsychological deficits, but negative neuro-radiological examination by CT and MRI, the situation is particularly problematic when it comes to: (a) diagnosing, (b) predicting long-term outcome, (c) deciding among therapeutic alternatives, and (d) making decisions about an individual's fitness to return to work. Indeed, it is not uncommon for many patients with psychological deficits subsequent to minor trauma to remain undiagnosed, or to be misdiagnosed as having a naturally occurring psychiatric illness (Lishman, 1988).

FUNCTIONAL BRAIN IMAGING

Given the relative inability of structural neurodiagnostic techniques (e.g., MRI and CT) to identify the neural consequences of mild head trauma, many clinical research centers have begun to explore the abilities of non-invasive functional procedures in this regard. Traditional techniques of interest include electroencephalography (EEG), single photon emission computed tomography (SPECT), and positron emission tomography (PET).

EEG measures the electrical activity of the brain through metal electrodes attached to the scalp surface. EEG is well documented to be useful in the assessment of severe head injury (Bauer, 1987; Rodin, 1967). For example, in comatose patients, analyses of the frequency and amplitude of the EEG, combined with an assessment of the reactivity of the EEG to external stimuli, provide insight into the depth of coma and the possibility of brain death. In patients who recover from coma, EEG techniques can be especially useful in long-term follow-up evaluation, and in the assessment of posttraumatic epilepsy, which develops in a percentage of trauma cases (Courjon, 1972; Jennet, 1975). Related EEG techniques for recording multimodality-evoked potentials are also useful, especially in the prognostic evaluation of cases with severe head injury (Greenberg, Newlon, Hyatt, Narayan, & Becker, 1981). Unfortunately, the diagnostic utility of EEG techniques in cases of mild head trauma has yet to be established. Even in cases with significant postconcussive neuropsychological changes, EEG only occasionally reveals epileptiform activity or slowing of normal spontaneous background rhythms—an abnormal EEG is the exception, not the rule (Courjon, 1972; Fisch, 1991). Advanced EEG techniques involving topographic mapping and quantitative and statistical evaluation of EEG power spectra are under development. At present, the sensitivity and specificity of these methods of analysis are low.

Metabolic and hemodynamic techniques such as SPECT and PET are beginning to show considerable promise in the evaluation of mild head trauma. However, both of these techniques are semi-invasive, each involving exposure to radioactive materials. In a recent series of studies by Reid and colleagues, HMPAO-SPECT was used to demonstrate that low cerebral perfusion is common in many cases of mild TBI, and that reduced perfusion soon after injury may be predictive of subsequent development of postconcussive headaches (Reid, Gulenchyn, Ballinger, & Ventureyra, 1990). In many cases, SPECT abnormalities are focal, with the locations consistent with expectations based on neuropsychological testing (Wiedmann, Wilson, Wyper, & Hadley, 1989).

A recent study by Ruff and colleagues (1994) suggested that the sensitivity of PET to the subtle consequences of mild head trauma is extremely high, with each of the study's nine patients demonstrating PET abnormalities. Other PET studies have also demonstrated a high degree of sensitivity in head trauma, although the specificity of the abnormal findings remains to be determined (Langfitt, Obrist, Alavi, & Grossman, 1986; Rao, Turski, Polcyn, & Nickels, 1984; Ruff, Buchsbaum, & Troster, 1989).

MAGNETIC SOURCE IMAGING—BASIC PRINCIPLES

The newest addition to the diagnostic armamentarium for evaluating neural consequences of head trauma is magnetic source imaging (MSI)—a technique that integrates functional information from magnetoencephalography (MEG) with structural data from MRI. MEG is similar to EEG in that it provides a direct measurement of the brain's electrophysiological activity, although it is based on slightly different biophysical principles (Lewine, 1990; Lewine & Orrison, 1994).

Just as current flow within a power line generates a surrounding magnetic field, current flow within brain cells generates a surrounding neuromagnetic field. The direction of the field is given by the "right hand rule." When the thumb of the right hand is pointing in the direction of current flow, the fingers of the hand curl in the direction of the surrounding magnetic field. Because of biophysical considerations, magnetic fields detectable outside of the head mostly reflect intracellular current flow within the apical dendrites of pyramidal cells, which are oriented parallel to the skull surface.

The extracranial magnetic field generated by activity in a single neuron is negligible, so many thousands of nearby cells must be synchronously active to produce a detectable signal. Still, even the largest neuromagnetic signals (those associated with epileptic spikes) are more than 1 billion times smaller than the earth's steady magnetic field and magnetic noise generated by even distant electrical equipment (e.g., computers, room lights) and moving metal objects (e.g., elevators, automobiles). The detection and isolation of neuromagnetic signals is hence a challenging problem. In many respects, measuring neuromagnetic signals is like trying to listen for the footsteps of an ant in the middle of a rock concert. The signals are very small, and the background noise is nearly overwhelming.

Magnetic fields are measured using induction coils made of wire loops. When a time-varying magnetic field passes through a wire loop, it induces a current within the loop. Because neuromagnetic fields are so small, most biomagnetometers use detection coils made of niobium wire. When immersed in a liquid helium bath at $-269°C$, niobium becomes superconducting (i.e., it loses its electrical resistivity). This allows small magnetic fields to induce significant currents that are not quickly dissipated as heat.

The detection coil is inductively coupled to a superconducting quantum interference device (SQUID). The SQUID acts as a low-noise, high-gain, current-to-voltage converter. The detailed physics of how SQUIDs operate are beyond the scope of this chapter (but see Lewine & Orrison, 1994). Suffice it to say that the SQUID, in conjunction with the superconducting detection coil, provides the system with the required sensitivity for detecting neuromagnetic signals.

External magnetic noise is a significant problem in neuromagnetic experiments. Two technological developments are employed to deal with this. The system is generally operated in a magnetically shielded room. Just as different materials have differing electrical resistivities, different materials have differing magnetic permeabilities. The magnetically shielded room is partly made of a high-permeability material known as mu-metal. The permeability of air is 1, whereas that of mu-metal is 80,000. External magnetic fields that impinge on the room mostly flow through the high-permeability walls of the chamber (around and away from the internally located sensor), rather than entering into the air-filled room. The typical shielded room provides a shielding factor of about 10,000. This amount of shielding is necessary for typical neuromagnetic experiments, but it is not sufficient.

One solution to the noise problem is use of a detector configured with two linked coil loops wound in opposite directions. In particular, most systems employ axial first-order gradiometers where the two loops are situated one above the other, with 5-cm separation (Fig. 1.1). In this gradiometer configuration, the total current flowing in the detection circuit reflects the difference in the magnetic field at the two coil locations. The magnetic field of an electric current decreases rapidly with increasing distance from the source (as a function of the square of the distance or higher, dependent on the exact current configuration). Near a magnetic source, the gradient of the magnetic field is steep. For example, the magnetic field at 6 cm is less than 3% of the field at only 1 cm. Far from a source, the gradient of the magnetic field is shallow. The

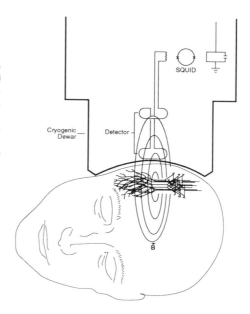

FIG. 1.1. Current flow within neurons (not drawn to scale) generates a surrounding magnetic field (B). Time variations in this field lead to the induction of currents within the niobium wire loops of the detector. The upper and lower loops are wound in opposite directions so that the net-induced current reflects the spatial gradient of the magnetic field. The detector is inductively coupled to a superconducting quantum interference device (SQUID). The detector and SQUID are contained within a cryogenic Dewar filled with liquid helium.

magnetic field at 1,006 cm is more than 99% of that at 1,001 cm. Hence, near the source, the output of the gradiometer is high (the two coils experience very different fields); far from the source, the output of the gradiometer is small even if the overall field strength at each coil is high. Consequently, the gradiometer is sensitive to magnetic signals generated by neurons a few centimeters below the sensor, but insensitive to magnetic fields generated by hospital equipment several meters outside of the shielded room. The output of the sensor unit is a time-varying voltage waveform that reflects local changes in magnetic flux as a function of time. These waveforms look similar to EEG signals that reflect time-varying changes in the scalp's electrical potential. There are several neuromagnetic signals of interest. For example, the various spontaneous brain rhythms well described in EEG (e.g., the alpha rhythm) are also seen in MEG. MEG is especially useful in the detection of several types of abnormal signals, including abnormal slow waves and epileptic spikes.

To date, the most extensive clinical experiments have been done using the 37-channel detector system of Biomagnetic Technologies incorporated (BTi; Fig. 1.2), although other large array systems by BTi and other manufacturers (e.g., Neuromag Ltd., CTF Inc.) are obtaining increased

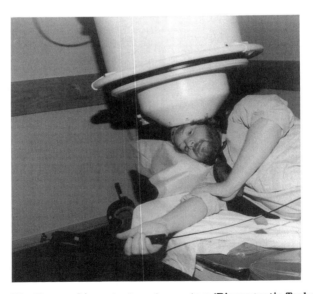

FIG. 1.2.   The Magnes biomagnetometer system (Biomagnetic Technologies Inc.) contains 37 first-order axial gradiometers of the type diagrammed in Fig. 1.1. The Dewar unit is easily positioned over regions of interest.

clinical exposure. In many biomagnetic experiments, the question of interest is identification of brain regions involved in processing specific types of sensory information. Signal averaging techniques are useful in this endeavor because they allow for isolation of time-locked information-processing signals. For example, consider a typical somatosensory mapping experiment. Here, a mechanical stimulus is repeatedly applied to one of the fingers of the hand (or an electrical stimulus is applied to the median nerve underlying the wrist) while signals are recorded over the contralateral parietal lobe. Epochs of neuromagnetic data spanning the stimulus event are averaged. Most of the activity in each epoch is unrelated to processing the sensory stimulus. However, a small portion of the signal does reflect activation of primary somatosensory cortex. The timing of this activation, relative to stimulus presentation, is relatively constant from trial to trial because of the fixed length of the neural conduction pathway from the finger to the brain. When the data epochs are averaged, the time-locked activity can be extracted from the background noise. Similar strategies can be used to evaluate auditory, visual, and motor organization.

During an experiment, a three-dimensional digitizer is used to define the exact spatial position of the detector coils within a head-centered coordinate frame. At each instant in time, the spatial pattern of the magnetic field is defined, providing critical information for localizing brain regions of interest.

The magnetic field that a prespecified neuronal current produces at a particular sensor location outside of the head can be exactly specified using Maxwell's equations and the Biot–Savart law. Unfortunately, the inverse problem of specifying the neuronal currents that generate a measured magnetic field pattern is ill posed because there are many intracranial configurations of current that all produce the same extracranial magnetic field pattern. The inverse problem can only be made mathematically tractable by making certain assumptions about the shape of the head and the nature of the underlying current configuration. Computer algorithms can be used to infer the location of the relevant activity.

The most common model used in the analysis of neuromagnetic data is that of a "dipole in a sphere." This model makes two fundamental assumptions: (a) the head can be modeled as a spherically symmetric volume conductor, and (b) the recorded magnetic field can be modeled as if it were generated by a point-source, current dipole. The spherical assumption is not really essential to the calculations; it is clearly correct only as a first-order approximation, but greatly simplifies the mathematics of inverse modeling. Realistic deviations from sphericity appear to generate only minimal errors in source modeling, except at anterior temporal regions where source location errors of more than 1 cm may be introduced. The assumption that the magnetic field pattern of interest can be modeled as if it were produced by a current dipole is important to making the inverse strategy tractable. Basically, the dipole provides a simplified biophysical representation of the actual currents that generate the recorded signal. The dipole model is only valid when the key neuronal currents are associated with the focal activation of a small cortical region, so one must be careful not to use this model in situations where it is not justified.

Given the previously discussed model, it is possible to employ computer algorithms that identify the location, orientation, and strength of the dipole that best accounts (in a statistical sense) for the measured magnetic field pattern. These algorithms work as follows. A dipole is hypothesized to exist at a particular position, orientation, and strength within the conductive volume, and the Biot–Savart law is used to forward calculate the magnetic signal that this hypothetical dipole would generate at each of the detectors. At each detector, the difference between the forward calculated signal and the actually measured signal is determined. The value of this mismatch term is squared and summated across all of the detectors to generate an overall error term. A new dipole is then postulated at a different position, and its error term calculated. Using iterative minimization procedures, the computer algorithm continues to hypothesize dipoles until it determines the position, orientation, and strength of the dipole that provides the smallest error term. The position, orientation, and strength of this "best-fitting" dipole are then taken as indicative of the position, orientation, and strength of the relevant neuronal currents (Fig. 1.3).

In considering the validity of the dipole model, it is important to avoid confusing the model (a dipole) with that which is being modeled (a complex pattern of neuronal currents). Provided that the external neuromagnetic field mostly reflects activation of a single cortical region, and provided that the spatial extent of the active region is small relative to the distance to the detector coil, localization of the best-fitting dipole provides for excellent localization of the activated region. However, if multiple, separated cortical regions simultaneously make significant contributions to the field pattern and a single-dipole model is used erroneously, the dipole solution will fail to accurately characterize the neuronal activity. Fortunately, in most of these cases, visual inspection of isofield contour maps, coupled with evaluation of the correlation between the dipole model and the field measurements, make it possible to recognize when the dipole model is inappropriate. Another limitation of the dipole model is seen when neuromagnetic signals of interest are generated by activity of an extended cortical sheet several square centimeters in area. Extended sheets often produce a dipolar-appearing magnetic field pattern. When a single-dipole model is used to describe this type of activity, the dipole may be erroneously localized deep into the white matter below the actual cortical site of activity. These partly inaccurate localizations may still provide useful diagnostic information on the hemisphere and lobe of the critical activity.

Given this, investigators must identify those circumstances under which the dipole model may be validly applied. Available empirical data indicate that the dipole model can be appropriately applied to neuromagnetic signals generated by the primary cortical regions involved in motor, somatosensory, and auditory processing. The model is also valid for the characterization of some epileptic spikes, sharp waves, and paroxysmal slow waves.

The head-centered MEG coordinate system in which dipole locations are specified is defined by left and right preauricular points and the nasion (located at the bridge of the nose). These fiducials are readily identified on MRIs. Using appropriate computer algorithms, it is possible to align MEG and MRI coordinate frames so that MEG sources can be plotted directly on the relevant anatomical images. The resulting magnetic source localization images provide graphic details on the spatial relationships among brain structure, function, and pathology.

APPLICATIONS: FUNCTIONAL MAPPING

The most common clinical use of MEG is in presurgical localization of functional brain regions (Benzel, Lewine, Bucholz, & Orrison, 1993). The central sulcus is the anatomical division between the precentral motor cortex and the postcentral somatosensory cortex. In normal subjects, this prominent sulcus can often be easily identified in MRIs. However, in neurosurgical patients with neoplasms and vascular malformations, the local neuroanatomy is often so distorted that the central sulcus cannot be identified. This is a significant problem because the possibility of a surgically induced hemiparalysis is considered a major risk for these patients. In many cases, surgeons are unwilling to perform these operations because hemiparalysis would significantly compromise the quality of a person's life. A short life without hemiparalysis is considered preferable to a longer life with hemiparalysis. Recent work with MEG indicates that neuromagnetic methods allow for accurate localization of sensorimotor cortex, even in the presence of significant structural pathology. Typically, a median nerve, somatosensory-evoked response is used to localize the somatosensory cortex, and a motor-evoked response associated with thumb movement is used to localize the motor cortex.

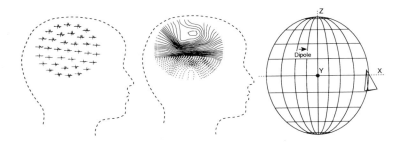

FIG. 1.3.   Each of the 37 channels measures time-varying changes in magnetic flux. The leftmost panel shows an averaged somatosensory-evoked signal. The vertical line in each trace represents the time of signal onset, a
mechanical tap delivered to the contralateral index finger. Waveforms show a
significant change in the magnetic field pattern at about 40 ms post-
stimulus. The middle panel shows an isofield contour map at the time of
maximal response. This map provides information on the spatial pattern of
the magnetic field. Solid lines indicate emerging flux, dashed lines indicate
entering flux. The field pattern is highly dipolar (characterized by single
regions of exiting and entering flux). The rightmost panel shows the location
of the best-fitting dipole source. It is located approximately midway between
the regions of maximal entering and exiting flux.

Figure 1.4 illustrates data from one of these critical cases. The patient
was a 58-year-old male with a high-grade astrocytoma resistant to both
chemo- and radiation therapy. From MRI, it is very difficult to determine
if sulcus "A" or "B" is the central sulcus. Several neuroradiologists examining the full set of this patient's sagittal, axial, and coronal MRIs
indicated that sulcus "B" was most likely the central sulcus. If this interpretation is correct, the tumor invades sensorimotor cortex, and it is not
unusual that three different neurosurgeons refused to operate on this
patient. After reading about the utility of MEG in an Arkansas news-
paper, the patient went to the Magnetic Source Imaging Facility at the
Albuquerque VA Medical Center, where a presurgical mapping examination was performed. The MEG data indicated sulcus "A" to be the
central sulcus. The patient was taken to surgery, where intraoperative
evaluation of the somatosensory-evoked potential and intraoperative
stimulation of the cortex confirmed that somatosensory and motor cortices were anterior to the tumor. The tumor was removed without induction of motor deficits.

   This type of functional mapping study also has utility in examining
how the brain compensates and reorganizes in response to injury. To
date, most of the work in this area has focused on reorganization in
response to stroke (Lewine et al., 1994), although applications in trauma
are beginning to be explored. Figures 1.5 and 1.6 show data from a case

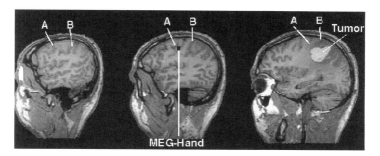

FIG. 1.4. Data are from a 58-year-old male with a rapidly growing astrocytoma. From MRI it is difficult to tell whether sulcus "A" or "B" demarcates
the sensorimotor region. MEG data obtained in response to stimulation of
the median nerve demonstrate that the hand representation of sensorimotor
cortex (indicated by the black square) is along sulcus "A." The tumor was
removed without inducing motor impairments. (From "Magnetic Source Imaging: A Review of the Magnes System by Biomagnetic Technologies Inc." by
E. C. Benzel, J. D. Lewine, R. Bucholz, and W. W. Orrison, 1993, *Neurosurgery, 33.* Adapted with permission.)

of neonatal stroke; these help illustrate how extensive brain reorganization can be. The patient was a 22-year-old male who suffered an infarct of
the left middle cerebral artery (LMCA) at approximately 1 month of age.
This caused loss of the entire left hemisphere territories supplied by the
LMCA, including primary and secondary somatosensory cortex. Despite
this massive loss of cortical tissue, the subject has an IQ only slightly
below normal, and he graduated from high school. He has reasonably
good language skills, and has fairly good somatosensation on the right
side of the body. Electrical stimulation of the left median nerve produced a
completely normal pattern of activity in the intact right hemisphere. This
was characterized by sequential activation of primary (SI) and secondary
(SII) somatosensory cortices (Fig. 1.5). Stimulation of the right median
nerve produced a very abnormal pattern of activation characterized by
early activity of inferior left temporal cortex and later activation of a
midline right parietal area (Fig. 1.6). These data indicate extensive brain
reorganization, some of which must have taken place at the thalamic
level, which is the only route via which somatosensory information could
reach the left temporal lobe in the requisite time frame (40 ms).

APPLICATIONS: EPILEPSY

Another major application of MEG technology is in the characterization
of epilepsy, especially in cases where other neuroimaging modalities fail
to provide conclusive data on the location of the epileptogenic zone

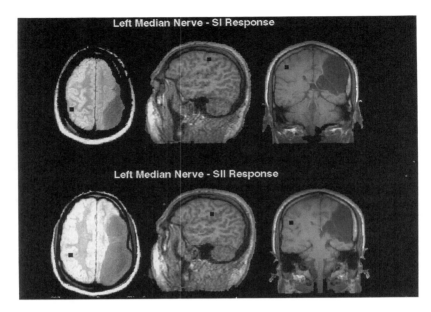

FIG. 1.5. Data are from a 22-year-old male who suffered a neonatal infarct of the left middle cerebral artery at approximately 1 month of age. Most of the brain tissue of the left hemisphere has been replaced by a porencephalic cyst. Stimulation of the left median nerve evokes sequential activation of primary (SI) and sencondary (SII) somatosensory cortex of the right hand, as indicated by the black boxes. (From "Cortical Organization in Adulthood Is Modified by Neonatal Infarct: A Case Study" by J. D. Lewine et al., 1994, *Radiology, 190.* Adapted with permission.)

(Lewine et al., 1994). Posttraumatic epilepsy is a common problem following moderate to severe trauma. For a proportion of these cases, seizures do not respond to medication, thus surgery is considered an option (provided that the region of pathology can be specified). Unfortunately, in many posttraumatic cases, neuroimaging by MRI and SPECT reveals multiple structural and metabolic abnormalities, and it is difficult to determine the primary source of the epilepsy. Because MEG provides good spatial and temporal resolution of brain activity, identification of epileptic trigger zones and pathways of propagation is possible, although technical factors typically limit examinations to the interictal rather than ictal period.

Figure 1.7 shows an example data set. The patient was an 18-year-old male who suffered significant trauma at age 5. The patient had frequent seizures, which were poorly controlled by medication. MRI revealed extensive bilateral cortical and subcortical abnormalities. MEG demon-

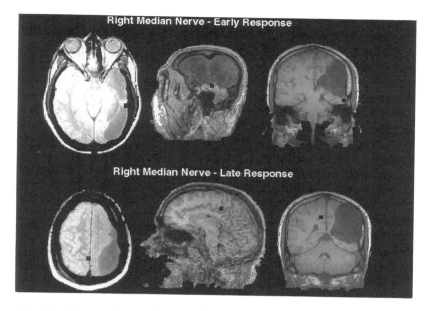

FIG. 1.6.   Data are from a 22-year-old male who suffered a neonatal infarct of the left middle cerebral artery at approximately 1 month of age. Most of the brain tissue of the left hemisphere has been replaced by a porencephalic cyst. Stimulation of the right median nerve evokes an abnormal pattern of cortical activity characterized by early activation of left temporal cortex and subsequent activation of midline right parietal areas, as indicated by the black boxes. (From "Cortical Organization in Adulthood Is Modified by Neonatal Infarct: A Case Study" by J. D. Lewine et al., 1994, *Radiology, 190.* Adapted with permission.)

strated that a fairly focal region of lateral right frontal cortex was responsible for generation of this patient's extensive interictal spiking.

APPLICATION: ABNORMAL LOW-FREQUENCY MAGNETIC ACTIVITY (ALFMA)

One of the most significant challenges in the diagnostic evaluation of trauma victims concerns patients with significant postconcussive syndromes after relatively minor head trauma. For many of these patients, structural brain imaging by CT and MRI fails to reveal gross structural pathology. As a consequence, many patients who claim to have symptoms are not believed, or they are misdiagnosed as having psychiatric dysfunction without a clear neurological basis.

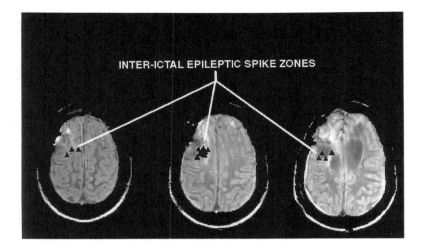

FIG. 1.7.   Data are from an 18-year-old male who suffered significant head trauma at age 5. The trauma caused bilateral MRI abnormalities, and the patient was experiencing uncontrolled posttraumatic epileptic seizures. MEG localized interictal spikes (black triangles) to the right frontal cortex. Surgical resection of this region alleviated the seizures.

Research at the Albuquerque Magnetic Source Imaging Facility indicates that MEG may help provide objective evidence of neurological dysfunction in a high percentage of these patients. For normal subjects, the magnetoencephalogram (also abbreviated as MEG) at most recording sites is dominated by an 8–13 Hz alpha rhythm, but the MEG of many mild trauma victims is dominated by abnormal low-frequency magnetic activity (ALFMA) in the theta and delta bands (Fig. 1.8). Furthermore, it has been demonstrated that individual "slow-wave" events often have dipolar field configurations with localizable sources (Lewine et al., 1994).

For the past 2 years, the Albuquerque facility has been equipped with a 37-channel biomagnetometer system. The detection coils and SQUIDs are contained within a liquid helium-filled Dewar that is readily positioned over various parts of the head. During the typical ALFMA experiment, 3 minutes of continuous data are collected at each of eight Dewar positions, providing for a whole head examination. The Dewar positions are over the following areas: (a) midline frontal; (b) midline occipital, (c) right and left parietal, (d) right and left anterior-temporal/inferior-frontal, and (e) the right and left temporal/parietal/occipital junctions. In these experiments, the data from each Dewar position are analyzed separately. The first step in the analysis procedure is to digitally filter the

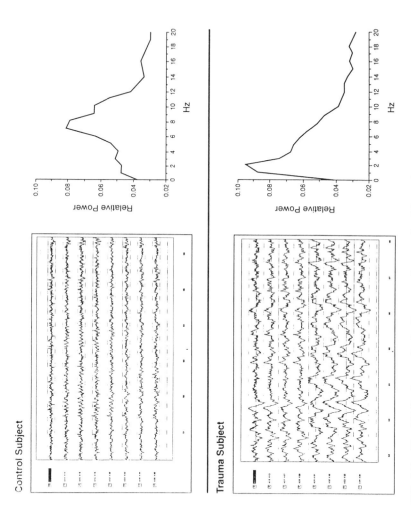

FIG. 1.8. The MEG of neurologically normal control subjects is characterized by frequent bursts of alpha activity in the 8–13 Hz band. The MEG of many trauma victims is characterized by a large-amplitude slow wave in the 1–6 Hz range. This patient shows significant abnormal low-frequency activity (ALFMA), mostly at about 2.5 Hz.

data from 1 to 6 Hz to better isolate abnormal low-frequency signals. The next step is to apply a peak-detection algorithm that identifies time points where the average magnetic signal is unusually large—greater than 200 femtoTesla. Dipole modeling is then applied to the instantaneous magnetic field pattern at these time points. Only dipole fits where the correlation between the forward calculated and measured field pattern exceeds 0.97 are considered in further analyses, and only one dipole fit is retained per slow-wave event. The final step in the analysis is to determine if multiple (15) slow-wave events can be traced to the same cortical region. If so, that cortical region is considered to be pathological, and the relevant dipoles are plotted on appropriate MRIs. These procedures eliminate more than 99.9% of the recorded data from further analysis, but nevertheless provide valuable clinical information.

In an initial series of experiments, the Albuquerque group studied 15 patients with postconcussive syndromes subsequent to mild head trauma. Each patient reported only a single episode of trauma, and none had evidence of neurological or psychiatric dysfunction prior to the incident. *Mild trauma* was defined as causing a loss of consciousness of less than 20 minutes. No patient was admitted to the hospital for more than 24 hours, and all had Glasgow Coma Scale (GCS) scores of 12 or higher when first examined by a physician. Each subject participated in MEG and MRI evaluations. The time between diagnostic evaluation and injury ranged from 24 hours to 2 years, with all patients complaining of symptoms at the time of MEG examination. Fifteen age- and sex-matched controls were also studied.

As summarized in Fig. 1.9, abnormal MEG findings were found for 10 of the patients, but none of the controls. Four of the patients also had MRI abnormalities (one case of subdural hematoma, two cases of contusion, one case of minor white matter changes). There was no significant correlation between abnormal examination and recency of injury. It is noteworthy that an abnormal MEG examination was apparent as early as 24 hours after trauma, as demonstrated by the data of Patient 231 in Figure 1.10. This patient, a neuroradiologist, hit his head during a basketball game 24 hours prior to examination. He spent a restless night and awoke with a headache and photophobia. Finding himself unable to concentrate on reading MRI films, he reported for an MEG examination. Extensive ALFMA was found. MRI examination was negative. Symptoms resolved throughout that day, and the following morning he was symptom free. Follow-up MEG examination revealed a normal MEG without ALFMA.

The data clearly suggest that the diagnostic sensitivity of MEG to the neural consequences of minor trauma is superior to that of MRI (66% vs. 27%), but the sample size was small. Another limitation of the initial

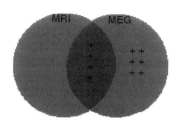

0 = Control Subject

+ = Trauma Patient With Symptoms

FIG. 1.9. Set diagram shows diagnostic results for 15 trauma patients and 15 age- and sex-matched controls. None of the controls showed any diagnostic abnormalities. Four patients had abnormal MRIs. Each of these, plus six others, were also abnormal by MEG examination.

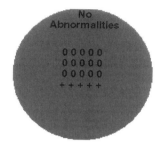

study was the possibility that EEG, a technology far less expensive than MEG, might also reveal similar changes. Therefore, a second study with a larger patient population and simultaneous MEG and EEG measurements was initiated.

The second study evaluated 30 patients with a history of a single episode of minor head trauma, and 30 age- and sex-matched controls (Lewine et al., 1994). Twenty-five of the patients had active postconcussive symptoms at the time of physiological evaluation, whereas five were symptom free. The MEG and MRI data collection and primary analysis strategies for Study 2 were identical to that for Study 1. Twenty channels of EEG data were collected simultaneously with the MEG. Data were collected at the standard locations of the 10–20 International EEG location system (Jasper, 1958), referenced to Cz. The data were visually inspected by a trained neurophysiologist for evidence of abnormal slowing. Additional spectral analyses involving calculations of regional values of the ratio between delta and theta power versus alpha power were performed.

Figure 1.11 summarizes the data from Study 2. Seventeen of the 25 trauma victims with symptoms, and 1 of the 5 without symptoms, had abnormal MEG findings. The false positive rate among the control sub-

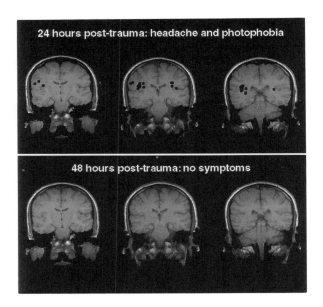

FIG. 1.10. Data are from a 41-year-old male. Upper panels show the presence of ALFMA (each black dot represents a dipole source associated with a large-amplitude slow-wave event) 24 hours after mild trauma, at a time when the patient was complaining of postconcussive headache and photophobia. Lower panels show complete resolution of the ALFMA by 48 hours, at a time when no symptoms were present. [Adapted from "Neuromagnetic Assessment of Pathophysiological Brain Activity induced by Minor Head Trauma" by Lewine et al., *Archives of Neurology*, 1996, submitted].

jects was low (3.3%). EEG abnormalities were found for only nine of the patients with symptoms, and MRI was abnormal for only six. That is, nine patients were abnormal only by MEG examination, as was the case for the patient whose MEG data are shown in Fig. 1.12. The diagnostic sensitivity of the MEG examination for patients with postconcussive syndromes was significantly better than that for EEG or MRI ($p < .01$, paired t tests). Together, the two studies indicated that MEG findings closely tracked symptomatology. Even more than 1 year after initial trauma, MEG examination was abnormal, as illustrated in the data in Fig. 1.13. Indeed, MEG abnormalities were quite stable in patients with stable postconcussive symptoms, as shown in Fig. 1.14. This particular patient showed significant posttraumatic attentional deficits. Approximately 1 year after initial trauma, the patient's physician prescribed Ritalin for this condition. Prior to his first dose, his MEG was still very abnormal; 30 minutes after medication, ALFMA was no longer present. Although a single dose of Ritalin clearly did not cure this patient, the

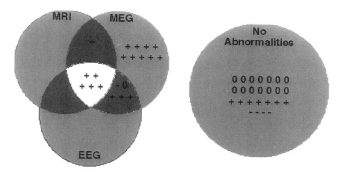

0 = Control Subject

+ = Trauma Patient With Symptoms

- = Trauma Patient Without Symptoms

FIG. 1.11.   Set diagram shows diagnostic results of Study 2, for 25 trauma patients with postconcussive symptoms, 5 patients without symptoms, and 30 age- and sex-matched controls. [Adapted from "Neuromagnetic Assessment of Pathophysiological Brain Activity Induced by Minor Head Trauma" by Lewine et al., *Archives of Neurology*, 1996, submitted].

data indicate that MEG may be useful in monitoring the short- and long-term effects that pharmacotherapies have on brain activity. The data also suggest a reasonable relationship between the locations of MEG abnormalities and specific neuropsychological symptoms. For example, patients with memory deficits typically display ALFMA in temporal regions, whereas those with attentional deficits display parietal abnormalities. It is noteworthy that few patients displayed frontal lobe

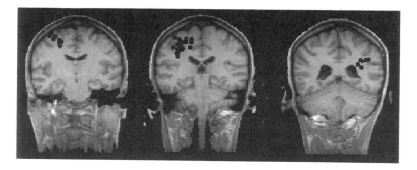

FIG. 1.12.   Data are from a 45-year-old female with postconcussive attentional deficits. Biparietal sources of ALFMA (black circles) are seen. Both EEG and MRI examinations were normal. [Adapted from "Neuromagnetic Assessment of Pathophysiological Brain Activity Induced by Minor Head Trauma" by Lewine et al., *Archives of Neurology*, 1996, submitted].

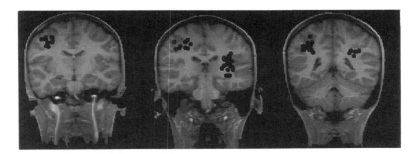

FIG. 1.13. Data are from a 14-year-old female with attentional, mnemonic, and emotional problems. The subject was involved in a car accident 1 year prior to MEG examination, which revealed extensive biparietal and left temporal sources of ALFMA. Both EEG and MRI examinations were normal. [Adapted from "Neuromagnetic Assessment of Pathophysiological Brain Activity Induced by Minor Head Trauma" by Lewine et al., *Archives of Neurology*, 1996, submitted].

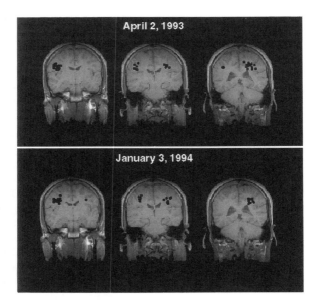

FIG. 1.14. Data are from an 18-year-old male with postconcussive attentional deficits. Initial examination at 3 months posttrauma revealed extensive biparietal sources of ALFMA. Follow-up examination 9 months later revealed MEG abnormalities to be stable. Interestingly, after the January 3, 1994, examination, the patient ingested a new prescription of Ritalin. Follow-up examination 30 minutes later was devoid of ALFMA. [Adapted from "Neuromagnetic Assessment of Pathophysiological Brain Activity Induced by Minor Head Trauma" by Lewine et al., *Archives of Neurology*, 1996, submitted].

ALFMA, even though neuropsychological testing revealed "frontal lobe deficits" in most. There are several possible explanations for this. The brain is a highly integrated organ, and frontal lobe dysfunction on neuropsychological examination might reflect primary pathology in other regions. However, the lack of frontal lobe MEG findings may reflect the technique's lack of sensitivity to currents oriented radial to the skull surface— the situation for pyramidal cell currents for much of the frontal cortex.

Whereas the sensitivity of MEG examinations for ALFMA is high, the specificity may be low; many patients having other neurological conditions (including stroke and dementia) also show ALFMA. However, there may be subtle differences in the characteristics (amplitude, periodicity) of the ALFMA for different conditions. The Albuquerque facility has just completed purchase of a whole-head biomagnetometer system that will reduce examination times from approximately 2 hours to 20 minutes. This system will also allow for better characterization of the interrelationships among brain regions. A main focus of research during the next year will be to determine if the trauma-specific MEG tests can be developed.

REFERENCES

Bauer, G. (1987). Coma and brain death. In E. Niedermeyer & F. Lopes da Silva (Eds.), *Electroencephalography—Basic principles, clinical applications and related fields* (2nd ed., pp. 391–404). Baltimore: Urban and Schwarzenberg.

Benzel, E. C., Lewine, J. D., Bucholz, R., & Orrison, W. W. (1993). Magnetic source imaging: A review of the Magnes system by Biomagnetic Technologies Incorporated. *Neurosurgery, 33,* 252–259.

Courjon, J. (1972). Traumatic disorders. In A. Redmond (Ed.), *Handbook of electroencephalography and clinical neurophysiology,* Vol. 14, pp. 1–95). Amsterdam: Elsevier.

Department of Health and Human Services. (1989). *Interagency Head Injury Task Force Report.* Washington, DC: U.S. Government Printing Office.

Fisch, B. J. (1991). *Spehlmann's EEG primer.* Amsterdam: Elsevier.

Fong, Y. T., Teal, J. S., & Hieshima, G. B. (1984). *Neuroradiology of head trauma.* Baltimore: University Park Press.

Gentry, L. R., Godersky, J. C., & Thompson, G. H. (1988). MR imaging of head trauma: Review of the distribution and radiopathologic features of traumatic lesions. *American Journal of Neuroradiology, 9,* 101–110.

Gentry, L. R., Godersky, J. C., Thompson, B., & Dunn, V. D. (1988). Prospective Comparative Study of Intermediate-field MR and CT in the Evaluation of Closed Head Trauma. *American Journal of Roentgenology, 150*(3), 673–682.

Greenberg, R. P., Newlon, P. G., Hyatt, M. S., Narayan, R. K., & Becker, D. P. (1981). Prognostic implications of early multimodal evoked-potentials in severely head injured patients. *Journal of Neurosurgery, 55,* 227–236.

Jasper, H. H. (1958). Report of the Committee on Methods of Clinical Examination in EEG: Appendix: The ten-twenty electrode system of the International Federation, *Handbook of Electroencephalography and Clinical Neurophysiology, 10,* 371–375.

Jennett, W. B. (1975). *Epilepsy after non-missile head injuries.* Chicago: Mosby Year Book.

Langfitt, T. W., Obrist, W. D., Alavi, A., Grossman, R. I. (1986). Computerized tomography, magnetic resonance imaging, and positron emission tomography in the study of brain trauma. *Neurosurgery, 64,* 760–767.

Levin, H. S., Benton, A. L., & Grossman, R. G. (1982). *Neurobehavioral consequences of closed head injury.* New York: Oxford University Press.

Lewine, J. D. (1990). Neuromagnetic techniques for the noninvasive analysis of brain function. In S. E. Freeman, E. Fukishima, & E. R. Greene (Eds.), *Noninvasive techniques, in biology and medicine* (pp. 33–73). San Francisco: San Francisco Press.

Lewine, J. D., Astur, R. S., Davis, L. E., Knight, J. E., Maclin, E. L., & Orrison, W. W. (1994). Cortical organization in adulthood is modified by neonatal infarct: A case study. *Radiology, 190,* 93–96.

Lewine, J. D., & Orrison, W. W. (1995). Magnetoencephalography and magnetic source imaging. In W. W. Orrison (Ed.), *Functional brain imaging* (pp. 369–418). St. Louis: Mosby Year Book.

Lewine, J. D., Orrison, W. W., Astur, R. S., Davis, L. E., Knight, J. D., Maclin, E. L., Reeve, A. (1995). Explorations of pathophysiological spontaneous activity by magnetic source imaging. In C. Baumgartner, L. Deecke, G. Stroink, & S. J. Williamson (Eds.), *Biomagnetism: Fundamental Research and Clinical Applications, Vol. 7* (pp. 55–59). Amsterdam: Elsevier.

Lewine, J. D., Orrison, W. W., Halliday, A., Morrell, R., Chuang, S., Hwang, P., & Sanders, J. A. (in press). MEG functional mapping in epilepsy surgery. In G. D. Cascino & C. R. Jack (Eds.), *Neuroimaging in epilepsy: Principles and practice.* Amsterdam: Butterworth and Heinemann.

Lewine, J. D., Orrison, W. W., Sloan, J. H., Kodituwakku, P. W., Hart, B. L., Davis, J. T., Spar, J., Baldwin, N. G., Benzel, E., & Sanders, J. A. (in press). Neuromagnetic assessment of pathophysiological brain activity induced by minor head trauma. *Archives of Neurology.*

Lishman, W. A. (1988). Physogenesis and psychogenesis in the "post-concussional syndrome." *Br J Psychiatry, 153,* 460–469.

Rao, N., Turski, P. A., Polcyn, R. E., Nickels, R. J., Matthews, C. G., & Flynn, M. M. (1984). F-18 positron emission computed tomography in closed head injury. *Archives of Physical Medicine Rehabilitation, 65,* 780–785.

Reid, R. H., Gulenchyn, K. Y., Ballinger, J. R., & Ventureyra, E. C. (1990). Cerebral perfusion imaging with Technetium-99m HMPAO following cerebral trauma: Initial experience. *Clinical Nuclear Medicine, 15,* 383–388.

Reider-Groswasser, I., Cohen, M., Costeff, H., & Groswasser, Z. (1993). Late CT findings in brain trauma: Relationship to cognitive and behavioral sequelae and to vocational outcome. *American Journal of Roentgenology, 160,* 147–152.

Rodin, E. (1967). Contributions of EEG to prognosis after head injury. *Diseases of the Nervous System, 28,* 598–601.

Ruff, R. M., Crouch, J. A., Troster, A. I., & Marshall, L. F. (1994). Selected cases of poor outcome following a minor brain trauma: Comparing neuropsychological and positron emission tomography assessment. *Brain Injury, 8,* 297–308.

Ruff, R. M., Buchsbaum, M. S., Troster, A. L., & Marshall, L. F. (1989). Computerized tomography, neuropsychology, and positron emission tomography in the evaluation of head injury. *Neuropsychiatry, Neuropsychology, and Behavioral Neurology, 2,* 103–123.

Wiedmann, K. D., Wilson, J. T. L., Wyper, D., & Hadley, D. M. (1989). SPECT cerebral blood flow, MR imaging and neuropsychological findings in traumatic head injury. *Neuropsychology, 3,* 267–281.

2

Neuropsychological Significance of Contusional Lesions Identified by MRI

J. T. L. Wilson
D. M. Hadley
L. C. Scott
A. Harper

Neuropathological work on head trauma has emphasized the distinction between focal and diffuse injury (Adams et al., 1989; Adams, Gennarelli, & Graham, 1980; Adams, Graham, Murray, & Scott, 1982). Focal injuries include hematomas and contusions, whereas neuropathological studies have shown the importance of microscopic diffuse axonal injury in patients dying after injury. Damage due to secondary hypoxia and ischemia can also cause focal and diffuse patterns of lesions. The distinction between focal and diffuse injury is often applied to survivors. Magnetic resonance imaging (MRI) is more sensitive to traumatic brain damage than computed tomography (CT; Jenkins, Hadley, Teasdale, Macpherson, & Rowan, 1986). Many head-injury survivors have multiple lesions in frontal and temporal regions (Gentry , Godersky, & Thompson, 1988; Hadley et al., 1988; Wilson, Hadley, Wiedmann, & Teasdale, 1992), suggesting severe contusions. Lesions in the brain stem and corpus callosum (Gentry et al., 1988; Jenkins et al., 1986) are also sometimes visualized on MRI, and are presumably signs of severe diffuse axonal injury (Adams et al., 1989).

The later psychological consequences of diffuse and focal injuries are not well understood and are a matter of debate. The neuropathological view stresses the overwhelming importance of diffuse axonal injury, rather than focal injury, in determining outcome after head injury (Adams, Graham, Gennarelli, & Maxwell, 1991). Patients with severe diffuse injuries often have prolonged coma. Adams and colleagues (1991) claimed that such injuries are responsible for a large part of the disability observed after head injury. In contrast, focal contusional injuries are often thought to result in little permanent impairment even if lesions in the acute stage are extensive (Gentry, 1991).

Wilson, Teasdale, Hadley, Wiedmann, and Lang (1994) recently reported an MRI study of 38 patients with severe closed head injuries imaged at the acute stage and followed up at 6 months. In the group as a whole, both coma and posttraumatic amnesia (PTA) were related to the number of areas in deep brain structures in which lesions were detected on acute MRI, but only PTA was significantly related to the number of hemispheric areas in which lesions were found. A subgroup of patients who had relatively short periods of coma (less than 6 hours), but prolonged PTA (1 week or more) was identified. These patients had extensive hemispheric lesions on MRI, were older, and had neuropsychological impairment at follow-up. An implication of the study is that patients with MRI patterns indicative of severe contusional injuries show significant impairment at follow-up.

The significance of contusional lesions after mild and moderate head injuries is less clear. Levin and colleagues (1992) performed serial MRI and neuropsychological testing in 50 patients with an admission Glasgow Coma Scale (GCS) score of 9–15. They showed that lesions had resolved substantially by 3 months postinjury, and that there was considerable recovery of psychological functions. They were unable to demonstrate relationships between performance on particular tests and lesions in specific locations. Despite the recovery observed on both MRI and psychological testing, the results presented by Levin et al. indicate that there were still residual lesions and persisting deficits at 3 months postinjury. The trends suggest that lesions may disappear by 6 months postinjury, but this issue remains to be addressed.

The present study focuses on a group of patients who had an admission GCS score of 13–15, and thus fulfilled GCS criteria for minor head injury (Rimel, Giordani, Barth, Boll, & Jane, 1981), but who nonetheless had positive findings on acute MRI. Our expectation was that these patients would form a group that had purely focal injuries, without significant diffuse axonal injury. We followed up these patients at 6 months postinjury, examining the relationship between early and late imaging and neuropsychological outcome. The three main issues addressed by the study were: (a) How do such lesions evolve over 6 months? (b) What is the psychological status of such patients at follow-up? (c) Do abnormalities on MRI relate to residual impairment in this group?

METHOD

Patients

One hundred and three head-injured patients were initially recruited to the study. Patients were excluded if they had previous head injury, history of psychiatric hospitalization, treatment for alcohol abuse, or history of epilepsy. All patients had been transferred to the regional neurosurgical unit after being admitted to a primary surgical unit. The level of consciousness on admission to hospital was assessed using the GCS (Teasdale & Jennett, 1974). For the current analysis, a subgroup of patients fulfilling the following additional criteria was selected: (a) GCS score on admission was 13–15, (b) there was a parenchymal abnormality on acute MRI T2-weighted imaging, (c) patients were not operated on for hematoma, and (d) data for follow-up MRI and neuropsychological testing were available. Twenty-three patients fulfilled these criteria.

Controls

A group of 16 orthopedic outpatients served as controls for neuropsychological testing.

Neuroimaging

MRI was carried out in a Picker "Vista 1100," 0.15 Tesla resistive system operating at 6.38 MHz. An initial 2-cm thick spin echo (SE200/40) pilot image in the sagittal or coronal plane was used to determine the positions of 16 slices each 8-mm thick, for a T2-weighted spin echo sequence (SE2000/80), and an 8-slice, T1-weighted inversion recovery sequence (IR1660/400/40) in the axial plane. Care was taken to align the orientation of follow-up and acute imaging using internal landmarks. For three patients, follow-up MRI was carried out on a Siemens Magnetom 1.5 Tesla system, using a similar protocol. Image analysis was conducted by an experienced neuroradiologist using software supplied by the manufacturer. Parenchymal lesions were identified on T2-weighted images and delineated using a joystick; lesion area was calculated automatically. The areas of lesions in specific brain regions were summed and multiplied by the slice thickness to give lesion volumes.

Neuropsychological Assessment

Patients were followed up at a median of 6 months postinjury (range 5–10 months). Neuropsychological assessment was carried out on the same occasion as follow-up MRI. The neuropsychological test battery consisted of the following procedures: (a) The National Adult Reading Test (NART) was used to estimate premorbid IQ (Nelson, 1982); (b) general intellectual abilities were measured using six subtests of the Wechsler Adult Intelligence Scale (WAIS; Wechsler, 1955); (c) verbal memory and learning were assessed using two subtests of the Wechsler Memory Scale (WMS; Wechsler, 1945): Logical Memory and Associate Learning; (d) visuoperceptual ability and visual memory were assessed by the Rey Figure Immediate Recall (Rey, 1941); and (e) a word fluency test (Borokowski, Benton, & Spreen, 1967) was used to assess expressive aspects of language. A measure of simple and choice reaction time (RT) was also included (Wilson, Wiedmann, Phillips, & Brooks, 1988).

RESULTS

The mean lesion volumes in the acute stage and at follow-up for the 23 patients are shown in Fig. 2.1. In line with previous studies, the most extensive lesions were found in frontal and temporal regions. Overall mean volume of lesions was 28.9 cc in the acute stage (SD = 21.9) and 9.2 cc at follow-up (SD = 11.1). Thus, on average, the lesion volume measured on T2-weighted imaging at follow-up was 31% of the volume in the acute stage.

The mean values mask a considerable amount of individual variation in the extent to which lesions resolved between the acute stage and follow-up. Figure 2.2 shows a scatterplot of acute and follow-up lesion

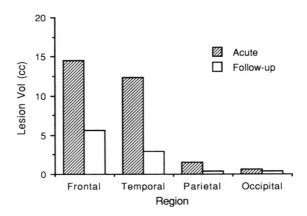

FIG. 2.1.   Mean volume of lesions in the acute stage and at 6-month follow-up in hemispheric regions. Lesions were measured from T2-weighted images.

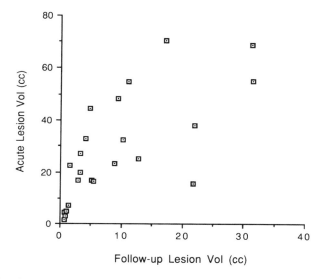

FIG. 2.2.   Scatterplot comparing the volumes of lesions in the acute stage and at 6-month follow-up. Each point represents a single patient; the number of patients was 23.

volumes in the 23 cases. Five patients with smaller lesions initially (less than 10 cc) showed small residual abnormalities at follow-up. However, in the 18 patients with larger lesions, there was a great deal of variability in the degree to which the size of lesions reduced over time. In several cases, quite extensive initial lesions reduced to 5 cc or less at follow-up, whereas others showed a much smaller reduction in lesion size; in one case, lesion size marginally increased.

Patients were compared with a control group to assess whether there was evidence of neuropsychological impairment. Patients and controls were matched for age and errors on the National Adult Reading Test (NART). Means and standard deviations for each group are shown in Table 2.1, together with the results of t testing. Although the performance differences between the groups were small, patients were significantly impaired on Digit Span, Digit Symbol, Word Fluency, and three measures from an RT test. Subjective complaints by patients are shown in Table 2.2.

The data were further analyzed to assess whether neuropsychological impairment was related to lesions in specific locations. Pearson correlation coefficients were calculated between neuropsychological test performance and lesion volume from follow-up MRI for the following areas: left frontal, right frontal, left temporal, right temporal, parietal, and occipital. The only correlation that reached a .01 level of significance was

TABLE 2.1
Means and Standard Deviations (in brackets) of Patients and Controls on Matching Variables and Neuropsychological Measures

Variable	Patients (N = 23)		Controls (N = 16)		t
Age (years)	34.3	(12.2)	34.4	(16.4)	
NART (errors)	23.1	(9.3)	21.7	(8.9)	
Similarities	17.4	(3.9)	17.2	(3.9)	
Digit Span	12.1	(2.4)	14.2	(1.4)	3.3**
Vocabulary	51.0	(13.5)	49.7	(15.6)	
Digit symbol	52.6	(11.9)	61.1	(8.6)	2.3*
Block Design	38.2	(7.2)	36.0	(6.8)	
Object Assembly	32.1	(5.8)	29.0	(6.8)	
Word Fluency	41.3	(8.7)	49.3	(9.5)	2.5*
Logical Memory	13.9	(3.3)	13.1	(3.5)	
Associate Learning	15.1	(3.3)	16.2	(3.3)	
Rey Recall	23.5	(7.1)	23.5	(5.2)	
Simple RT (msec):					
Decision Time	304	(42)	273	(38)	2.4*
Movement Time	242	(58)	220	(44)	
Choice RT (msec):					
Decision Time	345	(64)	306	(40)	2.1*
Movement Time	250	(67)	215	(48)	2.1*

* $p < .05$. ** $p < .01$.

TABLE 2.2
Percentages of Patients Complaining of Problems in Specific areas

Complaint	%
Tiredness	73
Irritability	60
Anxiety	53
Memory	53
Anger	47
Concentration	40
Hearing	40
Smell	40
Depression	40
Dizziness	40
Taste	27
Movement	27
Vision	20

TABLE 2.3
Unilateral Versus Bilateral Lesions: Means and Standard
Deviations (in brackets) of Two Groups of Patients

Variable	Unilateral (N = 13)		Bilateral (N = 10)		F
Age	30.7	(11.9)	39.0	(11.8)	
NART	22.7	(9.6)	23.9	(9.5)	
Similarities	18.1	(3.5)	16.5	(4.5)	
Digit Span	12.6	(2.3)	11.5	(2.5)	
Vocabulary	49.9	(15.0)	52.5	(11.9)	
Digit Symbol	57.7	(9.9)	46.5	(11.6)	5.2*
Block Design	37.2	(8.0)	39.6	(6.3)	
Object Assembly	31.7	(6.1)	32.6	(5.7)	
Word Fluency	43.4	(6.3)	38.7	(10.8)	
Logical Memory	14.9	(3.4)	12.5	(2.8)	
Associate Learning	16.4	(2.8)	13.5	(3.3)	5.0*
Rey Recall	24.2	(5.8)	22.6	(8.7)	
Simple RT (msec):					
Decision Time	298	(48)	312	(34)	
Movement Time	214	(38)	279	(60)	6.0*
Choice RT (msec):					
Decision Time	320	(39)	378	(79)	
Movement Time	215	(27)	297	(76)	8.4**

* $p < .05$. ** $p < .01$.

Associate Memory with the left frontal region ($r = .50$). Thus, there was no evidence of systematic relationships between performance on particular tests and lesions in specific cortical sites.

To establish whether there was a more general relationship between the extent of injury and psychological deficit, the patients were partitioned into two groups: (a) 13 with unilateral lesions at follow-up, and (b) 10 with bilateral lesions. The results of dividing the patients in this way are shown in Table 2.3. There was a difference in the age of patients with unilateral and bilateral lesions, the latter being older. Differences on the other measures were assessed using analysis of covariance (ANCOVA), controlling for the effects of age. Differences between groups that remained significant were found on Digit Symbol test, Associate Learning, and Movement Time components of the RT measures.

DISCUSSION

The results confirm other work, showing that patients with minor head injury by GCS criteria may nonetheless have extensive focal MRI lesions on acute imaging (Levin et al., 1992). Patients in the present study showed residual impairment of neuropsychological function at 6 months postinjury, and had a variety of subjective complaints. These findings are consistent with previous work, in which minor head injury was defined in a similar manner (Rimel et al., 1981).

A number of different definitions of minor head injury can be found in the literature, and this has led to some controversy. Williams, Levin, and Eisenberg (1990) suggested that patients should be classed as *moderate injuries* if they have positive findings on acute CT imaging. Based on this criterion, the present study included patients with moderate head injuries. Indeed, one might argue that any patient with a positive finding on acute MRI should be considered to have a moderate head injury. The present aim is not to enter the debate surrounding the definition of mild and moderate injuries. The goal of selecting patients with an admission GCS score of 13–15 was to exclude significant diffuse axonal injury and to highlight patients with focal lesions. These patients were not severely impaired, but nonetheless had persisting lesions and significant impairment.

The results show that, although there was a substantial reduction in the size of lesions on MRI by 6 months postinjury, there was still evidence of hemispheric abnormalities in these patients. A particular feature of the present study is the variability that was shown in individual recovery from focal lesions. It is not clear why such variability arises, but the results suggest that patients' age may play a role. We were unable to demonstrate a relationship between lesions in specific hemispheric areas and particular neuropsychological deficits. This finding is consistent with the report by Levin and colleagues (1992). We have suggested elsewhere that such relationships may be elusive in head injury because lesions tend to occur in patterns rather than singly (Wilson et al., 1992). Nonetheless, there was an overall relationship between the presence of bilateral lesions and cognitive impairment. Thus, the results add to the evidence that contusional lesions play a role in outcome, and suggest that they play a role in impairment even after mild to moderate injury.

ACKNOWLEDGMENT

The work described in this chapter was supported by a grant from the Wellcome Trust.

REFERENCES

Adams, J. H., Doyle, D., Ford, I., Gennarelli, T. A., Graham, D. I., & Mclellan, D. R. (1989). Diffuse axonal injury in head injury: Definition, diagnosis, and grading. *Histopathology, 15*, 49–59.

Adams, J. H., Gennarelli, T. A., & Graham, D. I. (1980). Brain damage in non-missile head injury: Observations in man and subhuman primates. In W. T. Smith & J. B. Cavanagh (Eds.), *Recent advances in neuropathology 2* (pp. 165–190). Edinburgh: Churchill Livingstone.

Adams, J. H., Graham, D. I., Gennarelli, T. A., & Maxwell, W. L. (1991). Diffuse axonal injury in non-missile head injury. *Journal of Neurology, Neurosurgery, & Psychiatry, 54,* 481–483.

Adams, J. H., Graham, D. I., Murray, L. S., & Scott, G. (1982). Diffuse axonal injury due to non-missile head injury in humans: An analysis of 45 cases. *Annals of Neurology, 12,* 557–563.

Borokowski, J. G., Benton, A. L., & Spreen, O. (1967). Word fluency and brain damage. *Neuropsychologia, 5,* 135–140.

Gentry, L. R. (1991). Head trauma. In S. W. Atlas (Ed.), *Magnetic resonance imaging of the brain and spine* (pp. 439–466). New York: Raven.

Gentry, L. R., Godersky, J. C., & Thompson, B. (1988). MR imaging of head trauma: Review of the distribution and radiopathologic features of traumatic lesions. *American Journal of Neuroradiology, 9,* 101–110.

Hadley, D. M., Teasdale, G. M., Jenkins, A., Condon, B., Macpherson, P., Patterson, J., & Rowan, J. O. (1988). Magnetic resonance imaging in acute head injury. *Clinical Radiology, 39,* 131–139.

Jenkins, A., Hadley, M. D. M., Teasdale, G., Macpherson, P., & Rowan, J. O. (1986). Brain lesions detected by magnetic resonance imaging in mild and severe head injury. *Lancet, ii,* 445–446.

Levin, H. S., Williams, D. H., Eisenberg, H. M., High Jr, W. M., & Guinto Jr, F. C. (1992). Serial MRI and neurobehavioural findings after mild to moderate closed head injury. *Journal of Neurology, Neurosurgery, & Psychiatry, 55,* 255–262.

Nelson, H. E. (1982). *National Adult Reading Test (NART): Test manual.* Windsor: NFER-Nelson.

Rey, A. (1941). L'examen psychologique dans le cas d'encéphalopathie traumatique. *Archives de Psychologie, 28*(112), 286–340.

Rimel, R. W., Giordani, B., Barth, J. T., Boll, T. J., & Jane, J. A. (1981). Disability caused by minor head injury. *Neurosurgery, 9,* 221–228.

Teasdale, G., & Jennett, B. (1974). Assessment of coma and impaired consciousness: A practical scale. *Lancet, ii,* 81–84.

Wechsler, D. (1945). A standardized memory scale for clinical use. *Journal of Psychology, 19,* 87–95.

Wechsler, D. (1955). *Manual for the Wechsler Adult Intelligence Scale.* New York: Psychological Corporation.

Williams, D. H., Levin, H. S., & Eisenberg, H. M. (1990). Mild head injury classification. *Neurosurgery, 27,* 422–428.

Wilson, J. T. L., Hadley, D. M., Wiedmann, K. D., & Teasdale, G. M. (1992). Intercorrelation of lesions detected by magnetic resonance imaging after closed head injury. *Brain Injury, 6,* 391–399.

Wilson, J. T. L., Teasdale, G. M., Hadley, D. M., Wiedmann, K. D., & Lang, D. (1994). Post-traumatic amnesia: Still a valuable yardstick. *Journal of Neurology, Neurosurgery, & Psychiatry, 57,* 198–201.

Wilson, J. T. L., Wiedmann, K. D., Phillips, W. A., & Brooks, D. N. (1988). Visual event perception in alcoholics. *Journal of Clinical & Experimental Neuropsychology, 10,* 224–234.

3

Factors Affecting Brain Injury in Subarachnoid Hemorrhage

Joshua L. Dowling
Ralph G. Dacey, Jr.

Subarachnoid hemorrhage, whether caused by the rupture of an aneurysm, arteriovenous malformation, or head trauma, can result in severe brain injury. Although much of this injury occurs with the initial event and is often fatal or irreversible, secondary factors also contribute significantly to morbidity and mortality. Attempts to improve outcome are generally designed to address these factors. Rehemorrhage is the most devastating complication following subarachnoid hemorrhage, and carries a high mortality. Additional brain injury can occur as a result of cerebral edema and intracranial hypertension. Cerebral ischemia resulting from vasospasm is another leading cause of delayed neurological deterioration. Hydrocephalus can result in either gradual or precipitous decline in neurological status. Some patients develop recurrent seizures. In addition, subarachnoid clots may have direct toxic effects on the brain. Recently, attention has focused on the role of free radicals, particularly the effects of membrane lipid peroxidation on the blood-brain barrier (BBB), cerebral edema, and vasospasm. Focus on the secondary causes of brain injury has led to the development of newer surgical, endovascular, and phamacological treatments in subarachnoid hemorrhage. Nevertheless, subarachnoid hemorrhage continues to be a significant cause of death and disability.

Subarachnoid hemorrhage can occur spontaneously or as a result of head trauma. Although head trauma is the most common etiology of subarachnoid hemorrhage (Martin et al., 1992), the associated cerebral trauma usually overshadows the direct effects of subarachnoid blood. Therefore, injury mechanisms are more easily discerned in spontaneous subarachnoid hemorrhage. Aneurysmal rupture is the most common etiology of spontaneous subarachnoid hemorrhage (Locksley, 1966).

Aneurysms can be of several varieties. Saccular aneurysms are most common. They develop at the bifurcations of the major cerebral arteries as a result of hemodynamic stress (Stehbens, 1989), and tend to occur in the sixth decade of life. Fusiform aneurysms are dilatations along the length of an artery, and usually do not present as rupture. The basilar artery is most commonly involved. Mycotic aneurysms form as a result of bacterial emboli, usually in the setting of subacute bacterial endocarditis. They tend to occur distally along the length of an artery, rather than at bifurcations, and can present with subarachnoid or intraparenchymal hemorrhage. Traumatic aneurysms are uncommon. They are classified as true, false, or mixed based on the degree of disruption of the media and adventitia. In true aneurysms the adventitia is intact, whereas in pseudoaneurysms the wall is formed by hematoma (Parkinson & West, 1980). A mixed traumatic aneurysm results when a true aneurysm ruptures and forms a pseudoaneurysm. Of the various types of aneurysms, saccular aneurysms account for the majority of aneurysmal ruptures. Much of what is known about subarachnoid hemorrhage has been learned in the setting of saccular aneurysmal rupture.

Upon rupture of a saccular aneurysm, several factors can contribute directly to brain injury. Blood escaping under high pressure can result in intracerebral hematoma or intraventricular hemorrhage. Intracerebral hematoma formation causes sudden disruption of brain tissue and can exert mass effect on the surrounding brain. Brain edema, increased intracranial pressure, midline shift, and herniation syndromes can all result. Intracerebral hematoma and intraventricular hemorrhage are both associated with increased intracranial pressure and poor outcome.

The immediate consequences of subarachnoid hemorrhage are usually reflected in the patient's initial clinical condition. The patient commonly presents with the sudden onset of severe headache accompanied by varying degrees of nuchal rigidity, photophobia, nausea, and vomiting. The patient may be neurologically intact or may have neurological deficits ranging from isolated cranial nerve palsies to deep coma. Diagnosis of subarachnoid hemorrhage is usually made by computed tomographic (CT) scanning. CT scanning demonstrates subarachnoid blood in greater than 95% of patients on the day of hemorrhage (Weir, 1987). The sensitivity of CT scanning declines over subsequent days to weeks. If the clinical setting is suggestive of subarachnoid hemorrhage, but the CT scan is negative, lumbar puncture should be performed. Angiography is required to determine the etiology of the subarachnoid hemorrhage and for surgical planning.

Several scales have been developed to clinically grade the severity of hemorrhage. The most widely used of these is the Hunt–Hess classification (Hunt & Kosnik, 1974; see Table 3.1). The World Federation of Neurological Surgeons scale (Drake, 1988), which incorporates the Glasgow

TABLE 3.1
The Hunt–Hess Classification of Patients
with Subarachnoid Hemorrhage

Grade	Description
0	Unruptured aneurysm
1	Asymptomatic, or mild headache and slight nuchal rigidity
1a	No acute meningeal or brain reaction, but with fixed neuro deficit
2	Moderate to severe headache, nuchal rigidity, cranial nerve palsy
3	Lethargy, confusion, or mild focal neurological deficit
4	Stupor, moderate to severe hemiparesis, early decerebrate rigidity
5	Deep coma, decerebrate rigidity, and moribund appearance

Note. One grade added for serious systemic disease (e.g., hypertension, diabetes mellitus, severe atherosclerosis, chronic obstructive pulmonary disease) or severe vasospasm on angiography. From "Timing and Perioperative Care in Intracranial Aneurysm Surgery" by W. E. Hunt and E. J. Kosnik, 1974, *Clinical Neurosurgery, 21,* p. 80. Copyright 1974 by The Congress of Neurological Surgeons. Adapted by permission.

Coma Scale (GCS), may more precisely reflect the patient's condition (see Table 3.2). These scales have been particularly important in classifying patients for cohort studies, but have also been used clinically to predict risk for different treatment approaches.

REHEMORRHAGE

The most devastating complication following subarachnoid hemorrhage is rehemorrhage. In a study examining the natural history of aneurysms, Jane, Kassell, Torner, and Winn (1985) found that the 6-month risk of rebleeding is 50% on Day 1 of the hemorrhage. This risk was found to

TABLE 3.2
World Federation of Neurological Surgeons Scale
for Subarachnoid Hemorrhage

Grade	Glasgow Coma Scale Score	Major Focal Deficit
0	15	No (unruptured aneurysm)
2	15	No
3	13–14	No
4	7–12	Yes or no
5	3–6	Yes or no

Note. From "Report of World Federation of Neurological Surgeons Committee on a Universal Subarachnoid Hemorrhage Grading Scale" by C. G. Drake, 1988, *Journal of Neurosurgery, 68,* p. 985. Copyright 1988 by American Association of Neurological Surgeons. Adapted by permission.

gradually decline up to 6 months, after which the risk stabilized to about 3% per year. In an earlier study, Jane, Winn, and Richardson (1977) demonstrated that, with a rehemorrhage rate of 3% per year, death occurred in 67% of late hemorrhages, thus comprising a 2% per year rate of fatal rehemorrhage.

Surgery is now the primary mode of preventing rerupture. The high rate of rehemorrhage and the severity of its consequences have led many to advocate early surgical intervention for ruptured cerebral aneurysms. Although some studies have supported this approach, others have failed to show the benefit of early surgery (Kassell et al., 1990; Ohman & Heiskanen, 1989). One study found that patients whose surgery was planned for Days 7–10 posthemorrhage fared worse than those operated on before or after that period (Haley et al., 1992). In addition, the advantages of early versus late surgery may be related to the clinical grade of the patient because poorer grade patients may be more susceptible to the trauma associated with surgery (Shucart & Wu, 1994). Therefore, many neurosurgeons will delay surgery in poorer grade patients. Nevertheless, although the timing of surgery for ruptured aneurysms may not be uniformly agreed on, aneurysm surgery clearly protects patients from the most devastating complication following subarachnoid hemorrhage.

VASOSPASM

Delayed cerebral ischemia due to vasospasm has become the leading cause of death and disability following subarachnoid hemorrhage, accounting for 14% of adverse outcomes (Kassel, Sasaki, Colohan, & Nazar, 1985). It can be demonstrated angiographically in 60%–70% of cases in the second week following subarachnoid hemorrhage, although only 20%–30% of patients will develop cerebral ischemia as a result. Onset of vasospasm is usually delayed, beginning around Day 3, becoming maximal by Days 6–8, and resolving in most cases by Day 12 (Weir, Grace, Hausen, & Rothbery, 1978). Although several therapies have been developed to prevent and treat vasospasm, none is effective in all cases. As a result, cerebral vasospasm continues to be a major focus of efforts to improve outcome after subarachnoid hemorrhage.

Although the exact pathophysiology of cerebral vasospasm following subarachnoid hemorrhage has not been fully defined, it is clearly related to the presence of blood and its breakdown products in the subarachnoid space surrounding the major arteries at the base of the brain. The risk for development of vasospasm correlates with the amount of subarachnoid clot (Fischer, Kistler, & Davis, 1980), and spasm usually occurs in the same distribution as the clot (Findlay, Macdonald, & Weir, 1991). Although earlier researchers considered vasospasm to be a proliferative angiopathy (Clower, Smith, Haining, & Lockard, 1981), arterial narrowing is now felt to be a result of sustained smooth muscle contraction (Findlay et al., 1991; Mayberg, 1990).

Several potential spasmogens have been implicated in cerebral vasospasm, including hemoglobin, eicosanoids, endothelin, and lipid peroxides. Hemoglobin released from extravasated erythrocytes in the form of oxyhemoglobin is probably the most significant cause of vasospasm (Findlay et al., 1991; Weir & Macdonald, 1993). The time course of vasospasm follows the release of oxyhemoglobin (Suzuki, 1979). Oxyhemoglobin has clearly been shown to produce vasospasm both in vitro (Findlay et al., 1991) and in vivo (Mayberg, Okada, & Bark, 1990). The spasmogenic effect of oxyhemoglobin may be related to the effects of superoxide anion and other free radicals that produce lipid peroxidation (Findlay et al., 1991), which is discussed in greater detail later.

Several risk factors associated with cerebral vasospasm have been identified. Fisher, Kistler, and Davis (1980) related the risk of vasospasm to the amount of blood seen on CT scanning (see Table 3.3). They found that of 18 patients with no blood or only diffuse blood (Groups 1 and 2), none developed clinical evidence of vasospasm, although several had angiographic evidence of spasm. Of 24 patients with subarachnoid clot or a thick layer of blood (Group 3), 23 had signs of severe vasospasm. Thus, the risk of vasospasm can usually be assessed when patients present because most will undergo CT scanning as part of their initial evaluation. Other factors associated with vasospasm include the use of antifibrinolytics or antihypertensives (Mayberg, 1990), dehydration, and fever (Weir et al., 1989).

Suspicion of vasospasm is usually raised because of a change in patients' neurological status within the typical time frame of 3–12 days

TABLE 3.3
Fisher Grading of Subarachnoid Hemorrhage on CT

Group	Description
1	No blood detected
2	Diffuse blood or thin layer with vertical layers < 1mm thick
3	Localized clot and/or vertical layers ≥ 1mm thick
4	Intraventricular or intracerebral clot with diffuse or no subarachnoid blood

Note. From "Relation of Cerebral Vasospasm to Subarachnoid Hemorrhage Visualized by Computerized Tomographic Scanning" by C. M. Fisher, J. P. Kistler, and J. M. Davis, 1980, *Neurosurgery, 6,* p. 6. Copyright 1980 by The Congress of Neurological Surgeons. Adapted by permission.

posthemorrhage. Patients typically become confused and disoriented with development or worsening of focal neurological deficits. Vasospasm can be confirmed by transcranial Doppler ultrasound or cerebral angiography. Transcranial Doppler ultrasound is a noninvasive technique that can measure flow velocities in the basal cerebral arteries. Patients with cerebral vasospasm have been shown to have flow velocities increased in proportion to the degree diameter of arterial narrowing (Aaslid, Huber, & Nornes, 1984). This technique has the advantages of being noninvasive and being possible at the bedside, however flow velocity values can be technician dependent. Cerebral angiography is the gold standard for confirming cerebral vasospasm and may provide the setting for treatment of spasm. Although vasospasm can be seen in 60%–70% of patients in the second week following hemorrhage, only 20%–30% will demonstrate delayed ischemia (Kassel et al., 1985). Therefore, angiography must be interpreted in light of patients' clinical condition.

Several therapies have been developed to prevent or treat cerebral vasospasm following subarachnoid hemorrhage. Calcium channel blockers and hypertensive, hypervolemic therapy have been widely used and are clearly beneficial. Newer endovascular techniques have been used to treat vasospasm refractory to medical treatment. In addition, experimental approaches, including the use of tissue plasminogen activator and 21-aminosteroids, show promise in actually preventing vasospasm.

Intravascular volume expansion and induced arterial hypertension have not been proved in randomized controlled trials. However, this approach has gained wide acceptance because of mounting clinical evidence of its efficacy, as well as a rationale consistent with present understanding of cerebral blood flow and vasospasm. In the presence of severe arterial spasm, the normal autoregulation of cerebral blood flow cannot function. Therefore, cerebral blood flow becomes a more direct function of systemic blood pressure and cardiac output (Findlay et al., 1991). Pharmacological agents such as dopamine and phenylepherine are used to raise cerebral perfusion pressure and increase cerebral blood flow. Volume expansion using blood, albumin, and intravenous fluids is directed at increasing cardiac output. Kassel et al. (1982) demonstrated that, in 58 patients with progressive neurological deterioration and angiographically proved vasospasm, volume expansion and induced hypertension resulted in reversal of neurological deterioration in 47 patients and permanent improvement in 43. Risks of this approach include cardiac ischemia, pulmonary edema, and hyponatremia. Moreover, in the presence of an unclipped aneurysm, hypertension increases the risk of rehemorrhage.

The calcium channel blocker nimodipine has been shown to decrease the incidence of fixed neurological deficit secondary to vasospasm following subarachnoid hemorrhage. The initial rationale behind the use of this agent was that it could interfere with the availability of calcium in smooth muscle cells necessary for arterial contraction. An early prospective, randomized, double-blind, controlled trial of nimodipine in good grade patients demonstrated a lower rate of severe neurological deficit in patients receiving nimodipine versus those receiving placebo (Allen et al., 1983). The authors attributed this to decreased arterial spasm. Other larger studies have confirmed the efficacy of this drug in poor grade patients (Hunt–Hess IV and V) as well as good grade patients (Hunt–Hess I–III; Petruk et al., 1988; Pickard et al., 1989). Nevertheless, these studies have not clearly demonstrated that nimodipine reduces angiographically evident vasospasm. Thus, nimodipine may have a direct cytoprotective effect on ischemic brain (Findlay et al., 1991). The calcium channel blocker nicardipine has also been tested in a large randomized, double-blind, placebo-controlled trial. This agent was shown to reduce both symptoms and radiographic evidence of vasospasm (Kassell, Haley, Torner, & Kongable, 1991). However, at 3 months, there was no difference in the incidence of either mortality or good result demonstrated (Haley et al., 1990).

In recent years, attention has focused on the role of free radicals in brain injury due to trauma, subarachnoid hemorrhage, and stroke. A new class of compounds—the 21-aminosteroids, also known as lazaroids—has been developed for its potent antioxidant effects. Tirilazad mesylate is the best studied of these compounds. It is currently being tested in clinical trials for its efficacy in improving outcome in head injury and subarachnoid hemorrhage.

Oxygen radical formation and lipid peroxidation have been studied for their role in central nervous system injury for many years. Free radicals cause cell damage by initiating a lipid peroxidation chain reaction, which progresses geometrically over the lipid bilayer of cell membranes and can lead to disruption of ionic gradiants and membrane lysis (Hall & Braughler, 1993; Watson & Ginsberg, 1989). Thus, free radicals can be directly toxic to neurons, glial cells, myelin, and vascular cell membrane (Hall & Braughler, 1993). In subarachnoid hemorrhage, free radical formation, especially the formation of the superoxide anion, is initiated by the release of hemoglobin from lysis of extravasated erythrocytes. Iron also creates superoxide anion through the reduction of oxygen. This leads to lipid peroxidation of vascular endothelium, with loss of integrity of the BBB (Hall & Braughler, 1993).

As mentioned earlier, oxyhemoglobin has been shown to play a major role in cerebral vasospasm. This effect may be mediated, in part, by the production of free radicals because the autooxidation of oxyhemoglobin results in the production of methemoglobin and superoxide anion. Several animal studies have demonstrated the efficacy of tirilazad mesylate in reducing cerebral vasospasm following subarachnoid hemorrhage (Kanamaru et al., 1990; Steinke et al., 1989). Clinical trials of tirilazad mesylate in humans are already underway.

The conclusion that a subarachnoid clot is responsible for vasospasm has led to investigations of the use of tissue plasminogen activator to dissolve a subarachnoid clot at the time of surgery. Earlier studies had shown that aggressive removal of a clot at the time of surgery could reduce the rate of vasospasm (Mizukami, Kawase, Usami, & Tazawa, 1982; Taneda, 1982). Nevertheless, aggressive clot removal at surgery increases the risk of damage to delicate perforating vessels. Also, a clot distant from the surgical site might not be accessible. Therefore, fibrinolytics seems a logical method to accelerate breakdown and reabsorbtion of the clot. A decreased rate of vasospasm due to subarachnoid hemorrhage in primates has been demonstrated following injection of recombinant tissue plasminogen activator into the basal cisterns, even when injected unilaterally (Findlay et al., 1989). Subsequent trials in human subarachnoid hemorrhage have shown promise, although clearly there are risks of hemorrhage associated with this therapy (Findlay et al., 1989; Ohman, Servo, & Heiskanen, 1991; Zabramski et al., 1991).

Endovascular techniques are now employed in many centers to treat symptomatic cerebral vasospasm. Percutaneous transluminal angioplasty, first introduced by Zubkov, Nikiforov, and Shustin in 1984, can be used to dilate spastic basal arteries. Moreover, the treatment is long lasting, often with immediate results. Intraarterial papaverine injection also appears to reverse angiographic spasm, although the effect is clearly not as permanent as angioplasty. Thus, angiography not only provides definitive diagnosis of vasospasm, but the setting for effective treatment of spasm as well.

HYDROCEPHALUS AND EPILEPSY

Following subarachnoid hemorrhage, hydrocephalus often develops and, if untreated, can result in neurological deterioration, brain injury, and even death. Hydrocephalus can be either acute or delayed. Acute hydrocephalus requiring intervention has an incidence of 15%–20% (Tresser, Selman, & Ratcheson, 1994). Intraventricular hemorrhage, diffuse subarachnoid clot, and hemorrhage from a posterior circulation aneurysm all contribute significantly to the development of acute hydrocephalus (Graff-Radford, Torner, Adams, & Kassell, 1989). A close association has been demonstrated between acute hydrocephalus and vasospasm, most likely reflecting the common etiology of blood in the basal cisterns (Black, 1986). Treatment for acute hydrocephalus usually involves the placement of an external ventricular drain. Ventriculostomy is often necessary after subarachnoid hemorrhage. However, a few reports have suggested that external drainage may increase the risk of vasospasm and the development of chronic hydrocephalus (Kasuya, Shimizu, & Kagawa, 1991). Release of intracranial pressure by ventriculostomy may be associated with rehemorrhage (Paré, Delfino, & LeBlanc, 1992). Nevertheless, the potential benefit of reducing intracranial pressure due to ventricular enlargement almost always exceeds the risk of rehemorrhage when a ventriculostomy is performed in this setting. Acute hydrocephalus is associated with poorer outcome after aneurysmal subarachnoid hemorrhage (van Gijn et al., 1985). Chronic hydrocephalus is caused by adhesions in the pia arachnoid interfering with cerebrospinal fluid absorption. It is treated by placement of a ventriculo-peritoneal or ventriculo-atrial shunt.

Epilepsy is another complicating factor in subarachnoid hemorrhage, developing in about 15% of patients (Rose & Sarner, 1965). Risk factors for the development of epilepsy include a large amount of cisternal blood, rebleeding, rupture of a middle cerebral artery (MCA) aneurysm, cerebral infarction due to vasospasm, and shunt-dependent hydrocephalus (Hasan et al., 1993; Rose & Sarner, 1965; Tresser et al., 1994).

CONCLUSION

Subarachnoid hemorrhage can clearly result in devastating brain injury. Because little can be done to prevent immediate injury, therapeutic efforts focus on the secondary effects of brain injury. Although rehemorrhage is potentially the most serious delayed complication, early surgery to clip aneurysms dramatically reduces that risk. As a result, delayed ischemia secondary to vasospasm has become the leading cause of death and disability in subarachnoid hemorrhage secondary to aneurysmal rupture. Several therapies have been developed to address vasospasm, including hypervolemic, hypertensive therapy; calcium channel blockers; 21-aminosteroids; tissue plasminogen activator; and endovascular techniques. Nevertheless, no treatment has effectively eliminated this major cause of morbidity. Hydrocephalus can also result in brain injury, either in the acute period or delayed by up to several weeks. Thus, subarachnoid hemorrhage, despite advances in treatment, continues to be a significant cause of brain injury.

REFERENCES

Aaslid, R., Huber, P., & Nornes, H. (1984). Evaluation of cerebrovascular spasm with transcranial Doppler ultrasound. *Journal of Neurosurgery, 60,* 37–41.

Allen, G. S., Ahn, H. S., Preziosi, T. J., Battye, R., Boone, S. C., Chou, S. N., Kelly, D. L., Weir, B. K., Crabbe, R. A., Lavik, P. J., Rosenbloom, S. B., Dorsey, F. C., Ingram, C. R., Mellits, D. E., Bertsch, L. A., Boisvert, D. P. J., Hundley, M. B., Johnson, R. K., Strom, J. A., & Transou, C. R. (1983). Cerebral arterial spasm—a controlled trial of nimodipine in patients with subarachnoid hemorrhage. *New England Journal of Medicine, 308,* 619–624.

Black, P. M. (1986). Hydrocephalus and vasospasm after subarachnoid hemorrhage from ruptured intracranial aneurysms. *Neurosurgery, 18,* 12–16.

Clower, B. R., Smith, R. R., Haining, J. L., & Lockard, J. (1981). Constrictive endarteropathy following experimental subarachnoid hemorrhage. *Stroke, 12,* 501–508.

Drake, C. G. (1988). Report of World Federation of Neurological Surgeons Committee on a Universal Subarachnoid Hemorrhage Grading Scale. *Journal of Neurosurgery, 68,* 985–986.

Findlay, J. M., Macdonald, R. L., & Weir, B. K. A. (1991). Current concepts of pathophysiology and management of cerebral vasospasm following aneurysmal subarachnoid hemorrhage. *Cerebrovascular and Brain Metabolism Reviews, 3,* 336–361.

Findlay, J. M., Weir, B. K. A., Gordon, P., Grace, M., & Bauman, R. (1989). Safety and efficacy of intrathecal thrombolytic therapy in a primate model of cerebral vasospasm. *Neurosurgery, 24,* 491–498.

Fisher, C. M., Kistler, J. P., & Davis, J. M. (1980). Relation of cerebral vasospasm to subarachnoid hemorrhage visualized by computerized tomographic scanning. *Neurosurgery, 6,* 1–9.

Graff-Radford, M. R., Torner, J., Adams, H. P., & Kassell, N. F. (1989). Factors associated with hydrocephalus after subarachnoid hemorrhage: A report of the cooperative aneurysm study. *Archives of Neurology, 46,* 744–752.

Haley, E. C., Kassell, N. F., Torner, J. C., & the participants. (1992). The International Cooperative Study on the timing of aneurysm surgery: The North American experience. *Stroke, 23,* 205–214.

Haley, E. C., Torner, J. C., Kassell, N. F. (1990). Cooperative randomized study of nicardipine in subarachnoid hemorrhage: Preliminary report. In K. Sano, K. Takakura, N. F. Kassell, & T. Sasaki (Eds.), *Cerebral vasospasm* (pp. 519–525). Tokyo, Japan: University of Tokyo Press.

Hall, E. D., & Braughler, J. M. (1993). Free radicals in CNS injury. *Research Publications—Association for Research Nervous and Mental Disease, 71,* 81–105.

Hasan, D., Schonck, R. S. M., Avezaat, C. J. J., Taughe, H. L. J., van Gijn, J., & van der Lugt, P. J. M. (1993). Epileptic seizures after subarachnoid hemorrhage. *Annals of Neurology, 33,* 286–291.

Hunt, W. E., & Kosnik, E. J. (1974). Timing and perioperative care in intracranial aneurysm surgery. *Clinical Neurosurgery, 21,* 79–89.

Jane, J. A., Kassell, N. F., Torner, J. C., & Winn, H. R. (1985). The natural history of aneurysms and arteriovenous malformations. *Journal of Neurosurgery, 62,* 321–323.

Jane, J. A., Winn, H. R., & Richardson, A. E. (1977). The natural history of intracranial aneurysms: Rebleeding rates during the acute and long term period and implication for surgical management. *Clinical Neurosurgery, 24,* 176–184.

Kanamaru, K., Weir, B. K. A., Findlay, J. M., Grace, M., & Macdonald, R. L. (1990). A dosage study of the effect of the 21-aminosteroid U74006F on chronic cerebral vasospasm in a primate model. *Neurosurgery, 27,* 29–38.

Kassell, N. F., Haley, E. C., Torner, J. C., & Kongable, G. (1991). Nicardipine and angiographic vasospasm [abstract]. *Journal of Neurosurgery, 74,* 341A.

Kassell, N. F., Peerless, S. J., Durward, Q. J., Beck, D. W., Drake, C. G., & Adams, H. P. (1982). Treatment of ischemic deficits from vasospasm with intravascular volume expansion and induced arterial hypertension. *Neurosurgery, 11,* 337–343.

Kassell, N. F., Sasaki, T., Colohan, A. R. T., & Nazar, G. (1985). Cerebral vasospasm following aneurysmal subarachnoid hemorrhage. *Stroke, 16,* 562–572.

Kassel, N. F., Torner, J. C., Jane, J. A., Haley, E. C., Adams, H. P., & participants. (1990). The International Cooperative Study on the Timing of Aneurysm Surgery: Part 2. Surgical results. *Journal of Neurosurgery, 73,* 37–47.

Kasuya, H., Shimizu, T., & Kagawa, M. (1991). The effect of continuous drainage of cerebrospinal fluid in patients with subarachnoid hemorrhage: A retrospective analysis of 108 patients. *Neurosurgery, 28,* 56–59.

Locksley, H. B. (1966). Report on the Cooperative Study of Intracranial Aneurysms and SAH. Section V. II. Natural history of SAH, intracranial aneurysms and AVM: Based on 6368 cases in the Cooperative Study. *Journal of Neurosurgery, 25,* 321–368.

Martin, N. A., Doberstein, C., Zane, C., Caron, M. J., Thomas, K., & Becker, D. P. (1992). Posttraumatic cerebral arterial spasm: Transcranial Doppler ultrasound, cerebral blood flow, and angiographic findings. *Journal of Neurosurgery, 77,* 575–583.

Mayberg, M. R. (Ed.). (1990). Cerebral vasospasm. *Neurosurgery Clinics of North America, 1,* 265–267.

Mayberg, M. R., Okada, T., & Bark, D. H. (1990). The role of hemoglobin in arterial narrowing after subarachnoid hemorrhage. *Journal of Neurosurgery, 72,* 634–640.

Mizukami, M., Kawase, T., Usami, T., & Tazawa, T. (1982). Prevention of vasospasm by early operation with removal of subarachnoid blood. *Neurosurgery, 10,* 301–307.

Ohman, J., & Heiskanen, O. (1989). Timing of operation for ruptured supratentorial aneurysms: A prospective randomized study. *Journal of Neurosurgery, 70,* 55–60.

Ohman, J., Servo, A., & Heiskanen, O. (1991). Effect of intrathecal fibrinolytic therapy on clot lysis and vasospasm in patients with aneurysmal subarachnoid hemorrhage. *Journal of Neurosurgery, 75,* 197–201.

Paré, L., Delfino, M. S., & LeBlanc, R. (1992). The relationship of ventricular drainage to aneurysmal rebleeding. *Journal of Neurosurgery, 76,* 422–427.

Parkinson, D., & West, M. (1980). Traumatic intracranial aneurysms. *Journal of Neurosurgery, 52,* 11–20.

Petruk, K. C., West, M., Mohr, G., Weir, B. K. A., Benoit, B. G., Gentili, F., Disney, L. B., Khan, M. I., Grace, M., Holness, R. D., Karwon, M. S., Ford, R. M., Cameron, G. S., Tucker, W. S., Purves, G. B., Miller, J. D. R., Hunter, K. M., Richard, M. T., Durity, F. A., Chan, R., Clein, L. J., Maroun, F. B., & Godon, A. (1988). Nimodipine treatment in poor-grade aneurysm patients: Results of a multicenter double-blind placebo-controlled trial. *Journal of Neurosurgery, 68,* 505–517.

Pickard, J. D., Murray, G. D., Illingworth, R., Shaw, M. D., Teasdale, G. M., Foy, P. M., Humphrey, P. R., Lang, D. A., Nelson, R., Richards, P., Sinar, J., Bailey, S., & Skene, A. (1989). Effect of oral nimodipine on cerebral infarction and outcome after subarachnoid haemorrhage: British aneurysm nimodipine trial. *British Medical Journal, 298,* 636–642.

Rose, C. F., & Sarner, M. (1965). Epilepsy after ruptured intracranial aneurysm. *British Medical Journal, 1,* 18–21.

Shucart, W., & Wu, J. (1994). Timing of operation for ruptured aneurysms: Delayed surgery. In R. A. Ratcheson & F. P. Wirth (Eds.), *Ruptured cerebral aneurysms: Perioperative management* (pp. 54–58). Baltimore, MD: Williams & Wilkins.

Stehbens, W. E. (1989). Etiology of intracranial berry aneurysms. *Journal of Neurosurgery, 70,* 823–831.

Steinke, D. E., Weir, B. K. A., Findlay, J. M., Tanabe, T., Grace, M., & Krushelnycky, B. W. (1989). A trial of the 21-aminosteroid U74006F in a primate model of chronic cerebral vasospasm. *Neurosurgery, 24,* 179–186.

Suzuki, J. (1979). Cerebral vasospasm: Prediction, prevention, and protection. In H. W. Pia, C. Langmaid, & J. Zierski (Eds.), *Cerebral aneurysms. Advances in diagnosis and therapy* (pp. 155–161). Berlin: Springer.

Taneda, M. (1982). Effect of early operation for ruptured aneurysm on prevention of delayed ischemic symptoms. *Journal of Neurosurgery, 57,* 622–628.

Tresser, S. J., Selman, W. R., & Ratcheson, R. A. (1994). Pathophysiological alterations following aneurysm rupture. In R. A. Ratcheson & F. P. Wirth (Eds.), *Ruptured cerebral aneurysms: Perioperative management* (pp. 23–45). Baltimore, MD: Williams & Wilkins.

van Gijn, J., Hijdra, A., Wijdicks, E. F. M., Vermeulen, M., & van Crevel, H. (1985). Acute hydrocephalus after aneurysmal subarachnoid hemorrhage. *Journal of Neurosurgery, 63,* 355–362.

Watson, B. D., & Ginsberg, M. D. (1989). Ischemic injury in the brain: Role of oxygen radical-mediated processes. *Annals of the New York Academy of Science, 559,* 269–281.

Weir, B. (1987). *Aneurysms affecting the nervous system.* Baltimore, MD: Williams & Wilkins.

Weir, B., Disney, L., Grace, M., & Roberts, P. (1989). Eaily trends in white blood count and temperature after subarachnoid hemorrhage from aneurysm. *Neurosurgery, 25,* 161–165.

Weir, B., Grace, M., Hausen, J., & Rothbery, C. (1978). Time course of vasospasm in man. *Journal of Neurosurgery, 18,* 173–178.

Weir, B., & Macdonald, L. (1993). Cerebral vasospasm. *Clinical Neurosurgery, 40,* 40–55.

Zabramski, J. M., Spetzler, R. F., Lee, K. S., Papadopoulos, S. M., Bovill, E., Zimmerman, R. S., & Bederson, J. B. (1991). Phase I trial of tissue plasminogen activator for the prevention of vasospasm in patients with aneurysmal subarachnoid hemorrhage. *Journal of Neurosurgery, 75,* 189–196.

Zubkov, Y. N., Nikiforov, B. M., & Shustin, V. A. (1984). Balloon catheter technique for dilatation of constricted cerebral arteries after aneurysmal SAH. *Acta Neurochirugie, 70,* 65–79.

4

Role of Excitatory Amino Acids in Neuronal and Glial Responses to Traumatic Brain Injury

Yoichi Katayama
Atsuo Yoshino
Tatsuro Kawamata
Takashi Tsubokawa

Following traumatic brain injury (TBI), many neuronal cells are metabolically deranged at the subcellular level, but are not primarily disrupted. Several studies employing experimental models have indicated that neuronal cells subjected to TBI are more vulnerable to a secondary ischemic insult (e.g., Jenkins et al., 1989), implying that these cells are dysfunctional metabolically. One major goal of therapies for TBI during the acute period is to provide an ideal milieu for the recovery of these cells. To establish appropriate therapies for TBI, it is crucial to delineate the sequence of cellular and subcellular events that lead traumatized neuronal cells to undergo metabolic derangements. This chapter discusses the events that naturally begin from the moment of injury.

EXPERIMENTAL MODELS

One major event observed at the moment of injury in neuronal cells is the occurrence of massive ionic fluxes across the plasma membrane (Katayama, Becker, Tamura, & Horda, 1990; Nilsson, Hillered, Olsson, Sheardown, & Hansen, 1993; Takahashi, Manaka, & Sano, 1981; Tsubokawa, 1983). The ionic perturbation involves influxes of Na^+, Ca^{2+}, and Cl^-, and efflux of K^+. This is indeed a unique event caused by traumatic insults to the neuronal cells, when compared to any other cells within the body. Changes in ionic permeability mediated by voltage-and ligand-dependent ion channels in response to neurotransmitter release are characteristic of the neuron as an excitable cell. If there is anything unique to the mechanism of TBI, it could be related to this ionic event.

We have shown that massive ionic fluxes involving wide areas of the brain are observed in the fluid-percussion (FP) injury model of the rat. We delivered a brief fluid-pressure pulse to the epidural space of the vertex through a craniotomy via a fluid-filled column (central FP) at the level of injury. This caused loss of righting response for 5–15 minutes without overt morphological damage to the cerebral parenchyma. Such a fluid pulse flows over both cerebral cortices (Dixon et al., 1987) and produces widespread mechanical deformation of the brain bilaterally without causing primary cellular disruption. Consequently, cere- brovascular and metabolic changes, and subcortical diffuse axonal injury are induced by compressive and tensile strains over relatively wide areas of the brain (Hayes, 1991; Hovda, Becker, & Katayama, 1991; Katayama, Becker, Tamura, & Hovda, 1990; Povlishock, Becker, Sullivan, & Miller, 1978). Thus, the FP injury mimics clinical closed head injury, in which an acceleration produces shear and tensile strains throughout the brain.

Previous studies have indicated that neuronal cells subjected to mild FP injury are more vulnerable to a secondary ischemic insult (Jenkins et al., 1989), implying that these cells are dysfunctional metabolically. The FP injury thus provides a useful model of TBI for investigating the functional consequences of ionic fluxes occurring in neuronal cells that are traumatized but not primarily disrupted. In addition, we have em- ployed a controlled cortical impact (CI) injury model (Dixon, Clifton, Lighthall, Yaghmai, & Hayes, 1991). The CI injury produces primary damage to the cerebral cortex, but as well as well-controlled deformation of the hippocampus. This model is useful for examining the effects of compressive and tensile strains, in comparison with the other side, without causing primary cellular disruption in the hippocampus.

We applied the brain microdialysis technique in the present series of studies. This technique enables one to monitor the neurochemical changes occurring in the extracellular space (ECS) simultaneously. More impor- tant, the technique provides a means to administer various agents into the ECS through the dialysis probe. Based on these advantages, the under- lying mechanism of the massive ionic fluxes and their causal relationships to the processes of metabolic derangement can be effectively examined.

MASSIVE IONIC FLUXES

The abrupt increase in extracellular concentration of potassium ($[K^+]_e$) occurring as a component of the massive ionic fluxes following FP injury can be detected by K^+-free microdialysis (Katayama, Cheung, Alves, &

Becker, 1989; Katayama, Becker, Tamura, & Hovda, 1990). Following the initiation of K^+-free microdialysis, a stationary level of dialysate concentration of potassium ($[K^+]_d$) is obtained within 5 minutes. Although a slow, progressive decrease takes place thereafter, the $[K^+]_d$ remains at approximately the same level for a considerable period of time. We naturally need to remove the dialysis probes at the moment of trauma and reposition them immediately after the trauma. Such procedures, however, led to only small changes in $[K^+]_d$. More interesting, a massive increase in $[K^+]_d$ was observed when the magnitude of trauma was increased above a certain threshold. The lack of large changes in baseline $[K^+]_d$ in response to repositioning of the probes or subthreshold FP injury indicates that $[K^+]_e$ is rigidly maintained by powerful mechanisms for ionic homeostasis (e.g., Nicholson, Phillips, & Gardner-Medwin, 1979). When the mechanical deformation of the brain is sufficiently severe, TBI causes a certain event that disrupts such mechanisms for ionic homeostasis completely.

Localized mechanical or potassium stimulation of the brain can cause a similar ionic flux termed *spreading depression*. However, there are three major differences between the massive ionic fluxes observed following FP injury and spreading depression. First, the ionic fluxes following FP injury occur over wide brain areas at the same time. Second, although the ionic shifts associated with spreading depression propagate to adjacent brain areas slowly, the ionic fluxes following FP injury do not spread. Finally, it takes 3–5 minutes for recovery from the ionic fluxes following FP injury. In contrast, the ionic shifts associated with spreading depression last for approximately 1 minute. Based on these differences, a distinction should be made between spreading depression and the ionic fluxes caused by widespread mechanical deformation of the brain. For the sake of convenience, the latter could be termed *traumatic depolarization*. Abrupt and rapid ionic fluxes are also observed at a minute or more after ischemia or anoxia induction as a consequence of energy failure. Such rapid ionic fluxes are termed *anoxic depolarization* (e.g., Hansen, 1977, 1985). The traumatic depolarization cannot be accounted for by energy failure, however, because it occurs immediately after the trauma. Mechanical deformation of the neuronal cell membrane could easily induce changes in electrical field and neuronal discharges, which would activate much more voltage-dependent ion channels and cause more ionic fluxes. However, the traumatic depolarization following FP injury is not attenuated by tetrodotoxin administered by microdialysis (Katayama, Becker, Tamura, & Hovda, 1990), suggesting that it is not due merely to activation of voltage-dependent ion channels associated with neuronal discharges.

Alternatively, the traumatic depolarization might be ascribable to an activation of the ligand-dependent ion channels, which could also produce enormous ionic fluxes if neurotransmitters are massively released. If the Ca^{2+}-dependent exocytotic release of neurotransmitters is responsible for the abrupt increase in $[K^+]_e$, inhibition of Ca^{2+} entry into the nerve terminals (e.g., Drejer, Benveniste, Deemer, & Schousboe, 1985) would be expected to alter the traumatic depolarization. In support of this hypothesis, the abrupt, large increase in $[K^+]_d$ following induction of ischemia is significantly attenuated by dialysis with Ca^{2+}-free perfusate containing Co^{2+}, which blocks Ca^{2+} entry (Katayama, Tamura, Becker, & Tsubokawa, 1991a). The increase in $[K^+]_d$ following FP injury is also partially Ca^{2+}-dependent (Katayama, Becker, Tamura, & Hovda, 1990), suggesting the involvement of Ca^{2+}-dependent exocytotic release of neurotransmitters in the traumatic depolarization.

EXCITATORY AMINO ACID RELEASE

The anoxic depolarization occurring during ischemia or anoxia is too rapid to be accounted for simply by failure of the energy-dependent ion pump activity alone. Sudden changes in ion permeability of the cellular membranes have therefore been postulated to take place, presumably through indiscriminative release of neurotransmitters (Moghaddam, Schenk, Stewart, & Hansen, 1987; Nicholson & Kraig, 1981; Van Harreveld, 1978). Excitatory amino acids (EAAs) are the most likely neurotransmitters that could produce such marked ionic shifts (Choi, 1987; Mayer & Westbrook, 1987; Olney, Price, Samson, & Lambuyere, 1986; Rothman & Olney, 1987). The dialysate concentration of glutamate ($[Glu]_d$) has been monitored during ischemia (e.g., Benveniste, Drejer, Schousboe, & Diemer, 1984). The elevation of $[Glu]_d$ occurring during ischemia begins concomitantly with the large increase in $[K^+]_d$ (Katayama, Kawamata, Tamura, Becker, & Tsubokawa, 1991). This finding is not surprising because the massive ionic fluxes at the moment of injury are associated with an increase in $[K^+]_e$ far above the level necessary for depolarization of the nerve terminals. Consistent with this inference, the earlier rapid increase in $[Glu]_d$ during ischemia is markedly attenuated by Ca^{2+}-free perfusate containing Co^{2+} (Drejer et al., 1985; Katayama, Kawamata, Tamura, et al., 1991).

The abrupt increase in $[K^+]_d$ following ischemia induction is significantly delayed by EAA antagonists administered by microdialysis (Katayama, Tamura, Becker, & Tsubokawa, 1992b). Among various EAA antagonists, kynurenic acid (KYN), a broad spectrum antagonist of EAA receptors (Ganong & Cotman, 1986; Ganong, Lanthorn, & Cotman, 1983; Perkins & Stone, 1982), causes the most profound effect. The delay in latency induced by KYN is comparable to the previously mentioned delay induced by Ca^{2+}-free dialysis with Co^{2+} or Mg^{2+}. Other investigators have failed to delay the sudden ionic shifts during ischemia or anoxia with EAA antagonists (Hernandez-Caceres, Macias-Gonzalez, Brozele, & Bures, 1987; Hansen, Lauritzen, & Wieloch, 1988; Marrannes, De Prins, Willems, & Wauquier, 1988a, 1988b). However, denervation of glutamatergic afferents has been reported to delay ionic changes in the hippocampus during ischemia (Benveniste, Jorgensen, Lundback, & Hansen, 1989). The disparity in results obtained for systemically administered EAA antagonists may reflect differences in the efficiency of elimination of the effect of EAAs. Together with the role of an elevated $[K^+]_e$ in the Ca^{2+}-dependent exocytotic release of EAAs, it appears that the sudden and rapid increase in $[K^+]_e$ occurring during ischemia represents the result of a malignant cycle between the K^+ flux and EAA release.

An increase in $[Glu]_d$ simultaneous with the increase in $[K^+]_e$ is also observed following FP injury (Katayama, Becker, Tamura, & Hovda, 1990). EAA release has been demonstrated further in other models of TBI (Bullock, Butcher, Chen, Kendall, & McCulloch, 1991; Faden, Demediuk, Panter, & Vink, 1989). Moreover, the traumatic depolarization following FP injury is effectively attenuated in an area perfused by EAA antagonists through microdialysis (Katayama, Becker, Tamura, & Ikezaki, 1990). Among various EAA antagonists, KYN again causes the most profound effect. Systemically administered EAA antagonists have been reported to inhibit spreading depression (Gorelova, Koroleva, Amemori, Pavlik, & Bures, 1987; Hansen et al., 1988; Hernandez-Caceres et al., 1987; Marrannes et al., 1988a, 1988b). These findings imply that involvement of EAA-operated ligand-dependent ion channels is a common feature of the sudden and rapid ionic fluxes, regardless of the cause. It appears that such ionic events may be initiated when a malignant cycle between the ionic fluxes and indiscriminative release of EAAs is triggered.

CELLULAR SWELLING

The massive ionic fluxes, together with other associated phenomena, result in cellular swelling. When rapid cellular swelling occurs, water moves from the ECS into the cells and causes shrinkage of the ECS (i.e., a decrease in water volume in the ECS). The occurrence of cellular swelling and resultant shrinkage of the ECS during spreading depression or anoxic depolarization has been repeatedly demonstrated and can be detected as an increase in concentration of ECS markers, such as tetraethylammonium, tetraethyltris-methylammonium, and choline, which do not move from the ECS into the cells (Hansen & Olsen, 1980; Phillips & Nicholson, 1979). These markers are introduced into the ECS by a superfusion technique. Changes in their ECS concentration are monitored by employing electrodes sensitive to ammonium ions.

Cellular swelling during anoxic depolarization can be detected by microdialysis based on similar principles (Katayama, Tamura, Becker, & Tsubokawa, 1990, 1991b, 1992a). ^{14}C-Sucrose is preperfused into the ECS through the dialysis probe. This substance has been widely employed in in vitro studies as an ECS marker. Changes in the ECS concentration of ^{14}C-sucrose ([^{14}C-sucrose]$_e$) are then determined from the dialysate using perfusate without ^{14}C-sucrose. Following termination of the perfusion of ^{14}C-sucrose, the dialysate concentration of ^{14}C-sucrose ([^{14}C-sucrose]$_d$) decreases rapidly during an initial period of a few minutes, and decreases slowly thereafter. Autoradiograms have demonstrated that an area approximately 1.5 mm from the probe is perfused by the ^{14}C-sucrose. The increase in [^{14}C-sucrose]$_d$ (approximately 1.4-fold) is generally smaller than the increase in ECS marker concentration detected by other methods. This difference may be due, in part, to a decreased recovery rate of the dialysis system in vivo during ischemia (Katayama, Tamura, Becker, & Tsubokawa, 1991a). Transient cellular swelling is also observed in association with the traumatic depolarization following FP injury (Katayama, Becker, Tamura, & Ikezaki, 1990; Katayama, Becker, & Tamura, 1993).

The cellular swelling occurring during anoxic and traumatic depolarization is again inhibited by KYN administered through the dialysis probe (Katayama, Tamura, et al., 1990, 1992a). Although ionic shifts may not be the sole cause of the cellular swelling, this finding indicates that Ca^{2+}-dependent exocytotic release of EAAs may play a major role in producing cellular swelling during the early period after ischemia induction and TBI. EAAs cause large fluxes of Na$^+$, K$^+$, Ca^{2+}, and Cl$^-$ across the cellular membrane in vitro, and these have been shown to generate cellular swelling (Choi, 1987; Mayer & Westbrook, 1987; Olney et al., 1986; Rothman & Olney, 1987). Among the various EAA antagonists, KYN attenuates such cellular swelling in vitro most effectively (Choi, Koh, & Peters, 1988). Pathological processes quite similar to the EAA-mediated ionic fluxes and cellular swelling, which are demonstrated in vitro, may underlie the early cellular swelling following TBI.

ACCELERATED GLYCOLYSIS

The energy metabolism of the brain increases during the period soon after TBI (Duckrow et al., 1981; Nelson, Lowry, & Passonneau, 1966;

Nilsson & Nordstrom, 1977a, 1977b; Nilsson & Ponten, 1977). A diffuse increase in glucose utilization is observed by ^{14}C-deoxyglucose autoradiography following FP injury (Yoshino, Hovda, Kawamata, Katayama, & Becker, 1991). Sudden ionic fluxes across the cellular membrane, such as those seen in spreading depression, strongly activate the energy-dependent ion pumps and adenosine triphosphate (ATP) hydrolysis for restoration of ionic homeostasis (e.g., Rosenthal & Somjen, 1973). During a single passage of spreading depression, almost parallel decreases in glucose content and pH, and elevation of the lactate concentration are detected (Csiba, Paschen, & Mies, 1985; Harris, Richards, Symon, Habib, & Rosenstein, 1987; Mutch and Hansen, 1984; Somjen, 1984). The observed increase in glucose utilization following FP injury may thus be caused by the traumatic depolarization discussed earlier. Because the major component of the ionic fluxes following FP injury appears to be mediated by EAA-coupled ion channels, KYN would tend to attenuate the increase in glucose utilization rate. Consistent with this hypothesis, the increase is clearly inhibited in areas perfused with KYN by microdialysis (Kawamata, Katayama, Hovda, Yoshino, & Becker, 1992). Removal of EAA-mediated afferents also prevents the increase in glucose utilization rate following FP injury (Yoshino, Hovda, Katayama, Kawamata, & Becker, 1992).

LACTATE ACCUMULATION

A sudden increase in ATP hydrolysis stimulates glycolysis and lactate formation, regardless of the energy substrates supply (e.g., Howse & Duffy, 1975; Paschen, Djuricic, Mies, Schmidt-Kostner, & Linn, 1987). As mentioned previously, elevation of the lactate concentration is observed during spreading depression. The anoxic depolarization during ischemia also appears to accelerate lactate accumulation. The dialysate concentration of lactate ($[lactate]_d$) increases dramatically, beginning at a few minutes after ischemia induction (Katayama, Kawamata, Kano, & Tsubokawa, 1992). The increase in $[lactate]_d$ during ischemia is clearly delayed by KYN administered through dialysis probes at doses that delay the anoxic depolarization (Katayama, Kawamata, Kano, et al., 1992). This finding indicates that the early increase in lactate during ischemia is caused by the anoxic depolarization. Such data suggest that the sudden ionic shifts occurring during ischemia may be mediated at their commencement by EAA-coupled ion channels, rather than being merely a result of energy depletion that terminates ion-pump activity.

The value of $[lactate]_d$ also increases following FP injury for 15–20 minutes (Kawamata, Katayama, Hovda, Yoshino, & Becker, 1994). It is not surprising that the traumatic depolarization that lasts for only 3–5 minutes exerts a more sustaining effect on the brain metabolism. Following the passage of a single wave of spreading depression, in which ionic perturbation lasts for approximately 1 minute, a recovery of pH and tissue lactate to their original levels is observed at 10 minutes after repolarization. The increase in [lactate]$_d$ following FP injury can also be inhibited by KYN administered by microdialysis (Kawamata, Katayama, Hovda, Yoshino, & Becker, 1995). Furthermore, inhibition of the energy-dependent ion pump by ouabain administered through dialysis probes can clearly attenuate the increase in [lactate]$_d$ (Kawamata et al., 1995). These findings indicate that strong activation of the energy-dependent ion pumps for the restoration of ionic homeostasis from the traumatic depolarization contributes to the lactate accumulation following FP injury.

Lactate accumulation is one of the most important factors affecting cell viability under pathological conditions such as ischemia and trauma (e.g., Ginsberg, Welsh, & Budd, 1980; Kalimo, Rehncrona, Soderfelt, Olsson, & Siesjo, 1981; Marmarou, 1992; Pulsinelli, Waldman, Rawlinson, & Plum, 1982; Welsh, Ginsberg, Rieder, & Budd, 1980). Earlier in vitro and in vivo studies have demonstrated deleterious effects of lactate accumulation on the brain tissue. It has been reported that, when lactate accumulates at higher concentrations, altered cell membrane structure and function, breakdown of the blood-brain barrier (BBB), brain edema, and widespread damage to the brain tissue are induced. Thus, the lactate accumulation appears to reflect subcellular dysfunctional states of traumatized neuronal cells, and is likely to be related to their vulnerability to a secondary ischemic insult.

FREE FATTY ACID LIBERATION

The tissue levels of free fatty acids become rapidly elevated after induction of ischemia (e.g., Aveldano & Bazan, 1975). This early and rapid increase in free fatty acids is a unique characteristic of the adult brain, and is not seen in neonates or other organs. A rapid increase in free fatty acid levels, superimposed on a continuous slow increase, is observed a few minutes after ischemia induction (Katayama, Kawamata, Masda, Ishikawa, & Tsubokawa, 1994). The early and rapid increase in free fatty acids can be profoundly inhibited by KYN administered through the microdialysis probe, suggesting that EAAs are critically involved in the early phase of free fatty acid liberation (Katayama et al., 1994). Because the development of anoxic depolarization can be delayed for several minutes by KYN administered by the same procedure, the observed inhibition of early free fatty acid liberation may be attributable to a delay in developing anoxic depolarization.

Free fatty acids, such as arachidonic acid, are also liberated rapidly following FP injury. The rapid increase in tissue free fatty acids is inhibited in areas perfused with KYN given by microdialysis (Kawamata et al., unpublished observations). This effect of KYN suggests that free fatty acid liberation may be attributable, at least in part, to neurotransmitter release, which may activate phospholipase C through mechanisms coupled to a guanosine triphosphate-binding protein. Arachidonic acid generates prostaglandins, leukotriens, and free radicals, and this process has been reported to occur in experimental models of TBI. It is possible that such events could also be attributable to the massive ionic fluxes and indiscriminative release of neurotransmitters.

CALCIUM-DEPENDENT DAMAGING PROCESSES

The massive ionic shifts inevitably accompany Ca^{2+} influxes through voltage-dependent Ca^{2+} channels and a decreased function of the Ca^{2+} antiport system. The phospholipase C activation results in an increase in inositol triphosphate-mediated Ca^{2+} mobilization from the intracellular store. Ca^{2+} entry can also occur through N-methyl-D-aspartate receptor-coupled ion channels by EAA release and depolarization. Thus, the free fatty acid liberation may be partially related to Ca^{2+}-dependent activation of phospholipase A_2. Elevation of the intracellular Ca^{2+} would also activate many Ca^{2+}-dependent enzymes, such as proteases and protein kinases (Yang et al., 1993). These enzymes are involved in the induction of immediate early genes and the degradation of cytoskeletal proteins. In fact, c-fos expression (Phillips & Belardo, 1992) and degradation of microtubule-associated protein II (Taft et al., 1992) have been observed in experimental models of TBI. It appears possible that the massive ionic fluxes and indiscriminative release of neurotransmitters are responsible for these subcellular events and their functional consequences (Miyazaki et al., 1992).

MICROGLIAL AND ASTROGLIAL REACTIONS

It has recently been found that microglial activation and astroglial reactions are induced in the hippocampus as early as 1 hour following CI injury (Koshinaga et al., unpublished observations). Microglial cells are identified by the presence of OX 42 immunoreactivity, and the astroglial reaction is evaluated by the glial fibrillary acidic protein (GFAP) immunoreactivity. The intensity of OX 42 immunoreactivity clearly increases in the hippocampus on the injured side, compared with the hippocampus on the other side. An enlargement of astrocytes and elaboration of their processes are noted at the same time. These responses are not dependent on neuronal necrosis. Although the precise functions of the microglia are not yet fully understood, they could play a role in the development of neuronal cell damage through the release of potentially cytotoxic mediators, such as cytokines, proteases, or oxygen radicals (e.g., Giulian & Robertson, 1990).

The microglial activation and astroglial reactions occurring after CI injury are strongly inhibited in areas perfused by KYN administered through the dialysis probe (Koshinaga et al., unpublished observations). This suggests that the initial ionic events and concomitant neurotransmitter release are responsible for these cellular responses as well. Because the microglial cell is sensitive to depolarizing events, in contrast to other glial cells (e.g., Kettenmann, Hoppe, Gottmann, Banati, & Kreutzberg, 1990), the traumatic depolarization may play an important role in microglial activation.

CONCLUSIONS

Based on the previous data, we postulate that important causal relationships exist between the traumatic depolarization, in which EAAs play a vital role, and subsequent subcellular and cellular events, which lead neuronal cells to undergo metabolic derangements. Similar relationships can be postulated in ischemic brain injury. In the case of severe ischemia, the anoxic depolarization develops rapidly and is associated with substantial elevations of the intracellular Na^+, Ca^{2+}, and Cl^-. Most neurons are irreversibly damaged by lactic acidosis, free radical generation, and overactivation of Ca^{2+}-sensitive mechanisms (e.g., Siesjo & Wieloch, 1985).

Among the patterns of brain damage following clinical TBI, diffuse ischemia-like damage is one of the dominant findings, even in cases without episodes of hypoxia (hypoxemia or hypotension) or elevated intracranial pressure (Graham et al., 1988, 1989). The ischemia-like damage after TBI can occur without boundary-zone ischemic damage, suggesting that it may not be caused merely by ischemic insults. Hippocampal ischemia-like damage is especially common, occurring in 50% of cases without episodes of hypoxia (hypoxemia or hypotension) or elevated intracranial pressure (Graham et al., 1988; Kotapka et al., 1991). The similarities between the cellular and subcellular events associated with traumatic depolarization and those associated with anoxic depolarization may underlie the ischemia-like damage observed in TBI.

There is, however, an essential difference in the processes of neuronal cell damage between ischemic brain injury and TBI. In ischemic brain injury, the normal ionic gradients maintained by the neuronal cells become compromised as a consequence of the depleted energy stores. In contrast, the ionic perturbation in TBI is directly initiated by mechanical deformation of the neuronal cells. Thus, depletion of the energy store does not occur primarily in TBI, which may be why the damage to neuronal cells after TBI varies greatly depending on the supply of energy substrates.

ACKNOWLEDGMENTS

The data reviewed in this chapter are derived from experiments conducted in collaboration with Drs. T. Tamura, M. Koshinaga, T. Kano, and T. Maeda (Department of Neurological Surgery, Nihon University, Tokyo), and Drs. D. A. Hovda and D. P. Becker (Department of Neurosurgery, University of California at Los Angeles). These investigations were supported by a grant from the National Institutes of Health of the U.S.A. (NS27544), a research grant for Cardiovascular Disease (2A-2) from the Ministry of Health and Welfare, and a research grant from the Ministry of Education and Culture (CO6671425) of Japan.

REFERENCES

Aveldano, M. I., & Bazan, N. G. (1975). Rapid production of diacylglycerols enriched in arachidonate and stearate during early brain ischemia. *Journal of Neurochemistry, 25,* 919–920.

Benveniste, H., Drejer, J., Schousboe, A., & Diemer, N. H. (1984). Elevation of the extracellular concentrations of glutamate and aspartate in rat hippocampus during transient cerebral ischemia monitored by intracerebral microdialysis. *Journal of Neurochemistry, 43,* 1369–1374.

Benveniste, H., Jorgensen, M. B., Lundbaek, J. A., & Hansen, A. J. (1989). Ionic changes in the normal and denervated hippocampus during ischemia. *Journal of Cerebral Blood Flow Metabolism, 9,* 46.

Bullock, R., Butcher, S. P., Chen, M.-H., Kendall, L., & McCulloch, J. (1991). Correlation of the extracellular glutamate concentration with extent of blood flow reduction after subdural haematoma in the rat. *J. Neurosurg, 74,* 794–802.

Choi, D. W. (1987). Ionic dependence of glutamate neurotoxicity. *Journal of Neuroscience, 7,* 369–379.

Choi, D. W., Koh, J.-Y., & Peters, S. (1988). Pharmacology of glutamate neurotoxicity in cortical cell culture: Attenuation by NMDA antagonist. *Journal of Neuroscience, 8,* 185–196.

Csiba, L., Paschen, W., & Mies, G. (1985). Regional changes in tissue pH and glucose content during cortical spreading depression in rat brain. *Brain Research, 336,* 167–170.

Dixon, C. E., Clifton, G. L., Lighthall, J. W., Yaghmai, A. A., & Hayes, R. L. (1991). A controlled cortical impact model of traumatic brain injury in the rat. *Journal of Neuroscience Methods, 39,* 253–262.

Dixon, C. E., Lyeth, B. G., Povlishock, J. T., Findling, R. L., Hamm, R. J., Marmarou, A., Young, H. F., & Hayes, R. L. (1987). A fluid-percussion model of experimental brain injury in the rat. *Journal of Neurosurgery, 67,* 110–119.

Drejer, J., Benveniste, H., Deemer, N. H., & Schousboe, A. (1985). Cellular origin of ischemia-induced glutamate release from brain tissue *in vivo* and *in vitro. Journal of Neurochemistry, 45,* 145–151.

Duckrow, R. B., LaManna, J. C., Rosenthal, M., Levasseur, J. E., & Patterson, J. L., Jr. (1981). Oxidative metabolism activity of cerebral cortex after fluid-percussion head injury in the cat. *Journal of Neurosurgery, 54,* 607–614.

Faden, A. I., Demediuk, P., Panter, S. S., & Vink, R. (1989). The role of excitatory amino acids and NMDA receptors in traumatic brain injury. *Science, 244,* 798–800.

Ganong, A. H., & Cotman, C. W. (1986). Kynurenic acid and quinolinic acid act at N-methyl-D-aspartate receptors in the rat hippocampus. *Journal of Pharmacology and Experimental Therapeutics, 236,* 293–299.

Ganong, A. H., Lanthorn, T. H., & Cotman, C. W. (1983). Kynurenic acid inhibits synaptic and acidic amino acid-induced responses in the rat hippocampus and spinal cord. *Brain Research, 273,* 170–174.

Ginsberg, M. S., Welsh, F. A., & Budd, W. W. (1980). Deleterious effect of glucose pretreatment on recovery from diffuse cerebral ischemia in the cat. *Stroke, 11,* 347–354.

Giulian, D., & Robertson, C. (1990). Inhibition of mononuclear phagocytes reduces ischemic injury in the spinal cord. *Annals of Neurology, 27,* 33–42.

Gorelova, N. A., Koroleva, V. I., Amemori, T., Pavlik, V., & Bures, J. (1987). Ketamine blockade of cortical spreading depression in rats. *Electroencephalography and Clinical Neurophysiology, 66,* 440–447.

Graham, D. I., Ford, I., Adams, J., Doyle, D., Teasdale, G. M., Lawrence, A. E., & McLellan, D. R. (1989). Ischemic brain damage is still common in fatal non-missile head injury. *Journal of Neurology Neurosurgery Psychiatry, 52,* 346–350.

Graham, D. I., Lawrence, A. E., Adams, J. H., Doyle, D., & McLellan, D. R. (1988). Brain damage in non-missile head injury without high intracranial pressure. *Journal of Clinical Pathology, 41,* 34–37.

Hansen, A. J. (1977). Extracellular potassium concentration in juvenile and adult rat brain cortex during anoxia. *Acta Physiologica Scandinavica, 99,* 412–420.

Hansen, A. J. (1985). Effect of anoxia on ion distribution in the brain. *Physiological Review, 165,* 101–148.

Hansen, A. J., Lauritzen, M., & Wieloch, T. (1988). MK-801 inhibits spreading depression but not anoxic depolarization. In J. Lehman & L. Turski (Eds.), *Recent advances in excitatory amino acid research.* New York: Allan Liss.

Hansen, A. J., & Olsen, C. E. (1980). Brain extracellular space during spreading depression and ischemia. *Acta Physiologica Scandinavica, 108,* 355–365.

Harris, R. J., Richards, P. G., Symon, L., Habib, A.-H. A., & Rosenstein, J. (1987). pH, K^+, and PO_2 of the extracellular space during ischemia of primate cerebral cortex. *Journal of Cerebral Blood Flow Metabolism, 7,* 599–604.

Hayes, R. L. (1991). Central nervous system trauma: Neurotransmitter mediated mechanisms of traumatic brain injury: Acetylcholine and excitatory amino acids. *Journal of Neurotrauma, 9*(Suppl. 1), 157–164.

Hernandez-Caceres, J., Macias-Gonzalez, R., Brozek, G., & Bures, J. (1987). Systemic ketamine blocks spreading depression but does not delay the onset of terminal anoxic depolarization in rats. *Brain Research, 437,* 360–364.

Hovda, D. A., Becker, D. P., & Katayama, Y. (1991). Central nervous system trauma: Secondary injury and acidosis. *Journal of Neurotrauma, 9*(Suppl. 1), 47–70.

Howse, D. C., & Duffy, T. E. (1975). Control of the redox state of the pyridine nucleotides in the rat cerebral cortex: Effect of electroshock-induced seizures. *J. Neurochem, 24,* 935–940.

Jenkins, L. W., Moszynski, K., Lyeth, B. G., Lewelt, W., DeWitt, D. S., Allen, A., Dixon, C. E., Povlishock, J. T., Majewski, T. J., Clifton, G. L., Young, H. F., Becker, D. P., & Hayes, R. L. (1989). Increased vulnerability of the mildly traumatized rat brain to cerebral ischemia: The use of controlled secondary ischemia as a research tool to identify common or different mechanisms contributing to mechanical and ischemic brain injury. *Brain Research, 477,* 211–224.

Kalimo, H., Rehncrona, S., Soderfelt, B., Olsson, Y., & Siesjo, B. K. (1981). Brain lactic acidosis and ischemic cell damage: 2. Histopathology. *Journal of Cerebral Blood Flow Metabolism, 1,* 313–327.

Katayama, Y., Becker, D. P., & Tamura, T. (1993). Changes in cerebrovascular permeability and excitatory amino acid-mediated cellular swelling in experimental concussive brain injury. In C. J. J. Avezaat, J. H. M. van Eijndhoven, A. I. R. Mass, J. Th. J. Tans (Eds.), *Intracranial pressure* (Vol. 8, pp. 484–487). Berlin: Springer.

Katayama, Y., Becker, D. P., Tamura, T., & Hovda, D. (1990). Massive increase in extracellular potassium and indiscriminative glutamate release after concussive brain injury. *Journal of Neurosurgery, 73,* 889–900.

Katayama, Y., Becker, D. P., Tamura, T., & Ikezaki, K. (1990). Early cellular swelling in experimental traumatic brain injury: A phenomenon mediated by excitatory amino acids. *Acta Neurochirurgica, 51,* 271–273.

Katayama, Y., Cheung, M. K., Alves, A., & Becker, D. P. (1989). Ion fluxes and cell swelling after experimental traumatic brain injury: The role of excitatory amino acids. In J. T. Hoff & A. L. Betz (Eds.), *Intracranial pressure* (Vol. 7, pp. 584–588). Berlin: Springer.

Katayama, Y., Kawamata, T., Kano, T., & Tsubokawa, T. (1992). Excitatory amino acid antagonist administered via microdialysis attenuates lactate accumulation during cerebral ischemia and subsequent hippocampal damage. *Brain Research, 584,* 329–333.

Katayama, Y., Kawamata, T., Maeda, T., Ishikawa, K., & Tsubokawa, T. (1994). Inhibition of the early phase of free fatty acid liberation during cerebral ischemia by excitatory amino acid antagonist administered by microdialysis. *Brain Research, 635,* 331–334.

Katayama, Y., Kawamata, T., Tamura, T., Becker, D. P., & Tsubokawa, T. (1991). Calcium-dependent glutamate release concomitant with massive potassium flux during cerebral ischemia in vivo. *Brain Research, 558,* 136–140.

Katayama, Y., Tamura, T., Becker, D. P., & Tsubokawa, T. (1990). Cellular swelling during cerebral ischemia demonstrated by microdialysis in vivo: Preliminary data indicating the role of excitatory amino acids. *Acta Neurochirurgica, 51,* 183–185.

Katayama, Y., Tamura, T., Becker, D. P., & Tsubokawa, T. (1991a). Calcium-dependent component of massive increase in extracellular potassium during cerebral ischemia as demonstrated by microdialysis *in vivo. Brain Research, 567,* 57–63.

Katayama, Y., Tamura, T., Becker, D. P., & Tsubokawa, T. (1991b). Detection of cellular swelling and subsequent increase in plasma membrane permeability during cerebral ischemia *in vivo* using microdialysis. *Journal of Cerebral Blood Flow Metabolism, 11,* 479.

Katayama, Y., Tamura, T., Becker, D. P., & Tsubokawa, T. (1992a). Early cellular swelling during cerebral ischemia *in vivo* is mediated by excitatory amino acids released from nerve terminal. *Brain Research, 584,* 329–333.

Katayama, Y., Tamura, T., Becker, D. P., & Tsubokawa, T. (1992b). Inhibition of rapid potassium flux during cerebral ischemia *in vivo* with excitatory amino acid antagonist. *Brain Research, 568,* 294–298.

Kawamata, T., Katayama, Y., Hovda, D. A., Yoshino, A., & Becker, D. P. (1992). Administration of excitatory amino acid antagonists via microdialysis attenuates the increase in glucose utilization seen following concussive brain injury. *Journal of Cerebral Blood Flow Metabolism, 12,* 12–24.

Kawamata, T., Katayama, Y., Hovda, D. A., Yoshino, A., & Becker, D. P. (1995). Lactate accumulation following concussive brain injury: The role of ionic fluxes induced by excitatory amino acids. *Brain Research, 674,* 196–204.

Kettenmann, H., Hoppe, D., Gottmann, K., Banati, R., & Kreutzberg, G. (1990). Cultured microglial cells have a distinct pattern of membrane channels different from peritoneal macrophages. *Journal of Neuroscience Research, 26,* 278–287.

Kotapka, M. J., Gennarelli, T. A., Graham, D. I., Adams, J. H., Thibault, L. E., Ross, D. T., & Ford, I. (1991). Selective vulnerability of hippocampal neurons in acceleration-induced experimental head injury. *Journal of Neurotrauma, 8,* 247–258.

Marmarou, A. (1992). Intracellular acidosis in human and experimental brain injury. *Journal of Neurotrauma, 9,* 551–562.

Marrannes, R., De Prins, E., Willems, R., & Wauquier, A. (1988a). NMDA antagonists inhibit cortical spreading depression but accelerate the onset of neuronal depolarization induced by asphyxia. In G. Somjen (Ed.), *Mechanisms of cerebral hypoxia and stroke* (pp. 303–304). New York: Plenum.

Marrannes, R., De Prins, E., Willems, R., & Wauquier, A. (1988b). Evidence for a role of the N-methyl-D-aspartate (NMDA) receptor in cortical spreading depression in the rat. *Brain Research, 457,* 226–240.

Mayer, M. L., & Westbrook, G. L. (1987). Cellular mechanisms underlying excitotoxicity. *TINS, 10,* 59–61.

Miyazaki, S., Katayama, Y., Lyeth, B. G., Jenkins, L. W., DeWitt, D. S., Goldberg, S. J., Newlon, P. G., & Hayes, R. L. (1992). Enduring suppression of hippocampal long-term potentiation following traumatic brain injury in rat. *Brain Research, 585,* 335–339.

Moghaddam, B., Schenk, J. O., Stewart, W. B., & Hansen, A. J. (1987). Temporal relationship between neurotransmitter release and ion flux during spreading depression and anoxia. *Canadian Journal of Physiology and Pharmacology, 54,* 1105–1110.

Nelson, S. R., Lowry, O. H., & Passonneau, J. V. (1966). Changes in energy reserves in mouse brain associated with compressive head injury. In W. F. Careness & A. W. Walker (Eds.), *Head injury* (pp. 444–447). Philadelphia: Lippincott.

Nicholson, C., & Kraig, R. P. (1981). The behavior of extracellular ions during spreading depression. In T. Zeuthen (Ed.), *The application of ion electrodes* (pp. 217–238). Amsterdam: Elsevier, North-Holland.

Nicholson, C., Phillips, J. M., & Gardner-Medwin, A. R. (1979). Diffusion from a iontophoretic point source in the rat brain: Role of tortuosity and volume fraction. *Brain Research, 169,* 580–584.

Nilsson, P., Hillered, L., Olsson, Y., Sheardown, M. J., & Hansen, A. J. (1993). Regional changes in interstitial K^+ and Ca^{2+} levels following cortical compression contusion trauma in rats. *Journal of Cerebral Blood Flow Metabolism, 13,* 183–192.

Nilsson, B., & Nordstrom, C. H. (1977a). Experimental head injury in the rat: Part 3. Cerebral blood flow and oxygen consumption after concussive impact acceleration. *Journal of Neurosurgery, 47,* 262–273.

Nilsson, B., & Nordstrom, C. H. (1977b). Rate of cerebral energy consumption in concussive head injury in the rat. *Journal of Neurosurgery, 47,* 274–281.

Nilsson, B., & Ponten, U. (1977). Experimental head injury in the rat: Part 2. Regional brain energy metabolism in concussive trauma. *Journal of Neurosurgery, 47,* 252–261.

Olney, J. W., Price, M. T., Samson, L., & Lambuyere, J. (1986). The role of specific ions in glutamate neurotoxicity. *Neuroscience Letters, 65,* 65–71.

Perkins, M. N., & Stone, T. W. (1982). An iontophoretic investigation of the actions of convulsant kynurenines and their interaction with the endogenous excitant quinolinic acid. *Brain Research, 247,* 184–187.

Phillips, J. M., & Nicholson, C. (1979). Anion permeability in spreading depression investigated with ion-sensitive microelectrodes. *Brain Research, 173,* 567–571.

Phillips, L. L., & Belardo, E. T. (1992). Expression of c-fos in the hippocampus following mild and moderate fluid percussion brain injury. *Journal of Neurotrauma, 9,* 323–334.

Povlishock, J. T., Becker, D. P., Sullivan, H. G., & Miller, J. D. (1978). Vascular permeability alterations to horseradish peroxidase in experimental brain injury. *Brain Research, 153,* 223–239.

Pulsinelli, W. A., Waldman, S., Rawlinson, D., & Plum, F. (1982). Moderate hyperglycemia augments ischemic brain damage: A neuropathologic study in the rat. *Neurology, 32,* 1239–1246.

Rosenthal, M., & Somjen, G. (1973). Spreading depression sustained potential shifts and metabolic activity of cerebral cortex in cats. *Journal of Neurophysiology, 36,* 739–745.

Rothman, S. M., & Olney, J. W. (1987). Excitotoxicity and the NMDA receptor. *TINS, 10,* 299–302.

Siesjo, B. K., & Wieloch, T. (1985). Molecular mechanisms of ischemic brain damage: Calcium related events. In F. Plum & W. Pulsinelli (Eds.), *Cerebrovascular diseases* (pp. 187–197). New York: Raven Press.

Taft, W. C., Yang, K., Dixon, C. E., Clifton, G. L., & Hayes, R. L. (1992). Microtubule-associated protein 2 levels decreases in hippocampus following traumatic brain injury. *Journal of Neurotrauma, 9,* 281–290.

Takahashi, H., Manaka, S., & Sano, K. (1981). Changes in extracellular potassium concentration in cortex and brain stem during the acute phase of experimental closed head injury. *Journal of Neurosurgery, 55,* 708–717.

Tsubokawa, T. (1983). Cerebral circulation and metabolism in concussion. *Neurological Surgery* (Tokyo), *11,* 563–573.

Van Harreveld, A. (1978). Two mechanisms for spreading depression in chicken retina. *Journal of Neurobiology, 9,* 419–431.

Welsh, F. A., Ginsberg, M. D., Rieder, W., & Budd, W. W. (1980). Deleterious effect of glucose pretreatment on recovery from diffuse cerebral ischemia in the cat. *Stroke, 11,* 355–363.

Yang, K., Taft, W. C., Dixon, C. E., Todaro, C. A., Yu, R. K., & Hayes, R. L. (1993). Alteration of protein kinase C in rat hippocampus following traumatic brain injury. *Journal of Neurotrauma, 10,* 287–295.

Yoshino, A., Hovda, D. A., Katayama, Y., Kawamata, T., & Becker, D. P. (1992). Hippocampal CA3 lesion prevents the post-concussive metabolic derangement in CA1. *Journal of Cerebral Blood Flow Metabolism, 12,* 996–1006.

Yoshino, A., Hovda, D. A., Kawamata, T., Katayama, Y., & Becker, D. P. (1991). Dynamic changes in local cerebral glucose utilization following fluid-percussion injury: Evidence of a hyper- and subsequent hypometabolic state. *Brain Res, 561,* 106–119.

5

Light and Electron Microscopic Studies of Fluid-Percussion Brain Injury in Rats: Posttraumatic Temperature Considerations

W. Dalton Dietrich

In many head-injured patients, the extent of neurological recovery may depend on the presence of posttraumatic secondary insults. In the clinical setting, such secondary injury consequences include posttraumatic hypotension, hypoxia, hyperglycemia, anemia, sepsis, and hyperthermia (Ellis, Chao, & Heizer, 1989; Hovda, Becker, & Katayama, 1992; Ishige et al., 1987; Young, 1988). Recent experimental evidence also indicates an increased susceptibility of the posttraumatic brain to secondary insults (Ishige et al., 1987; Jenkins et al., 1988, 1989; Tanno, Nockels, Pitts, & Noble, 1992). For example, Jenkins and colleagues (1989) showed that traumatic brain injury (TBI) produced sublethal selective neuronal vulnerability, especially within the CA1 hippocampus. In that study, mild levels of TBI not associated with CA1 damage preferentially enhanced the sensitivity of CA1 neurons to imposed secondary ischemia. In another fluid-percussion (FP) brain injury study, Tanno and colleagues (1992) demonstrated that secondary hypoxia exacerbated the blood-brain barrier (BBB) consequences of head trauma. Thus, a major goal of research on the traumatized brain is to determine the characteristics of these secondary processes, which may be attenuated by appropriate intensive care management and/or pharmacotherapy.

Small variations in brain temperature critically influence the histopathological and functional consequences of various types of brain injury (for reviews, see Dietrich, 1992; Dietrich, Alonso, Busto, Globus, & Ginsburg, 1994; Ginsberg, Sternau, Globus, Dietrich, & Busto, 1992). In models of brain ischemia, for example, mild intra- and postischemic

67

hypothermia improved ischemic outcome (Busto, Dietrich, Globus, & Ginsberg, 1989; Busto et al., 1987; Dietrich, Alonso, Busto, Globus, & Ginsberg, 1994a; Dietrich, Alonso, & Halley, 1994b; Dietrich, Busto, Globus, & Ginsberg, 1993; Dietrich, Busto, Halley, & Valdes, 1990a; Dietrich, Busto, Valdes, & Loor, 1990b; Dietrich, Halley, Valdes, & Busto, 1991; Green et al., 1992). In models of TBI, pre- and posttraumatic hypothermia improved behavioral recovery and histopathological outcome (Clifton et al., 1991; Dietrich et al., 1994a, 1994b; Lyeth, Jiang, & Shanliang, 1993; Palmer, Marion, Botsceller, & Redd, 1993; Jiang, Lyeth, Kapasi, Jenkins, & Povlishock, 1992). Recently, hypothermia has been used in the clinic to treat patients with brain trauma and subarachnoid hemorrhage (Clifton et al., 1993; Marion, Obrist, Carlier, Penrod, & Darby, 1993; Resnick, Marion, & Darby, 1994; Shiozaki et al., 1993). Thus, hypothermia may also be beneficial in the acute clinical setting.

In contrast to hypothermia, mild intra- and postinjury hyperthermia (40°C) has been shown to worsen outcome (Clifton et al., 1991; Dietrich, 1992; Dietrich, Alonso, Halley, & Busto, 1996; Dietrich, Busto, Halley, et al., 1990; Dietrich, Busto, Valdes, et al., 1990). Clinically, posttraumatic hyperthermia is commonly seen in head-injured patients and can be associated with poor outcome (Hayashi, Hirayama, & Ohata, 1993; Rousseaux, Scherpered, Bernard, Graftieaux, & Guyot, 1980). Recent studies, in which brain temperature was measured in patients, have documented transient periods of brain hyperthermia at variable periods following head injury (Hayashi et al., 1993; Sternau et al., 1991). In the laboratory, raising pretraumatic brain temperature to 40°C has been reported to worsen the behavioral consequences of TBI compared with 36°C (Clifton et al., 1991). Thus, posttraumatic hyperthermia is likely an important secondary insult that may retard recovery mechanisms. The purpose of this chapter is to review recent data regrading the early and more chronic histopathological consequences of TBI in the rat. Such studies describe pathophysiological events, which include both primary and secondary mechanisms that may be targeted for therapeutic consideration. In addition, recent data concerning the neuroprotective effects of posttraumatic hypothermia, as well as the detrimental consequences of delayed hyperthermia in a rat model of FP brain injury, are discussed.

ANIMAL MODELS

Various animal models of brain injury are currently in use to investigate the pathophysiology of head injury (see Gennarelli, 1994; Gennarelli & Thibault, 1985). Depending on the investigator's desires, different animal models and species can be chosen to investigate specific aspects of the injury process. The FP model has been used in cats, rats, and swine to produce brief behavioral unresponsiveness (e.g., coma) with variable degrees of histopathological damage (Cortez, McIntosh, & Noble, 1989; Dixon et al., 1987; Katayama, Becker, Tamura, & Hovda, 1990; McIntosh et al., 1989). Our laboratory has recently reported a consistent pattern of histopathological damage, including subcortical contusion and scattered ischemic neurons, in a rat model of TBI (Dietrich et al., 1994a, 1994b). For such studies, FP brain injury is induced in fasted Sprague–Dawley rats weighing between 250 and 300 g. One day prior to injury, rats are anesthetized with 1.5% halothane, 70% nitrous oxide, and 30% oxygen. Intubated rats are then placed in a stereotaxic frame and a 4.8-mm craniotomy made overlying the right parietal cortex. A plastic injury tube is then placed over the exposed dura, bounded by adhesive, and then plugged with a gelfoam sponge. The scalp is closed, at which time the animal is returned to its cage and allowed to recover overnight before TBI.

The FP device previously described is used the next day to produce brain injury. Rats are reanesthetized and maintained on 1.5% halothane, 70% nitrous oxide, and 30% oxygen. Temporalis muscle temperature is monitored and maintained at 37.5°C for 30 minutes prior to TBI. Mild to moderate injury ranging from 1.5 to 2.2 atmospheres is investigated. Following TBI, rats are immediately perfusion fixed for ultrastructural analysis, undergo brain temperature monitoring, or are returned to their cages and allowed to recover from the surgical procedures.

TEMPERATURE MANIPULATIONS

To determine the effects of posttraumatic hypothermia on histopathological outcome, brain temperature is reduced to 30°C after TBI by blowing cool air over the exposed skull. By using this methodology, brain temperature can be reduced to hypothermic levels in 1–2 minutes (Dietrich et al., 1994a). Brain temperature is monitored by a probe within the temporalis muscle because this procedure has been shown to accurately represent brain temperature (Busto et al., 1987; Jiang et al., 1991). After 3 hours of posttraumatic hypothermia, rats are returned to their cages prior to histopathological study.

To determine whether delayed posttraumatic hyperthermia worsens traumatic outcome, rats are reanesthetized 24 hours following TBI; brain temperature is elevated to 39°C for a 3-hour period by placing a heating lamp over the rat's head. Normothermic rats undergo similar procedures, but brain temperature is maintained at 37°C for the 3-hour period. Again, temporalis muscle temperature is used as an indirect measurement of brain temperature. Following the 3-hour temperature-monitoring period, rats are either perfusion fixed immediately for ultrastructural analysis or returned to their cages for a 3-day recovery period.

PATHOLOGICAL ASSESSMENT

For ultrastructural studies, rats are injected with the protein tracer horseradish peroxidase (HRP) 15 minutes prior to perfusion fixation (Dietrich et al., 1994b). This protein tracer is advantageous in studies where the ultrastructural correlates of BBB disruption are investigated. Brains are then cut with a Vibratome (50–100 um) and reacted for the visualization of HRP. Based on neuroanatomical landmarks or patterns of protein extravasation, sections are hand dissected and processed for plastic embedding. Thick plastic sections (1 um) are then stained for light microscopic analysis. Various morphometric procedures are used to quantitatively assess neuronal or vascular perturbations. For example, numbers of leaky blood vessels (Dietrich, Busto, Halley, et al., 1990) or swollen axons are counted per microscopic field, and regional abnormalities are assessed. These data are then compared with control or traumatized rats from the different temperature groups. Once these sections are analyzed, ultrathin sections are taken for ultrastructural analysis.

For paraffin embedding and subsequent light microscopic study, rats are anesthetized 3–4 days after TBI and are perfusion fixed for histopathological analysis. Semiserial sections are taken through the neuraxis and stained with hematoxylin and eosin. Quantitative assessment of histopathological injury includes the frequency of selective neuronal damage, as well as contusion area at several coronal levels (Dietrich, Alonso, Busto, Globus, et al., 1994).

POSTTRAUMATIC HYPOTHERMIA

Recent experimental studies have demonstrated that mild levels of pre- and posttraumatic hypothermia can provide significant protection in experimental models of TBI. In a study by Clifton et al. (1991), rats in which brain temperature was decreased to 30°C prior to injury demonstrated significantly less mortality after moderate TBI. In addition, hypothermia induced 5 minutes after TBI also reduced functional motor deficits. By using a controlled cortical impact (CI) model in rats, Palmer and colleagues (1993) showed that pretraumatic hypothermia (32°C–33°C) also significantly reduced infarct lesion volume. Recently, Lyeth, Jiang, and Liu, 1993 (1993) reported neurobehavioral protection by moderate hypothermia initiated after TBI. In that study, hypothermia (30°C) initiated 15 minutes but not 30 minutes after trauma improved beam balance and beam walking deficits on Days 3 and 4 compared with normothermic rats. To determine whether hypothermia would reduce the vascular permeability consequences of trauma, Jiang and colleagues (1992) investigated whether hypothermia induced prior to injury would protect the BBB. In hypothermic rats, albumin immunoreactivity was confined to the gray-white interface between the cortex and hippocampus, whereas normothermic rats demonstrated increased vascular permeability to albumin throughout the dorsal cortical gray and white matter structures, as well as the underlying hippocampus.

Our laboratory recently determined the effects of posttraumatic hypothermia on histopathological damage in the rat (Dietrich, Alonso, Busto, Globus, et al., 1994). In these studies, brain injury was produced by positioning the injury tube over the parasagittal right parietal cortex 3.8 mm posterior to bregma and 2.5 mm lateral to the midline. This injury site differs from the midline or lateral approach used by previous investigators (Cortez et al., 1989; Dixon et al., 1987; Faden, Demediuk, Panter, & Vink, 1989; Hayes et al., 1988; Hayes, Jenkins, & Lyeth, 1991; Jenkins et al., 1988; McIntosh et al., 1989). In normothermic rats, cortical areas lateral to the injury site contained necrotic neurons with eosinophilic cytoplasm and pynotic nuclei. Damaged neurons were most numerous within the deeper cortical layers, including Layers 5 and 6. Underlying the damaged cerebral cortex, a focal contusion was commonly seen at the gray-white interface. In most cases, the contused site was hemorrhagic, but the degree of hemorrhage varied among rats. Necrotic neurons were also detected within subcortical areas, including the ipsilateral hippocampus and thalamus. Within the hippocampus, the eosinophilic neurons were present within the CA3 and CA4 subsectors, as well as the dentate hilus. In the thalamus, necrotic neurons were seen in the lateral and dorsal nuclei.

These data document a consistent pattern of histopathological vulnerability after normothermic TBI. Neuronal damage within the gray-white interface remote from the impact site may primarily result from rotational forces that disrupt blood vessels. Recent ultrastructural studies have identified ruptured blood vessels within the subcortical white matter, which are responsible for early BBB perturbations (Dietrich, Alonso, & Halley, 1994). In this brain-injury model, shearing stress induced by the CI (Ribas & Jane, 1992) therefore leads to primary vascular damage and hemorrhagic contusion. Because the degree of cortical neuronal damage is related to contusion volume (Dietrich, Alonso, Busto, Globus, et al., 1994), cortical pathology may be a secondary consequence of acute microvascular damage within the contused region. Hippocampal damage may also be a secondary consequence of cortical damage.

Thus, the excessive activation of hippocampal circuits, leading to neuro-nal excitation and excitotoxic-mediated neuronal injury, may be in-volved in this pathology.

In contrast to these normothermic results, posttraumatic hypothermia significantly decreased the frequency of necrotic neurons, as well as decreasing contusion volume. Posttraumatic hypothermia also signifi-cantly reduced the incidence of selective neuronal necrosis within the hippocampus and thalamus. These results indicate that structural pro-tection may be possible in head-injured patients in whom early cooling is initiated. Recent clinical data supporting such a contention have been presented. In a Phase 2 study of moderate hypothermia in severe brain-injured patients, Clifton and colleagues (1993) reported the results of 46 patients with severe nonpenetrating brain injury who were randomized to standard management at 37°C and to standard management with systemic hypothermia at 30°C–32°C. In that study, cooling was begun within 6 hours of injury by the use of cooling blankets. Evidence of improved neurological outcome with minimum toxicity was reported in the moderately systemic hypothermic patients. In another study by Mar-ion and colleagues (1993), the potentially beneficial effects of post-traumatic hypothermia were assessed in 40 consecutively treated pa-tients with severe closed head injury. Patients in the hypothermic group were cooled to 32°C–33°C within a mean of 10 hours after injury. Hypo-thermia significantly reduced intracranial pressure (ICP) and cerebral blood flow (CBF) during the cooling period. In this study, a trend toward better outcome with hypothermia was also reported.

In a recent study by Resnick and colleagues (1994), no significant increase in the incidence of delayed traumatic intracerebral hemorrhage, prothrombin times, or platelet count abnormalities in hypothermic pa-tients with severe head injury was reported. Also, Shiozaki and col-leagues (1993) recently determined the effect of mild hypothermia on uncontrollable intracranial hypotension after severe injury. Their prelim-inary investigations suggest that mild hypothermia (34°C) is a safe and effective method to control traumatic intracranial hypertension and to decrease mortality and morbidity rates. Taken together, these studies indicate that posttraumatic hypothermia may increase survival rate and improve neurological recovery in patients, and therefore may be an important method for managing patients with severe head injury.

DELAYED POSTTRAUMATIC HYPERTHERMIA

Posttraumatic hyperthermia is a common consequence of TBI. Hayashi and colleagues (1993) reported brain tissue temperature elevations to 38°C–43.8°C during the first 17–30 hours after head injury. Sternau and colleagues (1991) reported a disparity between brain and body temperatures following brain injury in humans. In clinical settings where only core (i.e., bladder) temperature is monitored, degrees of brain hyperthermia may therefore be underestimated. Thus, posttraumatic brain hyperthermia may represent an important, yet clinically manageable, secondary injury mechanism. For this reason, our recent investigations have determined whether delayed posttraumatic hyperthermia would affect traumatic outcome. For ultrastructural studies, rats were perfusion fixed immediately following a 3-hour hyperthermic period initiated 24 hours after TBI. Figure 5.1 illustrates alterations in BBB permeability seen in posttraumatic rats where hyperthermia was secondarily induced. Compared with normothermic rats, delayed posttraumatic hyperthermia led to increased hemorrhage at the level of the gray-white interface underlying the lateral somatosensory cortex (Fig. 5.1a). At sites of increased hemorrhage, subcortical white matter tracts appeared severely swollen (Fig. 5.1b). Thus, an obvious consequence of delayed posttraumatic hyperthermia is increased hemorrhage and brain swelling.

Thick plastic sections of cortical and striatal regions demonstrated a higher frequency of abnormal myelinated axons from posttraumatic hyperthermia rats compared with normothermic rats (Figs. 5.1c and 5.1d). Within the cerebral cortex (Fig. 5.1c), swollen axons were predominantly seen within the deeper layers of cortical Layer 6. In the striatum, swollen axons were also seen in white matter fascicles (Fig. 5.1d). In addition to these axonal changes, luminal white blood cells with and without associated red blood cell stasis were observed in cortical and subcortical areas (Fig. 5.1e).

Ultrastructural examination of these sites revealed a high frequency of myelinated axons showing a range of abnormal features (Figs. 5.2a–5.2d). Reactive axonal swelling was seen in fields of unaltered axons (Fig. 5.2a). Reactive axons occasionally contained a core of clumped neurofilaments surrounded by an accumulation of organelles (Fig. 5.2b). This type of axonal change has been described previously in several models of diffuse axonal injury (Povlishock, 1992). In addition to these reactive changes, large numbers of swollen axons were observed. In these axons, the myelin sheath appeared thin, and the filamentous ultrastructure of normal axoplasm was replaced by a flocculent precipitate, or with no observable cytoskeleton. In addition, few membranous organelles were seen in swollen segments. Ultrastructural identification of white blood cells identified mono- and polynuclear white blood cells adhering to relatively intact endothelium (Figs. 5.2e and 5.2f). In addition, extravasated polymorphonuclear leukocytes (Fig. 5.2f) were frequently observed within a relatively normal-appearing brain parenchyma.

The early structural consequences of posttraumatic hyperthermia in-

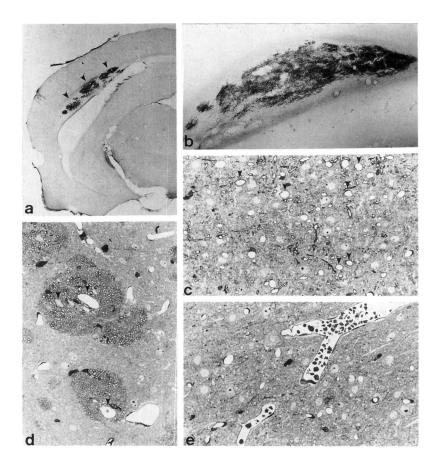

FIG. 5.1. Light microscopic findings from posttraumatic hyperthermic rats.
(a) Vibratome section reacted for horseradish peroxidase (HRP) histo-
chemistry from a rat that underwent 3 hours of posttraumatic hyperthermia
(39°C) 24 hours after fluid-percussion (FP) brain injury. Note abnormal staining within the subarachnoid space as well as the site of hemorrhage overlying the gray-white interface (arrowheads) of lateral cortex. (b) Higher magnification showing hemorrhagic contusion with brain swelling at the gray-white
interface. (c) One um-thick plastic section stained with toluidine blue showing swollen myelinated axons (arrowheads) in Layer 6 of the somatosensory
cortex. (d) Swollen axons (arrowheads) are also present in white matter bun-
dles within the striatum. (e) Within the cerebral cortex, blood vessels contain luminal leukocytes and erythrocytes.

FIG. 5.2. Transmission electron micrographs taken from posttraumatic hyperthermic rats. (a) Reactive axon contains a core of clumped neurofilaments
surrounding a lucent zone and myelin sheath. (b) Reactive axonal changes
include an accumulation of organelles surrounding a neurofilamentous
mass. (c) Myelinated axon with abnormal axoplasm. (d) Swollen axon containing a thin myelin sheath and lucent axoplasm with single mitochondrion
(arrowhead). (e) Leukocyte adhering to endothelial (E) cell. (f) Extravasated
polymorphonuclear leukocyte within normal-appearing brain parenchyma.

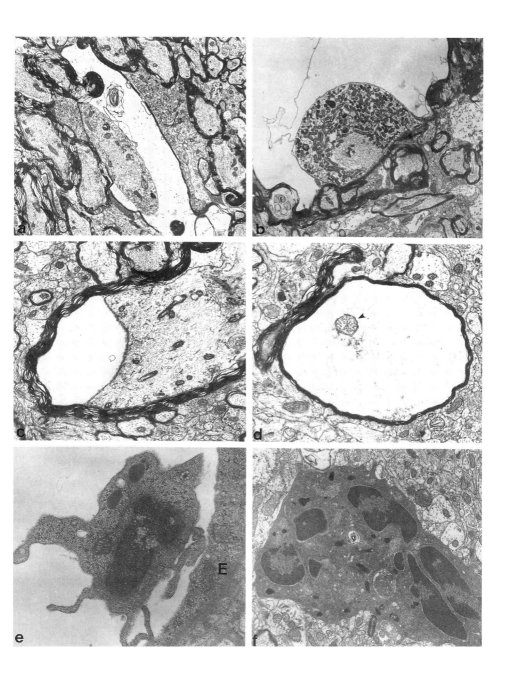

75

dicate that delayed heating may influence outcome by affecting both vascular and neuronal events. Compared with normothermic rats, increased brain swelling and hemorrhage were seen in heated rats 24 hours after TBI. Increased BBB breakdown leading to the extravasation of blood-borne factors could therefore contribute to the injury process (Chan, Schmidley, Fishman, & Longar, 1984; Dietrich et al., 1991; Povlishock, Becker, Sullivan, & Miller, 1978; Povlishock & Dietrich, 1992). In addition, increased brain swelling might produce increased ICP. Diffuse axonal damage is commonly reported in head-injured patients and in models of FP brain injury (Christman, Grady, Walker, Holloway, & Povlishock, 1994; Gennarelli et al., 1982; Grady et al., 1993; Povlishock, 1992; Povlishock, Becker, Cheng, & Vaughan, 1983; Yaghmai & Povlishock, 1992). Our present findings with posttraumatic hyperthermia indicate that delayed heating leads to increased axonal swelling. Thus, TBI enhanced the sensitivity of myelinated axons to secondary hyperthermia. Hyperthermia-induced axonal perturbations may therefore contribute to the increased mortality rate previously seen with posttraumatic hyperthermia (Dietrich, Alonso, Halley, & Busto, 1996).

In addition to the early ultrastructural consequences of delayed posttraumatic hyperthermia, chronic histopathological damage was also aggravated by secondary hyperthermia (Fig. 5.3). Compared with normothermic animals, posttraumatic hyperthermia enlarged the area of the subcortical contusion within the lateral cortex. In addition, more severe cortical damage was also seen compared with normothermic rats. In three out of five rats, evidence for cortical contusion in contrast to selective neuronal necrosis was seen (Fig. 5.3c). A high frequency of ischemic neurons was also observed within the CA3 hippocampus (Fig. 5.3d). More inconsistent findings in the hyperthermic group included infarction of white matter tracts, including the fimbria of the hippocampus and the intramural hemorrhages within cerebral arterioles (Figs. 5.3e and 5.3f).

SUMMARY

Clinical and experimental data indicate that variations in posttraumatic brain and body temperatures may critically influence traumatic outcome. Mild degrees of hypothermia appear to be neuroprotective, whereas delayed elevations in temperature significantly worsen outcome. In the clinic, whole-body hypothermia may be a means to control some of the detrimental consequences of TBI, including uncontrollable elevations in intracranial pressure or elevations in brain and body temperatures. Experimental evidence also has demonstrated that post-

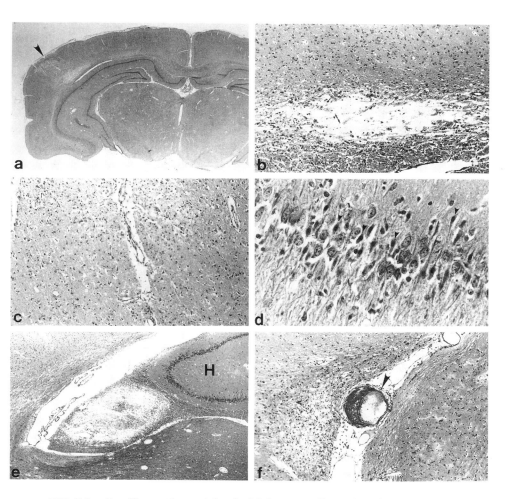

FIG. 5.3.   Paraffin sections stained with hematoxylin and eosin from post-traumatic rats that underwent delayed hyperthermia (39°C) 3 days prior to perfusion fixation. (a) Intracerebral contusion is present at the gray-white interface of the lateral cortex. The overlying cerebral cortex appears necrotic (arrowhead). (b) Higher magnification of subcortical contusion. (c) Lateral cerebral cortex appears infarcted. (d) Necrotic neurons are present within the CA3 hippocampus. (e) Necrosed fimbria of the hippocampus. (f) Arteriole within cerebrospinal fluid space showing intramural hemorrhage.

77

traumatic cooling improves histopathological outcome, whereas delayed hyperthermia worsens both the neuronal and vascular consequences of head trauma. Based on experimental data, it appears that TBI produces sublethal injury to both vascular and neuronal components, and is aggravated by delayed postischemic hyperthermia. Future experimental studies are necessary to clarify mechanisms by which posttraumatic temperature manipulations may affect traumatic outcome.

ACKNOWLEDGMENTS

This study was supported by USPHS Grants NS 30291 and NS 27127. The author thanks Helen Valkowitz for typing the manuscript.

REFERENCES

Busto, R., Dietrich, W. D., Globus, M. Y.-T., & Ginsberg, M. D. (1989). Postischemic moderate hypothermia inhibits CA1 hippocampal ischemic neuronal injury. *Neuroscience Letters, 101*, 299–304.

Busto, R., Dietrich, W. D., Globus, M. Y.-T., Valdes, I., Scheinberg, P., & Ginsberg, M. D. (1987). Small differences in intraischemic brain temeprature critically determine the extent of ischemic neuronal injury. *Journal of Cerebral Blood Flow and Metabolism, 7*, 729–738.

Chan, P. H., Schmidley, J. W., Fishman, R. A., & Longar, S. M. (1984). Brain injury, edema, and vascular permeability changes induced by oxygen-derived free radicals. *Neurology, 34*, 315–320.

Christman, C. W., Grady, M. S., Walker, S. A., Holloway, K. L., & Povlishock, J. T. (1994). Ultrastructural studies of diffuse axonal injury in humans. *Journal of Neurotrauma, 11*, 173–186.

Clifton, G. L., Allen, S., Barrodale, P., Plenger, P., Berry, J., Koch, S., Fletcher, J., Hayes, R. L., & Choi, S. G. (1993). A phase II study of moderate hypothermia in severe brain injury. *Journal Neurotrauma, 10*, 263–271.

Clifton, G. L., Jiang, J. Y., Lyeth, B. G., Jenkins, L. W., Hamm, R. J., & Hayes, R. L. (1991). Marked protection by moderate hypothermia after experimental traumatic brain injury. *Journal of Cerebral Blood Flow and Metabolism, 11*, 114–121.

Cortez, S. C., McIntosh, T. K., & Noble, L. J. (1989). Experimental fluid percussion brain injury: Vascular disruption and neuronal and glial alterations. *Brain Research, 482*, 272–282.

Dietrich, W. D., (1992). The importance of brain temperature in cerebral injury. *Journal of Neurotrauma, 9*(Suppl. 2), 476–485.

Dietrich, W. D., Alonso, O., Busto, R., Globus, M. Y.-T., & Ginsberg, M. D. (1994). Posttraumatic brain hypothermia reduces histopathological damage following concussive brain injury in the rat. *Acta Neuropathologica, 87*, 250–258.

Dietrich, W. D., Alonso, O., & Halley, M. (1994). Early microvascular and neuronal consequences of traumatic brain injury: A light and electron microscopic study in rats. *Journal of Neurotrauma, 11*, 289–301.

Dietrich, W. D., Alonso, O., Halley, M., & Busto, R. (1996). Delayed post-traumatic brain hyperthermia worsens outcome after fluid percussion brain injury: A light and electron microscopic study in rats. *Neurosurgery 38*, 533–541.

Dietrich, W. D., Busto, R., Globus, M. Y.-T., & Ginsberg, M. D. (1993). Intraischemic but not postischemic brain hypothermia protects chronically following forebrain ischemia in rats. *Journal of Cerebral Blood Flow and Metabolism, 13*, 541–549.

Dietrich, W. D., Busto, R., Halley, M., & Valdes, I. (1990). The importance of brain temperature in alterations of the blood-brain barrier following cerebral ischemia. *Journal of Neuropathology and Experimental, 49*, 486–497.

Dietrich, W. D., Busto, R., Valdes, I., & Loor, Y. (1990). Effects of normothermic versus mild hyperthermic forebrain ischemia in rats. *Stroke, 21*, 1318–1325.

Dietrich, W. D., Halley, M., Valdes, I., & Busto, R. (1991). Interrelationships between increased vascular permeability and acute neuronal injury damage following temperature controlled brain ischemia in rats. *Acta Neuropathologica, 81*, 615–625.

Dixon, C. E., Lyeth, B. G., Povlishock, J. T., Findling, R. L., Hamm, R. J., Marmarou, A., Young, H. F., & Hayes, R. L. (1987). A fluid percussion model of experimental brain injury in the rat. *Journal of Neurosurgery, 67*, 110–119.

Ellis, E. F., Chao, J., & Heizer, M. L. (1989). Brain kininogen following experimental brain injury: Evidence for a secondary event. *Journal of Neurosurgery, 71*, 437–442.

Faden, A. I., Demediuk, P., Panter, S. S., & Vink, R. (1989). The role of excitatory amino acids and NMDA receptors in traumatic brain injury. *Science, 244*, 798–800.

Gennarelli, T. A. (1994). Animate models of human head injury. *Journal of Neurotrauma, 11*, 357–368.

Gennarelli, T. A., & Thibault, L. E. (1985). Biological models of head injury. In D. P. Becker & J. T. Povlishock (Eds.), *Central nervous system status report* (pp. 391–404).

Gennarelli, T. A., Thibault, L. E., Adams, J. H., Graham, D. I., Thompson, C. J., & Marcincin, R. P. (1982). Diffuse axonal injury and traumatic coma in the primate. *Annals of Neurology, 12*, 564–574.

Ginsberg, M. D., Sternau, L. L., Globus, M. Y.-T., Dietrich, W. D., & Busto, R. (1992). Therapeutic modulation of brain temperature: Relevance to ischemic brain injury. *Cerebrovascular and Brain Metabolism Reviews, 4*, 189–225.

Grady, M. S., McLaughlin, M. R., Christman, C. W., Valadka, A. B., Fligner, C. L., & Povlishock, J. T. (1993). The use of antibodies targeted against the neurofilament subunits for the detection of diffuse axonal injury in humans. *Journal of Neuropathology and Experimental Neurology, 52*, 143–152.

Green, E. J., Dietrich, W. D., van Dijk, F., Busto, R., Markgraf, C. G., McCabe, P. M., Ginsberg, M. D., & Schneiderman, N. (1992). Protective effects of neural hypothermia on behavior following global cerebral ischemia. *Brain Research, 580*, 197–204.

Hayashi, N., Hirayama, T., & Ohata, M. (1993). The computed cerebral hypothermia management technique to the critical head injury patients. *Advances in Neurotrauma Research, 5*, 61–64.

Hayes, R. L., Jenkins, L. W., Lyeth, B. G., Balster, R. L., Robinson, S. E., Miller, L. P., Clifton, G., & Young, H. F. (1988). Pretreatment with phencyclidine, an N-methyl-D-aspartate receptor antagonist, attenuates long-term behavioral deficits in the rat produced by traumatic brain injury. *Journal of Neurotrauma, 5*, 287–302.

Hayes, R. L., Jenkins, L. W., & Lyeth, B. G. (1991). Neurotransmitter-mediated mechanisms of traumatic brain injury: Acethycholine and excitatory amino acids. *Journal of Neurotrauma, 9*(Suppl. 1), 173–187.

Hovda, D. A., Becker, D. B., & Katayama, Y. (1992). Secondary injury and acidosis. *Journal of Neurotrauma, 9*(Suppl. 1), S47–S60.

Ishige, N., Pitts, L. H., Berry, I., Carlson, S. G., Nishimura, M. C., Moseley, M. E., & Weinstein, P. R. (1987). The effect of hypoxia on traumatic head injury in rats: Alterations in neurologic function, brain edema, and cerebral blood flow. *Journal of Cerebral Blood Flow Metabolism, 7,* 759–767.

Jenkins, L. W., Lyeth, B. G., LeWelt, W., Moszynski, K., DeWitt, D. S., Balster, R. L., Miller, L. P., Clifton, G. L., Young, H. F., & Hayes, R. L. (1988). Combined pre-trauma scopolamine and phencyclidine attenuates post-traumatic increased sensitivity to delayed secondary ischemia. *Journal of Neurotrauma, 5,* 275–287.

Jenkins, L. W., Moszynski, K., Lyeth, B. G., Lewelt, W., DeWitt, D. S., Allen, A., Dixon, C. E., Povlishock, J. T., Majewski, T. J., Clifton, G. L., Young, H. F., Becker, D. P., & Hayes, R. L. (1989). Increased vulnerability of the mildly traumatized brain to cerebral ischemia: The use of controlled secondary ischemia as a research tool to identify common or different mechanisms contributing to mechanical and ischemic brain injury. *Brain Research, 477,* 211–224.

Jiang, J. Y., Lyeth, B. G., Clifton, G. L., Jenkins, L. W., Hamm, R. J., & Hayes, R. L. (1991). Relationship between body and brain temperature in traumatically brain-injured rodents. *Journal of Neurosurgery, 74,* 492–496.

Jiang, J. Y., Lyeth, B. G., Kapasi, M. Z., Jenkins, L. W., & Povlishock, J. T. (1992). Moderate hypothermia reduces blood-brain barrier disruption following traumatic brain injury in the rat. *Acta Neuropathologica, 84,* 495–500.

Katayama, Y., Becker, D. P., Tamura, T., & Hovda, D. A. (1990). Massive increases in extracellular potassium and the indiscriminate release of glutamate following concussive brain injury. *Journal of Neurosurgery, 73,* 889–900.

Lyeth, B. G., Jiang, J. Y., & Liu, S. (1993). Behavioral protection by moderate hypothermia initiated after experimental traumatic brain injury. *Journal of Neurotrauma, 10,* 57–64.

Marion, D. W., Obrist, W. D., Carlier, P. M., Penrod, L. E., & Darby, J. M. (1993). The use of moderate therapeutic hypothermia for patients with severe head injuries: A preliminary report. *Journal of Neurosurgery, 79,* 354–362.

McIntosh, T. K., Vink, R., Noble, L., Yamakami, I., Soares, H., & Faden, A. L. (1989). Traumatic brain injury in the rat: Characterization of a lateral fluid-percussion model. *Neuroscience, 28,* 233–244.

Palmer, A. M., Marion, D. W., Botsceller, M. L., & Redd, E. E. (1993). Therapeutic hypothermia is cytoprotective without attenuating the traumatic brain injury-induced elevations in interstitital concentrations of aspartate and glutamate. *Journal of Neurotrauma, 10,* 363–372.

Povlishock, J. T. (1992). Traumatically induced axonal injury: Pathogenesis and pathobiological implications. *Brain Pathology, 2,* 1–12.

Povlishock, J. T., Becker, D. P., Cheng, C. L. Y., & Vaughan, G. W. (1983). Axonal changes in minor head injury. *Journal of Neuropathology and Experimental Neurology, 42,* 225–242.

Povlishock, J. T., Becker, D. P., Sullivan, H. G., & Miller, J. D. (1978). Vascular permeability alterations to horseradish peroxidase in experimental brain injury. *Brain Research, 153,* 223–239.

Povlishock, J. T., & Dietrich, W. D. (1992). The blood-brain barrier in brain injury: An overview. In M. Y.-T. Globus & W. D. Dietrich (Eds.), *The role of neurotransmitters in brain injury* (pp. 265–269). New York: Plenum.

Resnick, D. K., Marion, D. W., & Darby, J. M. (1994). The effect of hypothermia on the incidence of delayed traumatic intracerebral hemorrhage. *Neurosurg, 34,* 252–256.

Ribas, G. C., & Jane, J. A. (1992). Traumatic contusions and intracerebral hematomas. *Journal of Neurotrauma, 9*(Suppl. 1), S265–S275.

Rousseaux, P., Scherpered, B., Bernard, M. H., Graftieaux, J. P., & Guyot, J. F. (1980). Fever and cerebral vasospasm in ruptured intracranial aneurysms. *Surgical Neurology, 14,* 459–465.

Shiozaki, T., Sugimoto, H., Taneda, M., Yoshida, H., Iwai, A., Yoshioka, T., & Sugimoto,

T. (1993). Effect of mild hypothermia on uncontrollable intracranial hypertension after severe head injury. *Journal of Neurosurgery, 79*, 363–368.

Sternau, L., Thompson, C., Dietrich, W. D., Busto, R., Globus, M. Y.-T., & Ginsberg, M. D. (1991). Intracranial temperature: Observations in human brain. *Journal of Cerebral Blood Flow Metabolism, 11* (2), S123.

Tanno, H., Nockels, R. P., Pitts, L. H., & Noble, L. J. (1992). Breakdown of the blood-brain barrier after fluid percussion brain injury in the rat: Part 2. Effect of hypoxia on permeability to plasma proteins. *Journal of Neurotrauma, 9*, 335–347.

Yaghmai, A., & Povlishock, J. (1992). Traumatically induced reactive change as visualized through the use of monoclonal antibodies targeted to neurofilament subunits. *Journal of Neuropathology and Experimental Neurology, 51*, 158–176.

Young, W. (1988). Secondary CNS injury. *Journal of Neurotrauma, 5*, 219–221.

6

Chronic Brain Stimulation as a Restorative Treatment for Brain Damage

Takashi Tsubokawa

The impact of the research carried out in the late 1960s derived largely from the demonstration that "sprouting" of an axon could culminate in the formation of a new synapse on denervated neurons (Land & Lune, 1971; Raisman, 1969). Furthermore, the comparative studies that have been undertaken suggest that such growth is certainly not limited to lower mammals (Steward & Mesenheimer, 1978).

Based on what is now known regarding the phenomenon of post-lesion neural growth, it seems that trauma involving the central nervous system, even in humans, is often followed by at least some neuronal growth and reorganization. Because such growth and reorganization of the neural circuits are likely to have functional consequences, these processes may eventually provide new insights into the outcome of traumatic damage of the central nervous system. However, loss of neuronal function caused by brain injury is not only difficult to reverse fully through a natural course, inevitably giving rise to neurological deficits, but also induces new troublesome syndromes caused by inadequate new synaptic connections, such as seizures, involuntary movements, or central deafferentation pain within several months after the insult to the brain (Lin & Chamber, 1958; McCouch et al., 1958; Tsubokawa, 1992). These clinical findings following damage to the central nervous system may indicate that damaged nerve cells do not have sufficient power of regeneration to recover their normal functions. In addition, regeneration or reorganization gives rise to some inadequate mal regeneration, which can induce certain kinds of seizure, involuntary movements, and central deafferentation pain during the recovery period after brain injury. Attempts must be made to facilitate an adaptive regeneration at the injured site in order to secure a more favorable clinical outcome from the brain injury.

For this purpose, transplantation of neural tissue offers the possibility of replacing lost neurons. Such a procedure is feasible and, in some situations, efficacious for restoring the lost function without spontaneous maladaptive regeneration (Bjorklund & Stenevi, 1979; Sladek & Gash, 1984). Transplants can form connections with the host tissue. Many such connections are strikingly similar to the patterns of projection in normal animals (Bjorklund & Stenevi, 1977; Stenevi, Bjorklund, & Kromer, 1984), if adequate immature neural tissues of the certain kinds as the injured brain tissue are transplanted using some form of guide system (Katayama et al., 1991).

For over a decade, the major impetus driving the development of neural transplantation techniques has been the hope of treating patients who are afflicted with neurotrauma, vascular disease, and degenerative disease. Nevertheless, huge difficulties still remain. Resolution of the graft problems must await improved cell technology (Flandaca & Gash, 1991), and effective guidance techniques governing the growth direction of the neuronal processes of the imparted cells need to be developed (Aguayo et al., 1982).

As a restorative treatment for brain injury, nerve growth factors that induce extensive axonal outgrowth and cellular hypertrophy and that promote neural survival may be of use for facilitating either naturally occurring reactive growth or regeneration of damaged brain tissue (Berg, 1984; Thoenen & Edgar, 1985). Some facilitation of the spontaneous reactive growth process in the injured area has been observed following direct application of nerve growth factors (Berg, 1984). It is difficult, however, to achieve changes likely to create a physiological neuronal network or to contribute in some way to normal function.

New therapies for brain-injured patients need to be developed on the basis of knowledge gained from both transplantation and the use of nerve growth factors. Nevertheless, from the clinical standpoint, it is difficult to apply them effectively in restorative treatment. Until such a restorative surgical procedure can be developed, chronic deep brain stimulation must be regarded as one of the more propitious treatments. This is so because chronic brain stimulation of some systems facilitates spontaneous reactive neuronal growth and controls the abnormal firing caused by maladaptive regeneration following brain damage at the target area of the stimulated system (Tsubokawa, 1992, 1993). This view is supported by experimental animal studies (Tsubokawa, 1992). In fact, we have applied chronic brain stimulation therapy to treat persistent vegetative state, involuntary movements, and central deafferentation pain (i.e., as an alternative surgical procedure to tissue transplantation or nerve growth factor therapy).

In this chapter, the methods and results of chronic brain stimulation for relief of the persistent vegetative state, involuntary movements, and central deafferentation pain caused by brain injury are outlined in the context of providing useful restorative surgery for the injured brain.

PERSISTENT VEGETATIVE STATE

At more than 3 months after sustaining the initial insult of head injury, patients fail to show verbal responses, actions or movements including food intake, or signs of expressing their own will. Such specific unconsciousness at the chronic stage after the insult is described as a *persistent vegetative state,* and the accompanying mental state has been termed *wakefulness without awareness* (Jennett & Plum, 1972). Among the head-injured cases suffering from prolonged coma, 30%–40% fall into a persistent vegetative state (Groswasser & Sazbon, 1990; Pazzaglia et al., 1975; Tsubokawa, Yamamoto, & Katayama, 1990a). The severity and location of the brain damage are known to differ among persistent vegetative patients, but the main lesions tend to be observed in the diffuse ascending system, including the brain stem, medial thalamus, and cortex. Thus, it is difficult to assess the severity of persistent vegetative patients. The neurobehavioral signs are evaluated using our prolonged coma scale (Table 6.1). The score is counted on the basis of the number of

TABLE 6.1
Neurobehavior Score for Evaluation
of Prolonged Coma Patients

Neurobehaviour Score
1. Alive with spontaneous respiration
2. Withdrawal response to pain
3. Spontaneous eye opening and closing
4. Sontaneous movement of extremities
5. Pursuit by eye movement
6. Emotional expression
7. Oral intake
8. Producing sounds
9. Obeying orders
10. Verbal response

Note. A grading is made by adding each positive item. Persistent vegetative state is ranged 2–4 points.

instances of abnormal function among 10 items. Persistent vegetative patients tend to show 2–4 points, which corresponds to the persistent vegetative state as outlined by Jennett and Plum (1972).

Therapies for the persistent vegetative state, pharmacological treatment to activate the ascending activating system (Di Rocco, 1974; Van Woerkom et al., 1982), and rehabilitation by sensory stimulation therapy to induce an arousal state (Ansell & Keenan, 1989; Weber, 1984) have been performed to enhance the spontaneous neural plasticity of the damaged brain. However, the results have fallen short of expectations. It may be necessary to induce a more vigorous regeneration within the damaged brain. Chronic brain stem stimulation in experimental animals with lesions of the thalamus or brain stem has been found to elicit arousal responses. It also has induced an increase in nerve growth factors, an increase in amount of sprouting and new synaptic contacts (Maejima et al., 1993) with an elevated cerebral blood flow, and an increase in oxygen level and glucose uptake (Tsubokawa, 1992, 1993). Chronic deep brain stimulation therapy has thus been applied in patients suffering from the persistent vegetative state (Sturm et al., 1979; Tsubokawa et al., 1990).

Method of Clinical Application

As the first step in the surgical procedure, a chronic stimulation electrode, comprising a flexible, platinum-iridium electrode (Medtronic DBS Lead Kit Model 3380), is inserted into the target by stereotaxic surgery under local anesthesia (Tsubokawa, 1993). The target is the mesencephalic reticular formation (i.e., the nucleus cuneiformis; Olszewski & Baxter, 1981), or nonspecific medial thalamic nuclei (CM-Pf complex) (AP: -7--9 mm, LR: 5–6 mm, H: 0–1 mm). After implantation of the electrode, bipolar stimulation between the tip active point and fourth active point is applied at various frequencies and strengths to check the threshold of the arousal response for both electroencephalography (EEG) and behavior. As the second step in the surgical procedure, internalization of the entire stimulation system (Medtronic X-TREL Transmitter system Model) is performed.

Stimulation is applied for 30 minutes every 2 hours in the daytime. The stimulation is completely stopped at night, with the aim of creating cycles at sleep and awake. The frequency of stimulation usually ranges from 25 to 50 Hz; the intensity is controlled at slightly higher than the threshold, inducing an arousal response in both the EEG and behavior (Tsubokawa et al., 1990).

Results

Patients diagnosed as being in a persistent vegetative state at more than 3 months after the brain-injury insult with neurobehavioral scores of 2–4 points were selected as candidates for chronic deep brain stimulation therapy. As an immediate effect of the stimulation, arousal responses in the EEG and behavior were observed as early as at the start of the stimulation. The patients opened their eyes with dilated pupils, their mouths also opened widely with meaningless vocalizations, and a slight increase in systemic blood pressure was detected during the stimulation in all treated cases with neurobehavioral scores of 2–4 points. Moreover, some cases demonstrated slight movements of the extremities. The EEG revealed desynchronization during the stimulation.

There was not much disparity in the appearance of such arousal responses between the different stimulation groups involving the midbrain reticular formation and the CM-Pf complex. The appearance of arousal responses did not display any relation with the severity of the neurobehavioral score.

At every stimulation application, the regional cerebral blood flow (r-CBF) increased from 10% to 72%. The regional cerebral oxygen consumption rate ($CMRO_2$) also increased from 10% to 40% of the prestimulation value without any obvious changes in the oxygen extraction rate (OER). The regional glucose uptake increased to two to three times the prestimulation value. These increments in both oxygen and glucose uptake were observed mainly at the stimulation site, as well as in both sides of the cortex and contralateral thalamic area (Table 6.2; Tsubokawa et al., 1990).

Improvement of the neurobehavioral score was evident at 3–4 months after the beginning of the chronic stimulation if the stimulation was effective. Thus, 35% of the treated cases were able to recover to 8–10 points on the neurobehavioral score (which represented an almost normal cognitivity) and to take food by themselves, whereas 10% of the treated cases showed incomplete recovery (7 points on the neurobehavioral score) by 1 year after stimulation therapy. The remaining 55% of the treated cases demonstrated arousal responses in their EEG and behavior as immediate effects of the stimulation, but their cognitivity and neurobehavioral scores did not recover to more than 6 points (Fig. 6.1).

There were no differences in the prestimulation neurobehavioral scores between the effective group, which emerged from the persistent vegetative state, and the noneffective group, but the results of prestimulation neurophysiological tests were quite different between the two groups. In the effective cases, auditory brainstem-evoked responses were clearly

TABLE 6.2

Alternation of r-CBF, r-CMRO$_2$, OEF, and r-Glucose Uptake Rate on Positron Emission CT Before and During r-Thalamic Stimulation*

	CBF (ml/100ml/min)		OER (%)		CMRO$_2$ (ml/100ml/min)		Glucose (%: tissue/blood)	
	Nonstimulation	Stimulation	Nonstimulation	Stimulation	Nonstimulation	Stimulation	Nonstimulation	Stimulation
Frontal lobe								
Right	37.3	48.4	55.4	60.6	1.60	2.16	45.3	118.4
Left	49.4	54.4	55.6	52.7	1.45	2.16	50.7	126.6
Parietal lobe								
Right	58.8	66.3	46.8	50.4	2.94	3.98	45.8	120.7
Left	61.5	58.8	57.7	57.6	2.33	3.15	51.6	125.2
Occipital lobe								
Right	29.4	42.9	60.4	60.2	1.28	1.93	39.4	103.4
Left	35.5	42.1	62.8	61.6	1.87	1.16	42.9	108.6
Thalamus								
Right	63.5	70.6	63.5	61.5	3.41	4.00	61.1	123.7
Left	45.4	78.3	57.4	60.7	3.94	5.40	62.6	114.5

Note. CBF, cerebral blood flow; CMRO$_2$, regional cerebral oxygen consumption rate; OER, oxygen extraction rate.
*Mean value of three cases who get r-thalamic stimulation

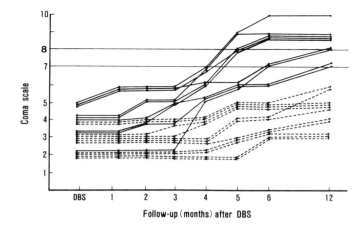

FIG. 6.1. Changes of the neurobehavior score following chronic deep brain stimulation. The solid line indicates the time course recovered from a persistent vegetative state on effective cases; the dotted line indicates the time course of changes of the neurobehavioral score on noneffective cases. The increase of the neurobehavior score by chronic stimulation is observed at least 3–4 months after beginning the stimulation on the effective or non-effective cases.

recorded with elongation of the latency; the N_{20} wave of the somatosensory-evoked potential was also recorded, but it was of low amplitude and longer latency. The EEG revealed a desynchronization pattern or a slight desynchronization pattern of a changeable spectrum on continuous EEG frequency analysis (Tsubokawa et al., 1990). Further, the amplitude of pain, related P_{250} (Katayama, Tsukiyama, & Tsubokawa, 1985; Katayama, Tsubokawa, & Yamamoto, 1991), was recorded with a value of over 8 μV in all effective cases.

These electrophysiological findings in effective cases following chronic deep brain stimulation provide useful information for the selection of candidates to receive treatment by chronic deep brain stimulation therapy. They also indicate that effective cases of stimulation must be left a minimum fundamental function in the injured brain to induce arousal responses in both the brain stem and the cortex. The injured brain must show a responsiveness involving increased levels of dopamine, prostaglandin E_2, and prostaglandin D_2 after chronic deep brain stimulation (Yamamoto et al., 1993). The deep brain stimulation must be applied over a period of more than 4 months to provide a chance of recovery from the persistent vegetative state, even if the patients had changeable spectrum on continuous EEG frequency analysis, a fifth wave on the auditory brain stem response, an N_{20} wave of the somatosansory-evoked potential and an amplitude of 8 μV for the pain-related potential, without any relation to the severity of the neurobehavioral score, whenever the score is 2–4 points.

These facts demonstrate that chronic stimulation, when applied to the ascending reticular formation in persistent vegetative patients, is able to induce an increased regeneration and reorganization within the lesion area. However, it is necessary to leave the minimal amount of brain tissue that can function to induce electrophysiological arousal response.

INVOLUNTARY MOVEMENTS CAUSED BY BRAIN DAMAGE

Head injury and stroke can cause a variety of involuntary movements. Tremor, hemiballism, and hemichorea have been identified as late sequelae of brain damage (Koller, Wong, & Lang, 1989). Such involuntary movements are induced by neuronal damage with maladaptive regeneration in the striatum, subthalamic nucleus, and cerebellum, leading to an imbalance between facilitation and inhibition of the extrapyramidal neural circuits' activities.

Tremor or intention tremor caused by brain injury has been controlled in 85% of cases treated by thalamotomy at the nucleus ventralis lateralis (VL) (Mundinger, 1965). Hemiballism was also controlled in 35%–70% of cases treated by either lateral pallidotomy (Tsubokawa & Moriyasu, 1975) or thalamotomy at the nucleus ventralis oralis posterior (Vop) (Bullard & Nashold, 1984). However, such stereotaxic lesion-making procedures led to a considerable new risk of persistent morbidity, including dysarthria or new involuntary movements in 38%–68% of the treated cases (Bullard & Nashold, 1984; Krauss et al., 1994), because the new stereotaxic lesions induced further maladaptive regeneration, which is a cause of such involuntary movements. To prevent this type of postsurgical abnormality, chronic thalamic stimulation has been attempted; the expectation is that such stimulation would inhibit abnormal facilitation of the thalamic activities to induce involuntary movements and adaptive neuroplastic reorganization of the initially damaged brain (Maejima et al., 1993; Tsubokawa, 1992, 1993).

Method of Clinical Application

The surgical procedure consists of two steps. First, the chronic stimulation electrode (Medtronic DBS Lead Kit Model 3380) is inserted into the target by stereotaxic surgery under local anesthesia. For hemiballism, the target is 6–7 mm in front of the posterior commissure, 14–15 mm lateral to the midline, and +1–0 mm to the bicommissural line. The electrode is oriented in the anterodorsal direction at an angle of 45 degrees to the intercommissural line. The tip of the electrode is inserted into the Vim, while at 15 mm up from the tip, the third active point of the electrode is situated in the Vop of the thalamus. These two points are stimulated bipolarly. For tremor, the electrode is inserted into the Vim 6–7 mm in front of the posterior commissure, 13–14 mm lateral to the midline, and +1 mm to the bicommissural line; the second active point of the electrode at 5 mm up from the tip is also located in the Vim. Both the tip and the second active point were selected for bipolar stimulation.

Second, internalization of the entire stimulation system (Medtronic X-TREL Transmitter system Model 3425) is performed. This is done after checking the stimulation effect on the involuntary movements over a test stimulation period of 1–3 days after insertion of the electrode. During the test stimulation, the most effective stimulation parameters must be evaluated for each case. They are usually a frequency of 60–100 Hz with a duration of 0.5 msec, and a slightly higher intensity than the sensory threshold for control of both tremor and hemiballism.

After internalization of the entire stimulating system, the patients have control of the stimulation period themselves. This allows them to live without trouble from their involuntary movements. However, they are not allowed to apply stimulation during the night. The stimulation period per day was checked monthly until 1 year following the stimulation therapy.

Results

Among six cases suffering from hemiballism, the causative lesion was located in the subthalamic nucleus in three cases and in the stratum in two cases; the remaining case was a head-injury patient whose causative lesion was difficult to identify by both computed tomography (CT) and magnetic resonance imaging (MRI). During the initial 2–3 weeks after the beginning of stimulation therapy, control of the involuntary movements was incomplete in some cases, but all cases were able to return to society without involuntary movements during application of the stimulation. Hemiballistic movement quickly reappeared when stimulation was terminated near the beginning of stimulation therapy. However, several months after stimulation, complete disappearance of the hemiballistic movement continued for more than 1 hour after turning off the stimulation. The duration of the stimulation application time to stop involuntary movements then became progressively shorter (Fig. 6.2).

One year after stimulation, the stimulation period to ensure freedom from ballistic movement in the daytime became quite short, because the

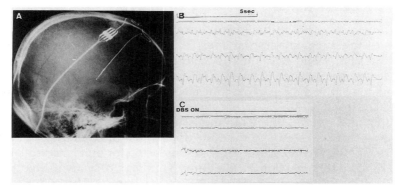

FIG. 6.2. The implanted electrode in the Vop-Vim of the thalamus on craniogram (A) and immediate effect to stop the involuntary movement is shown on the surface EMG (top: recording at the dertoicleus muscle); middle: recording at triceps muscle; bottom: recording at ant. tibial muscle; B: before stimulation, hemiballistic movement; C: complete stop of ballistic movement during thalamic stimulation.

after affect of stimulation increased markedly. Further, 1 year after application of chronic stimulation, in cases with the causative lesion in the striatum, the stimulation period was much shorter than in cases with lesions in the subthalamic nucleus (Fig. 6.3).

Among seven cases suffering from tremor or intention tremor, four cases had suffered from stroke and had a lesion involving cerebellar

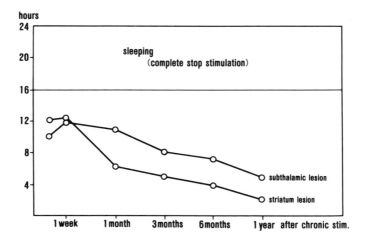

FIG. 6.3. The time course of the stimulating period (per day) to completely stop hemiballistic movement is shown. There is a slightly different time course of the effectiveness after the stimulation for hemiballism caused by subthalamic lesion and striatum lesion.

hemorrhage, subthalamic hemorrhage, and brainstem infarction. The other three cases had suffered from head injury and demonstrated cerebellar hematoma or diffuse brain injury.

Overall, 72% of the patients achieved an excellent effect for stopping the tremor during stimulation application. However, the other 28% revealed only a moderate effect, and their initial lesion was brainstem infarction or diffuse brain injury. At the beginning of the chronic stimulation course, tremor reappeared when the stimulation was terminated. However, the stimulation period per day to stop the tremor completely in the daytime decreased month by month because the after effect of the stimulation lengthened. Such a phenomenon was difficult to discern in Parkinson's tremor created by chronic Vim stimulation (Fig. 6.4).

The chronic stimulation did not induce any severe complications or untoward side effects in all cases, apart from wound infection in one case and electrode disconnection in another. There was also no change for the worse in the neurological deficits caused by the original diseases and no mortality during the follow-up period.

These results are almost identical to those of Cooper, Upton, and Amin (1982), who reported that a clinically useful improvement was observed following thalamic stimulation in six cases with unspecified poststroke involuntary movements. Andy (1983) described a case in which poststroke thalamic syndrome with choreiform movement was successfully treated by thalamic stimulation. Unlike thalamotomy, chronic thalamic stimulation can be employed to control the extent of electro-

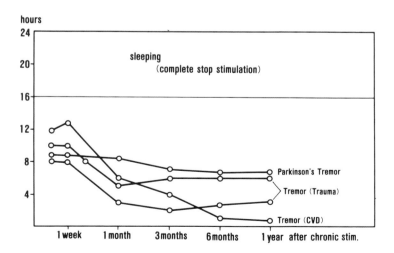

FIG. 6.4. The time course of the stimulating period (per day) to completely stop tremors is shown. There is a difference between Parkinson's disease and the other symptomatic tremor.

physiological ablation, as a desynchronization on abnormal synchroniz-ation of the thalamocortical system, which induces involuntary move-ments as an immediate effect, and also certain neuroplastic effects, which are indicated by a lengthening of the after effect of the stimulation on the involuntary movements (Tsubokawa, 1993).

The follow-up results also suggest that the stimulation period for complete stoppage of the involuntary movements became progressively shorter after the beginning of application of the chronic stimulation. Such elongation of the stimulation's after effect is in sharp contrast to the case of Parkinson's tremor treated by chronic stimulation (Fig. 6.3; Tsubokawa, 1993). The underlying mechanism of the progressive in-crease in efficiency in controlling the involuntary movements caused by head injury or stroke may be this: A readjustment of the imbalance in neural abnormal activities in the extrapyramidal system is induced by the immediate effect of the stimulation, and long-term application of the stimulation gives rise to certain neuroplastic effects at the lesion site due to the chronic stimulation, as suggested in several experimental studies (Maejima et al., 1993; Tsubokawa, 1993).

CENTRAL DEAFFERENTATION PAIN

Central deafferentation pain is caused by brain damage at the pain-conducting pathways, which consist of the spinothalamic and thalamocortical tracts within the brain. Further, many abnormal deaf-ferentation hyperactive neurons exist one or two synapses above the brain-damaged area on the pain-afferent pathways (Koyama et al., 1993; Lenz et al., 1989) due to maladaptive regeneration at the lesion site (Koyama et al., 1993). Chronic stimulation of the motor cortex inhibits such abnormal hyperactivity (Koyama et al., 1993), and increases the levels of growth factors, sprouting, and gliosis at the lesion site (Maejima et al., 1993). Because central deafferentation pain can subside in associa-tion with inhibitory effects on the abnormal hyperactivities at the pain pathways, it has been treated by chronic motor cortex stimulation.

Method of Clinical Application

For the motor cortex stimulation, a burr hole was made in the frontal part of the central sulcus and a plate electrode (Medtronic Resume Mod-el 3587) was inserted into the epidural space under local anesthesia. The location of the precentral gyrus was confirmed from phase reversal of the N_{20} wave of the somatosensory-evoked potential recorded from the electrode, and also on the basis of muscle contraction in response to stronger stimulation with the electrode. Bipolar stimulation, employing two appropriate active points from among four, was performed. Each suitable stimulating point was selected according to the observation of an induced abnormal sensation or motor responses at the painful area by stronger stimulation (Tsubokawa et al., 1993). After internalization of the stimulating system (Medtronic X-TREL Transmitter System Model 3425), the motor cortex was stimulated. A stimulus with a duration of 0.2 msec, a frequency of 50–100 Hz, and a strength slightly higher than the sensory threshold and less than the motor threshold was continuously applied for 10–20 minutes whenever the patients felt pain; no stimulation was given at night.

Results

Twenty cases suffering from central deafferentation pain—including those with superthalamic lesions (3 cases), thalamic lesions (12 cases), brainstem lesions (3 cases), and spinal cord lesions (2 cases)—were treated by motor cortex stimulation. The cases caused by superthalamic, thalamic, and midbrain lesions achieved excellent pain relief in 72% of the treated cases. However, relief of central pain caused by spinal cord injury was less effective (50% of the treated cases), which compared with the cases with causative lesions in the superspinal neural tissue.

Ten percent of all cases treated by motor cortex stimulation for the relief of central deafferentation pain were able to enjoy pain relief without stimulation at 1 year after application of the chronic stimulation. However, the other 90% still required stimulation several times per day after more than 1 year. In most of the treated cases, spasticity-associated deafferentation pain also subsided with this stimulation therapy.

These findings suggest that stimulation not only inhibits the hyperactive firing neurons at one synapse above the causative lesion site, as on immediate effect, but it also exerts an influence on new synaptic transformation, an increase in nerve growth factors, activation of the resting synapses, and induction of sprouting at the causative lesion as chronic effects (Tsubokawa, 1993).

CONCLUSION

As a restorative treatment for brain damage, neurotransplantation could be the most appropriate. It could yield excellent results if it were possible for the transplanted neural cells to induce adaptive regeneration in the reorganized damaged brain, leading to the recovery of original functions. However, such well-organized neural reconstruction by neural tissue implantation cannot yet be expected, except in the case of some specific chronic cells transplanted to certain kinds of tissues with cell defects caused by special diseases (Bjorklund & Stenevi, 1977; Katayama et al., 1991), or through application of peripheral nerve co-implantation methods (Aguayo et al., 1982; Benfrey & Aguayo, 1982). An alternative treatment to neurotransplantation is chronic brain stimulation, which affords direct facilitation or inhibition of the pathological cellular activities following brain injury. It also increases the levels of nerve growth factors and sprouting in the injured brain associated with increases in r-CBF, $CMRO_2$, and CMGlucose. Chronic brain stimulation has been applied for treatment of the persistent vegetative state, involuntary movements, and central deafferentation pain caused by brain injury. Indeed, the follow-up results are sufficient to justify the use of this procedure as a restorative treatment without any serious complications.

REFERENCES

Aguayo, A. J., David, S., Richardson, P. M., & Bray, G. M. (1982). Axonal elongation studied in periperal and central nervous system transplants. In S. Fedoroff and L. Hertz (Eds.), *Advances in cellular neurobiology 3*, (pp. 215–234). New York: Academic Press.

Andy, O. J. (1983). Thalamic stimulation for control of movement disorders. *Applied Neurophysiology, 46*, 107–111.

Ansell, B., & Keenan, L. (1989). The Western neurosensory stimulation profile: Tool for assessing slow-to-recover head-injured patients. *Archives of Physical Medicine and Rehabilitation, 70*, 104–108.

Benfey, M., & Aguayo, A. J. (1982). Extensive elongation of axons from rat brain into peripheral grafts. *Nature, 296*, 150–152.

Berg, D. K. (1984). New neuronal growth factors. *Annual Review of Neuroscience, 7*, 149–170.

Bjorklund, A., & Stenevi, U. (1977). Reformation of the severed septohippocampal cholinergic pathway in the adult rat by transplanted septal neurons. *Cell and Tissue Research, 185*, 289–302.

Bjorklund, A., & Stenevi, U. (1979). Reconstruction of nigrostriatal dopamine pathways by intracerebral nigral transplants. *Brain Research, 177*, 444–450.

Bullard, D. E., & Nashold, B. S., Jr. (1984). Stereotaxic thalamotomy for treatment of posttraumatic movement disorders. *Journal of Neurosurgery, 61*, 316–321.

Cooper, I. S., Upton, A. R. M., & Amin, I. (1982). Chronic cerebellar stimulation (CCS) and deep brain stimulation (DBS) in involuntary movement disorder. *Applied Neurophysiology, 45*, 209–217.

Di Rocco, C. (1974). L-DOPA treatment of comatose states due to cerebral lesions. *Journal of Neurosurgical Sciences, 7*, 169–176.

Flandaca, M., & Gash, D. M. (1991). New insights and technological brain grafting. *Clinical Neurosurgery, 39*, 482–508.

Groswasser, Z., & Sazbon, L. (1990). Outcome in 134 patients with prolonged post-traumatic unawareness: Part 1. Parameters determining late recovery of consciousness. *Journal of Neurosurgery, 72*, 75–80.

Jennett, B., & Plum, F. (1972). Persistent vegetative state after brain damage. *Lancet, 1,* 734–737.

Katayama, Y., Tsukiyama, T., & Tsubokawa, T. (1985). Thalamic negativity associated with endogenous late positive components (P300) of cerebral evoked potentials: Recordings using discriminative aversive conditioning in humans and rats. *Brain Research Bulletin, 14,* 223–226.

Katayama, Y., Tsubokawa, T., Koshinaga, M., & Miyazaki, S. (1991). Temporal pattern of survival and dendritic growth of fetal hippocampal cells transplanted into ischemic lesion of the adult rat hippocampus. *Brain Research, 562,* 352–355.

Katayama, Y., Tsubokawa, T., & Yamamoto, T. (1991). Characterization and modification of brain activity with deep brain stimulation in patients in a persistent vegetative state; Pain-related late positive component of cerevral evoked potential. *Pace, 14,* 116–121.

Koller, W. C., Wong, G. F., & Lang, A. (1989). Posttraumatic movement disorders: A review. *Movement Disorder and Disability, 4,* 20–36.

Koyama, S., Katayama, Y., Maejima, S., Hirayama, T., Fujii, M., & Tsubokawa, T. (1993). Thalamic neuronal hyperactivity following transection of the spinothalamic tract in the cat: Involvement of N-methyl-D-asparate receptor. *Brain Research, 612,* 345–350.

Krauss, J. K., Mohadjer, M., Nobbe, F., & Mundinger, F. (1994). The treatment of posttraumatic tremor by stereotactic surgery. *Journal of Neurosurgery, 80,* 810–819.

Land, R. D., & Lune, J. S. (1971). Synaptic adjustment after deafferentation of the superior colliculus of the rat. *Science, 171,* 804–807.

Lenz, F. A., Kwan, H. C., Dostrovsky, J., & Tasker, R. R. (1989). Characteristics of the bursting pattern of action potentials that occurs in the thalamus of patients with central pain. *Brain Research, 496,* 357–396.

Liu, C. N., & Chamber, W. W. (1958). Intraspinal sprouting of dorsal root axons. *Archives of Neurological Psychiatry, 79,* 46–61.

Maejima, S., Koshinaga, M., Koyama, Y., Katayama, Y., & Tsubakawa, T. (1993). Thalamic stimulation facilitates microglial and astroglial reactions in the cortex following spinal cord injury. *Advances in Neurotrauma Research, 5,* 144–146.

McCouch, G. P., Austin, G. M., Liu, C. N., & Liu, C. Y. (1958). Sprouting as a cause of spasticity. *Journal of Neurophysiology, 21,* 205–216.

Mundinger, F. (1965). Stereotaxic interventions on the zona incerta area for treatment of extrapyramidal motor disturbances and their results. *Confinia Neurologia, 26,* 222–230.

Olszewski, J., & Baxter, D. (1981). Cytoarchitecture of the human brain stem (2nd ed.). New York: Karger.

Pazzaglia, P., Frank, G., Frank, F., & Gaist, G. (1975). Clinical course and prognosis of acute post-traumatic coma. *Journal of Neurology, Neurosurgery and Psychiatry, 38,* 149–154.

Raisman, G. (1969). Neuronal plasticity in the septal nuclei of the adult rat. *Brain Research, 14,* 25–48.

Sladek, J. R., & Gash, D. M. (1984). Morphological and functional properties of transplanted vasopressin neurons. In J. R. Sladek & D. M. Gash (Eds.), *Neural transplants: Development and function* (pp. 243–280). New York: Plenum.

Stenevi, U., Bjorklund, A., & Kromer, L. F. (1984). Use of CNS implants to promote regeneration of central axons across denervating lesions in the adult rat brain. In J. R. Sladek & D. M. Gash (Eds.), *Neural transplants: Development and function* (pp. 325–337). New York: Plenum.

Steward, O., & Mesenheimer, J. A. (1978). Histochemical evidence for a post-lesion reorganization of cholinergic afferents in the hippocampal formation of the mature cat. *Journal of Comparative Neurology, 178,* 697–710.

Sturm, V., Kühner, A., Schmitt, H. P., Assmus, H., & Stock, G. (1979). Chronic electrical stimulation of the thalamic unspecific activating system in a patient with coma due to midbrain and upper brain stem infarction. *Acta Neurochirurgica, 47,* 235–244.

Thoenen, H., & Edgar, D. (1985). Neurotrophic factors. *Science, 229,* 238–242.

Tsubokawa, T. (1992). *Modern functional stereotaxy: Moderator P. Gildenberg.* Sixtieth annual meeting of the American Association of Neurological Surgery, San Francisco, CA.

Tsubokawa, T. (1993). *State of the art neurosurgery for movement this order: Moderator P. Gildenberg.* Sixty-first annual meeting of the American Association of Neurological Surgery, Boston, MA.

Tsubokawa, T., & Moriyasu, N. (1975). Lateral pallidotomy for relief of ballistic movement: Its basic evidences and clinical application. *Confernia Neurologica, 37,* 10–15.

Tsubokawa, T., Yamamoto, T., & Katayama, Y. (1990a). Deep brain stimulation for persistent vegetative state: Follow-up results and criteria for selection of candidates. *Functional Neurosurgery,* (Tokyo), *29,* 171–179.

Tsubokawa, T., Yamamoto, T., & Katayama, Y. (1990b). Prediction of the outcome of prolonged coma caused by brain damage. *Brain Injury, 4,* 329–337.

Tsubokawa, T., Yamamoto, T., Katayama, Y., Hirayama, T., Maejima, S., & Moriya, T. (1990). Deep-brain stimulation in a persistent vegetative state: Follow-up results and criteria for selection of candidates. *Brain Injury, 4,* 315–327.

Tsubokawa, T., Katayama, Y., Yamamoto, T., Hirayama, T., & Koyama, S. (1993). Chronic motor cortex stimulation in patients with thalamic pain. *Journal of Neurosurgery, 78,* 393–401.

Van Woerkom, T., Minderbound, J. M., Gottsschal, T., & Nicolai, G. (1982). Neurotransmitters in the treatment of patients with severe head injuries. *European Journal of Neurology, 21,* 227–234.

Weber, P. (1984). Sensorimotor therapy: Its effect on electroencephalogram of acute comatose patients. *Archives of Physical and Medical Rehabilitation, 65,* 457–462.

Yamamoto, T., Tsubokawa, T., Katayama, Y., & Hirayama, T. (1993). Changes of prostaglandin E_2, D_2 and monoamines in CSF: Comparison between deep brain stimulation and spinal cord stimulation. *Advances in Neurotrauma Research, 5,* 101–103.

7

Pharmacological Strategies in the Management of Cognition and Behavior Following Traumatic Brain Injury

Warren E. Lux

In recent years, the rehabilitation community has shown increasing interest in a therapeutic role for pharmacological interventions that might have beneficial effects on higher cerebral functions following traumatic brain injury (TBI). Advances in acute surgical trauma care, combined with increasingly sophisticated rehabilitative interventions, have led to improved patient treatment. However, uniformly satisfactory cognitive and behavioral outcomes for patients and families remain elusive. In an attempt to bring additional tools to bear on this problem, appropriate attention has begun to be directed toward pharmacotherapy. Major goals of a pharmacological approach in TBI patients include the following:

1. Amelioration of disturbances in psychological/behavioral function.
2. Enhancement of cognitive capabilities.
3. Promotion of neurological recovery.

The first and second goals, of course, relate to primary pharmacological effects on the functions in question. The third goal concerns secondary effects on cognitive and behavioral function that result from the administration of drugs whose primary effects are to prevent evolving neuronal death in the aftermath of injury and/or affect the return to function of those neurons that do survive. The purpose of this chapter is to examine pharmacotherapy as a direct and primary mediator and/or modulator of cognitive and behavioral function as expressed by the first and second goals. The indirect effects covered in the third goal are beyond the chapter's scope, although recent advances in the molecular biology of neural injury—some of which are discussed elsewhere in this volume—have made this an area of great potential clinical interest for the future. The concept that cytoprotective drugs (whose development is based on knowledge of molecular mechanisms of neuronal injury) can, by promoting neurological recovery, have secondary beneficial effects on long-term cognitive and behavioral outcomes for patients is at the forefront of evolving modern neuroscience research.

However, many kinds of secondary effects can occur whenever pharmacotherapy is utilized. In some instances, as in the example of cytoprotective drugs, there is the potential for these secondary effects to be beneficial. Moreover, several other favorable indirect drug effects, some of them commonly seen in clinical practice settings, come readily to mind as well. For example, when behavioral control is improved, it can allow for enhanced cognition—an observation that is made on a daily basis in brain-injury programs across the country. Likewise, a patient's improved ability to cognitively deal with his or her environment is often observed by clinicians to have beneficial secondary effects on behavioral function. On the more speculative side, it could be postulated that improvements in cognition or behavior, or both, might also be associated with the establishment of a physiological or biochemical cerebral milieu, which could facilitate the neuronal reorganization process, if not other aspects of neurological recovery.

It is equally clear that secondary drug effects may not always be so favorable. Indeed, even the idea that the promotion of neurological recovery will necessarily result in improved cognition and behavior later in the clinical course has not been fully established. For example, the imbalance created by a positive effect on cell survival in some limbic structures in the absence of a similar effect in frontal structures could theoretically have detrimental, rather than beneficial, effects on long-term behavioral function in some patients. Thus, there is no substitute for careful and rigorously scientific clinical testing. A more practical and familiar example of detrimental secondary drug effects, however, and one that is faced by experienced clinicians on a regular basis, is the propensity of some behaviorally active drugs to impair cognition at the same time that a net beneficial effect on a primary target behavior is emerging. This is seen particularly with drugs with sedative properties, although the resulting cognitive changes may be reversible at a later time following drug withdrawal.

There is perhaps a greater concern, however, because of the potential for irreversibility: Drugs that affect cognition and/or behavior favorably may also impair or impede the underlying neurological recovery process. For example, there is an emerging line of evidence implicating cholinergic mechanisms in the pathogenesis of cell damage following neurological injury (Hayes, Stonnington, Lyeth, Dixon, & Yamamoto, 1986). Yet acetylcholine is also a critical neurotransmitter for memory function—a function that is commonly impaired after TBI. Thus, the potential for a cholinergic agent to have beneficial effects on memory may be counterbalanced at some points during early recovery by the risk of an irreversible adverse effect on neuronal survival. A more clearly established example of a conceptually related phenomenon that is familiar to all behavioral pharmacologists is tardive dyskinesia. Indeed, whenever one uses a centrally acting drug, whether the primary goal is to affect cognition, behavior, or neuronal survival, it is also clear that secondary effects can occur in either target neurons or neurons elsewhere in the brain, and that these secondary effects can be either beneficial or detrimental, transient or irreversible.

Despite all of these caveats, there is reason for optimism. The pathological anatomy and distribution of axonal damage following closed head injury has a firm scientific base (Gennarelli, 1986; Ommaya & Gennarelli, 1974), which suggests vulnerability of projection systems utilizing neurotransmitters, particularly monoamines, known to play a role in cognition and behavior. Moreover, alterations of these neurotransmitters have been demonstrated following TBI (Bareggi et al., 1975; van Woerkom, Teelken, & Minderhoud, 1977; Vecht, van Woerkom, Teelken, & Minderhoud, 1975). If TBI patients' cognitive and behavioral deficits result, at least in part, from this loss of neurochemical homeostasis, then there exists the potential to remediate them pharmacologically with existing agents that affect such systems. In his comprehensive review, Gualtieri (1988) recognized this possibility and discussed in depth the classes of agents that might be so utilized. Although at that time he accurately pointed out that "there is no research to speak of in the neuropharmacology of TBI," he reviewed the inferences that might be drawn from the known neuropharmacological effects in other brain disorders of some of the agents of interest. Subsequently, an increasing number of neuropharmacological studies with TBI patients as subjects have begun to appear. This chapter examines the studies in this area that have been published to date, and thus provides a current review of the pharmacotherapy of the cognitive and behavioral sequelae of TBI as based on direct observation in TBI patients, insofar as data permit.

COGNITIVE PHARMACOLOGY STUDIES

Psychostimulant drugs have been a major focus of interest among investigators seeking to enhance cognition in patients following TBI. The earliest study in this area is a single case report of a patient with a chronic, stable traumatic encephalopathy who was treated with dextroamphetamine (Lipper & Tuchman, 1976). Institution of dextroamphet-amine in this patient was associated with an increase in memory and a decrease in confusion, as measured by clinical examination. No specific formal cognitive measures were reported. Cognitive function worsened when dextroamphetamine was discontinued. The authors also reported an enhanced therapeutic effect when amitriptyline was added to the therapeutic regimen while the patient was taking dextroamphetamine.

A number of other investigators have examined psychostimulants further. The cognitive effects of dextroamphetamine have been examined in double-blind, placebo-controlled, single case studies by two different groups (Bleiberg, Garmoe, Cederquist, Reeves, & Lux, 1993; Evans, Gualtieri, & Patterson, 1987). In each of these studies, dextroamphetamine showed beneficial effects on specific formal measures of attention, memory, and cognitive processing. In the study by Bleiberg et al., moreover, a computer-assisted cognitive test paradigm was utilized, which allowed for repeated-measures testing of the functions in question. Thus, a separate measure of variability of cognitive performance was derived from the data. This suggested that the improvement in cognition seen on dextroamphetamine was accompanied by a decrease in the variability of the subject's cognitive performance.

Another psychostimulant drug commonly used in clinical practice is methylphenidate. In addition to examining dextroamphetamine in their patients, Evans et al. (1987) also studied methylphenidate utilizing the same double-blind, placebo-controlled methodology. A similar positive effect on cognitive function was demonstrated. These investigators also utilized multiple doses of both methylphenidate and dextroamphetamine in their study. They established some classical dose-response data for each agent, thus providing further support for a true pharmacological effect. In a more extensive study, Gualtieri and Evans (1988) examined methylphenidate utilizing a double-blind, placebo-controlled, crossover design in a case series of 15 TBI patients. Again, the drug appeared to have a beneficial cognitive effect, but this was only striking in a subset of patients. Analysis of the data from the entire group was reported to be disappointing, and a clear overall benefit could not be concluded with certainty. This naturally raised questions about the homogeneity of the experimental group—something that frequently confounds research in this disorder of remarkable variability from patient to patient across a broad spectrum of possible lesions each time an injury occurs.

In another study of methylphenidate, group data were again examined in a case series utilizing a double-blind, placebo-controlled, crossover design (Speech, Rao, Osmon, & Sperry, 1993). These investigators found no statistically significant group differences between drug and placebo conditions on any of their measures of attention, learning, or cognitive processing speed. In their study group of 12 patients with a TBI at least 1 year prior to study, loss of consciousness varied from 0 to 33 days, and posttraumatic amnesia (PTA) varied from 3 to 270 days. Apparent drug responses, if any, in individual patients or in subsets of patients were not reported.

Methylphenidate has also been used in combination with parenteral physostigmine, a drug that increases cholinergic activity in the brain (Weinberg, Auerbach, & Moore, 1987). A positive effect on cognition was noted with methylphenidate alone, and this appeared to increase when physostigmine was added. However, the study was a single case report and was uncontrolled.

Although not a classical psychostimulant, the tricyclic agent protriptyline has been used as an alternative in some clinical settings. Because of this, one group of investigators examined its effects in TBI (Wroblewski, Glenn, Cornblatt, Joseph, & Suduikis, 1993). They reported a series of eight individual cases that appeared to respond favorably to this agent. However, cognitive function was assessed clinically and functionally without the benefit of standardized cognitive assessments common to all eight patients, and the study was uncontrolled.

The mechanism of action of psychostimulants in TBI, insofar as they are effective at all, remains unknown. However, their monoaminergic actions may be critical. Other classes of agents with monoaminergic agonist properties, moreover, have also been examined in TBI. Chief among these are agents with specific dopaminergic activity—most notably levodopa/carbidopa and bromocriptine. Levodopa is a dopamine precursor, and is therefore dependent on intact dopamine-forming neurons in the brain for its dopaminergic activity. Bromocriptine is a direct dopamine receptor agonist. Both have been studied in TBI. Lal, Merbtiz, and Grip (1988) examined levodopa/carbidopa in an uncontrolled case series of 12 patients with head injury with diffuse brain damage who had plateaued in rehabilitation prior to institution of the drug. Data were reported on 11 patients. All 11 patients improved in the majority of the areas evaluated, and, in particular, all improved in alertness and concentration. Ten of the 11 showed improvements in memory, and none worsened in any area of evaluation. Subsequently, Haig and Ruess (1990) reported another case in which there was an apparent response to levodopa/carbidopa. This case was striking in that the patient was in a vegetative state that had persisted for 6 months prior to the initiation of drug therapy, and he became conversant and responsive within days of the institution of levodopa/carbidopa. The authors argued that a spontaneous change of that magnitude in that time frame was unlikely, although the study was unblinded and uncontrolled.

Because of levodopa/carbidopa's dependence on intact dopamine-forming neurons for its activity, it has been suggested that a more rational way to approach dopaminergic therapy might be to administer a primary dopamine receptor agonist, such as bromocriptine (Eames, 1989). This avoids the problem of injury to the primary cells of origin of dopamine in the brainstem, and it avoids what may be the more likely problem of injury to the ascending axons projecting from these cells. In that regard, Eames reported that bromocriptine appeared to be effective in his hands in (presumably) unblinded and uncontrolled clinical situations, although he noted that the effects were predominantly on initiation and motor findings, rather than on arousal and cognitive function. He also noted that not all patients responded, thus confirming the experience of most other investigators and clinicians examining pharmacological interventions in this disorder, with its inherent problem of anatomic—and probably physiological and biochemical—heterogeneity.

Bromocriptine as a single agent has also been examined for its effect on speech dysfunction in patients with TBI, with particular attention to the syndrome of akinetic mutism. Crismon, Childs, Wilcox, and Barrow (1988) reported that unblinded institution of bromocriptine was associated with increased vocalization and verbal output in three brain-injured individuals who were either mute or had severely impaired verbal output on admission to their center. Verbal output in this uncontrolled study was assessed by clinical examination.

In addition to the single agent studies of dopaminergic agents, there is a report of combination pharmacotherapy with levodopa/carbidopa and bromocriptine in a TBI patient in an attempt to recruit both pre- and postsynaptic dopaminergic effects (Starr, Zafonte, & Bond, 1992). This single case report described the unblinded administration of levodopa/carbidopa, followed by the addition of bromocriptine, to an individual with persistent posttraumatic unconsciousness several months after injury. The cognitive response to levodopa/carbidopa was described as minimal, but the patient was reported to have become alert and responsive to commands shortly after the addition of bromocriptine. The authors did not include a period of treatment with bromocriptine alone in their report of this case.

A variety of other agents have been examined for their cognitive effects in TBI patients. McIntyre and Gasquoine (1990) studied two patients in an unblinded trial of clonidine, a centrally acting alpha-2 adrenergic receptor agonist that has been reported to have varying effects on memory in several different clinical and experimental situations. A battery of neuropsychological memory tests was administered to each patient prior to the institution of clonidine, and this battery was repeated on Day 15 of drug treatment. No differences in cognitive function on any of the measures utilized were demonstrated in either patient.

Levin et al. (1986) examined the central cholinergic system in a study of the effects of oral physostigmine and lecithin on memory and attention. Their report described a double-blind, placebo-controlled, crossover study in 16 TBI patients in which lecithin alone was compared with the physostigmine–lecithin combination. In general, no differences were observed, although the investigators did find that sustained attention on the continuous performance test was better under physostigmine than placebo when the drug condition occurred first in the crossover design.

Bohnen, Twijnstra, and Jolles (1993) reported on a neuropeptide, the vasopressin analogue desglycinamide-arginine[8]-vasopressin (DGAVP), in mild brain injury. They studied 32 patients for 3 months in a double-blind, placebo-controlled, matched-pairs design, and demonstrated no measurable cognitive benefit of DGAVP in their study group. Finally, McLean, Cardenas, Burgess, and Gamzu (1991) examined a nootropic drug, pramiracetam, in four patients utilizing a double-blind, placebo-controlled design. They reported improvement in memory, particularly delayed recall, under drug conditions, and they regarded the improvement as clinically significant. They also noted that improvement was maintained during an 18-month open-trial period that followed.

BEHAVIORAL PHARMACOLOGY STUDIES

Several of the previously cited studies of the cognitive effects of pharmacological agents in TBI utilized subjects who also showed behavioral abnormalities. In each instance, behavioral data were reported as well. These included four studies of psychostimulants (Evans et al., 1987; Gualtieri & Evans, 1988; Lipper & Tuchman, 1976; Speech et al., 1993), one study of an alternative stimulant, protriptyline (Wroblewski et al., 1993), and one study of a dopaminergic agent, levodopa/carbidopa (Lal et al., 1988). In all instances, the behavioral data were consistent with the cognitive data. The single report that did not demonstrate a cognitive benefit of the drug in question—the study of methylphenidate by Speech et al. (1993)—did not demonstrate behavioral benefit either. In all of the other studies, apparent behavioral and cognitive benefits were reported. Whether the cognitive and behavioral effects in the positive studies were simultaneous and independent, or whether one was primary and the other secondary, was uniformly difficult to determine.

Studies of psychostimulants and dopaminergic agents examining primarily behavioral target signs and symptoms have also been done.

Mooney and Haas (1993) reported a therapeutic effect of methylphenidate on anger in 38 brain-injured subjects utilizing a randomized, placebo-controlled, single-blind study design. Although anger was the primary variable being examined, this study also looked at measures of attention and memory. Again, some degree of consistency between cognitive and behavioral data was demonstrated: Significant improvement in memory occurred in the treated group. However, a similar therapeutic effect on attention was not shown in this study. In a case study of agitation, the administration of the dopaminergic agent, amantadine, was associated with a reduction in agitated and aggressive behavior in two cases (Chandler, Barnhill, & Gualtieri, 1988).

Agitation is a particularly problematic behavioral manifestation following TBI. When present, it can disrupt rehabilitation significantly. Thus, a number of agents other than amantadine have been examined for their effects on agitated behavior. Because seritonergic mechanisms have been invoked in the regulation of behavior in a variety of clinical and experimental settings, seritonergic agents have been of interest to clinicians for some time, particularly because of the potential for beneficial effects on attention as well. Jackson, Corrigan, and Arnett (1985) reported a single case in which the administration of the seritonergic tricyclic, amitriptyline, was associated with a marked reduction in agitated behavior in a 32-year-old woman who had persistent agitation more than 6 months after TBI. Improvements in attention and concentration accompanied the behavioral changes. The drug was administered in an unblinded fashion without placebo control. Subsequently, an unblinded case series of agitated patients treated with amitriptyline was reported (Mysiw, Jackson, & Corrigan, 1988). Again, an association between institution of drug treatment and reduction in agitation was noted. When the data were examined further, an apparent behavioral response to amitriptyline was more common in patients still in PTA and most common in patients at the Rancho IV level of cognitive functioning.

Another agent thought to affect seritonergic systems is the anxiolytic drug buspirone. Levine (1988) reported a case in which the unblinded institution of this agent was followed by a reduction in agitated behavior sufficient to permit renewed participation in a rehabilitation program. Two additional cases, also unblinded and uncontrolled but with a similar beneficial result, were reported by Ratey, Leveroni, Miller, Komry, and Gaffar (1992). Their cases both failed neuroleptics, anticonvulsants, and beta blockers prior to the institution of buspirone. Gualtieri (1991) also reported an unblinded experience with buspirone in TBI patients who had failed other agents. He found both responders and nonresponders, but felt that the drug worked better overall in restless, irritable, mildly injured patients than it did in frankly agitated patients with severe TBI.

In addition to its use as a single agent, buspirone, in combination with the anticonvulsant carbamazepine, has been reported for agitated delirium during the early posttraumatic period following TBI (Pourcher, Filteau, Bouchard, & Baruch, 1994). These authors described four cases without matched controls, in which the unblinded administration of this combination of drugs was followed within 12–36 hours by lessening or resolution of agitation.

Carbamazepine alone (Lewin & Sumners, 1992), or in combination with other agents (Rupright, Cantrell, & Kidman, 1992), has also been reported to be of benefit in agitation associated with TBI. In the report of Lewin and Sumners, a patient with episodic dyscontrol experienced a complete cessation of violent and aggressive outbursts following initiation of treatment with carbamazepine 2 years after a TBI; this remission persisted for a full year of follow-up. Rupright et al. reported the use of carbamazepine in combination with lithium carbonate in a series of 10 severely agitated patients in a rehabilitation setting. This case series was unblinded and uncontrolled, but a rapid reduction in agitation was seen in all 10 patients when the lithium/carbamazepine combination was instituted.

Other data support the positive effect of lithium carbonate alone in posttraumatic agitation. Haas and Cope (1985) reported a case of a belligerent, agitated TBI patient whose agitation persisted on benzodiazepines, neuroleptics, and beta blockers. Agitation worsened on methylphenidate, but improved notably on lithium. This improvement was sufficient to permit productive completion of an inpatient rehabilitation program and a safe discharge home. Glenn et al. (1989) reported on an open-label trial of lithium carbonate in a heterogeneous group of 10 patients with aggressive behavior or affective instability. Five of the 10 had a significant improvement in behavioral control as observed by clinicians, and a sixth had a moderate response. Not all of these patients were on lithium alone, however, although some were.

The use of other agents to control agitated behavior following TBI was reported in a randomized, double-blind, placebo-controlled study of the beta blocker, propranolol, in 21 brain-injured subjects (Brooke, Patterson, Questad, Cardenas, & Farrel-Roberts, 1992). Although the number of agitation episodes in the treatment and control groups was similar, the intensity of agitation was reported to be significantly lower in the treatment group. In addition, the use of physical restraint was significantly lower in the group that received propranolol.

Neuroleptic or antipsychotic medication has long been used to treat agitation in a variety of clinical settings. Rehabilitation physicians are familiar with TBI patients who arrive at their centers on haloperidol or other neuroleptics that were started in acute care to suppress agitated behaviors that could not be tolerated in an intensive care unit (ICU) or an acute ward. However, there is strikingly little literature on the specific efficacy of such treatment in TBI patients, despite its widespread use and the clear clinical impression that if all behaviors are sufficiently suppressed pharmacologically, the unwanted, agitated behaviors will be suppressed with them. Clozapine, a new antipsychotic drug used to treat schizophrenics unresponsive to other agents, has been examined in a TBI population (Michals, Crismon, Roberts, & Childs, 1993). These investigators reported an uncontrolled, unblinded series of nine patients, in whom the therapeutic response, particularly in terms of decreased agitation and aggression, was marked in three, mild in three, and indeterminate in three. However, they also noted a high incidence of side effects, with seizures occurring in two of the nine patients.

In addition to agitation, a few other behavioral syndromes following TBI have been the subject of reports examining the effects of pharmacological interventions. In general, these reports have focused on disorders of mood and affect. Bakchine et al. (1989) reported a maniclike state after bilateral orbitofrontal and right temporoparietal injury, and examined the effects of several agents in a careful, placebo-controlled, single case study design. Clonidine, a centrally acting alpha-2 adrenergic receptor agonist that has shown activity in psychiatric patients with mania, was associated with a rapid reduction in mania scores on the measures used in this study both times it was introduced in the sequence of agents studied. After the second introduction, the drug was continued, and the effect persisted throughout the follow-up period of approximately 150 days. Placebo and carbamazepine had no effect, and levodopa was associated with worsening. Bipolar disorder has also been reported as a posttraumatic phenomenon by Yassa and Cvejic (1994). These authors described an 83-year-old man with recurrent manic and depressive attacks dating to an episode of head trauma 22 years earlier. They reported that control of his symptoms occurred after treatment with the anticonvulsant valproate.

Because both bipolar disease and isolated mania have been reported following TBI, it is not surprising that unipolar depression, a disorder not uncommon in clinical practice, has been the subject of a pharmacological report as well. Dinan and Mobayed (1992) reported a series of 13 patients, with unipolar depression following minor head injury, who were matched to 13 controls with functional depression. All were treated with amitriptyline, a classical tricyclic antidepressant, in a open-label trial. Eleven of the functional patients, but only four of the head-injured patients, improved during the 6-week trial, thus suggesting a relative treatment resistance in the posttraumatic group.

Although not a true disorder of mood, emotional lability or emotional incontinence can occur after TBI. This disorder can also occur in a variety of other states, including multiple bilateral subcortical infarcts. It is characterized by outbursts of excessive involuntary emotional expression (e.g., weeping) that are incongruent with the actual emotions being felt by the patient at the time. Because tricyclic antidepressants have been reported to improve this condition in stroke patients, Sloan, Brown, and Pentland (1992) examined fluoxetine, a new selective serotonin reuptake inhibitor with antidepressant properties, in an open-label trial in six patients with this syndrome. Five had vascular brain injuries, but one— a victim of an assault—had severe TBI. All six, including the traumatically brain-injured individual, improved within 1 week of beginning fluoxetine.

SUMMARY AND CONCLUSIONS

Neuropsychopharmacological data specific to TBI patients are finally becoming increasingly available, as evidenced by the numbers and recency of the papers cited in this chapter. However, our current state of knowledge is still limited, and problems abound. Many of the papers cited here are case reports or case series in which agents were administered in uncontrolled and/or unblinded study designs. The validity of the conclusions derived from such reports is necessarily uncertain. Moreover, the studies reviewed here were not always positive, particularly in cases where more rigorous study designs were used. There are a number of possible explanations for this, including (a) ineffective drugs or drugs given at ineffective doses, (b) measures that are insufficiently sensitive to the drug effects even when true pharmacological effects occur, and (c) the previously mentioned problem with the heterogeneity of TBI, which can dilute the positive findings if only some patients respond, particularly in some of the more rigorous study designs in which only randomized group data are analyzed.

Yet the situation is not wholly gloomy, and there is much that is positive. New drug development continues, and more can be done to study promising old drugs in study designs that systematically examine a range of doses. The computer revolution has facilitated the development of computer-assisted, repeated-measures cognitive testing, which has been demonstrated to be highly sensitive to drug effects in TBI (Bleiberg, Lux, Garmoe, & Reeves, 1992). Rigorous single case study designs utilizing double blinding, placebo controls, and crossover strategies are available to help address the problem of heterogeneity.

If nothing else, the current evidence reviewed here suggests that at least some TBI patients derive cognitive and/or behavioral benefits from a pharmacological approach at least some of the time. In some instances, the benefits may be dramatic. Although increasingly rigorous and systematic studies are required if we are to achieve even more specific and effective pharmacological treatment of TBI patients, the tools to do so are at hand. Although more than pharmacology may be needed in many patients, they and their families are likely to welcome the additional benefits that an improved pharmacological approach may be able to provide.

REFERENCES

Bakchine, S., Lacomblez, L., Benoit, N., Parisot, D., Chain, F., & Lhermitte, F. (1989). Manic-like state after bilateral orbitofrontal and right temporoparietal injury: Efficacy of clonidine. *Neurology, 39,* 777–781.

Bareggi, S. R., Porta, M., Selenati, A., Assael, B. M., Calderini, G., Collice, M., Rossanda, M., & Morselli, P. L. (1975). Homovanillic acid and 5-hydroxyindole-acetic acid in the CSF of patients after a severe head injury. *European Neurology, 13,* 528–544.

Bleiberg, J., Garmoe, W., Cederquist, J., Reeves, D., & Lux, W. (1993). Effects of dexedrine on performance consistency following brain injury. *Neuropsychiatry, Neuropsychology, and Behavioral Neurology, 6,* 245–248.

Bleiberg, J., Lux, W. E., Garmoe, W. S., & Reeves, D. (1992). A procedure for assessing and monitoring cognitive enhancement and cognitive degradation secondary to pharmacotherapy. *Archives of Physical Medicine and Rehabilitation, 73,* 994.

Bohnen, N. I., Twijnstra, A., & Jolles, J. (1993). A controlled trial with vasopressin analogue (DGAVP) on cognitive recovery immediately after head trauma. *Neurology, 43,* 103–106.

Brooke, M. M., Patterson, D. R., Questad, K. A., Cardenas, D., & Farrel-Roberts, L. (1992). The treatment of agitation during initial hospitalization after traumatic brain injury. *Archives of Physical Medicine and Rehabilitation, 73,* 917–921.

Chandler, M. C., Barnhill, J. L., & Gualtieri, C. T. (1988). Amantadine for the agitated head-injury patient. *Brain Injury, 2,* 309–311.

Crismon, M. L., Childs, A., Wilcox, R. E., & Barrow, N. (1988). The effect of bromocriptine on speech dysfunction in patients with diffuse brain injury (akinetic mutism). *Clinical Neuropharmacology, 11,* 462–466.

Dinan, T. G., & Mobayed, M. (1992). Treatment resistance of depression after head injury: A preliminary study of amitriptyline response. *Acta Psychiatrica Scandinavica, 85,* 292–294.

Eames, P. (1989). The use of Sinemet and bromocriptine. *Brain Injury, 3,* 319–320.

Evans, R. W., Gualtieri, C. T., & Patterson, D. (1987). Treatment of chronic closed head injury with psychostimulant drugs: A controlled case study and an appropriate evaluation procedure. *Journal of Nervous and Mental Disease, 175,* 106–110.

Gennarelli, T. A. (1986). Mechanisms and pathophysiology of cerebral concussion. *Journal of Head Trauma Rehabilitation, 1*(2), 23–29.

Glenn, M. B., Wroblewski, B., Parziale, J., Levine, L., Whyte, J., & Rosenthal, M. (1989). Lithium carbonate for aggressive behavior or affective instability in ten brain-injured patients. *American Journal of Physical Medicine & Rehabilitation, 68,* 221–226.

Gualtieri, C. T. (1988). Pharmacotherapy and the neurobehavioral sequelae of traumatic brain injury. *Brain Injury, 2,* 101–129.

Gualtieri, C. T. (1991). Buspirone: Neuropsychiatric effects. *Journal of Head Trauma Rehabilitation*, 6(1), 90–92.

Gualtieri, C. T., & Evans, R. W. (1988). Stimulant treatment for the neurobehavioral sequelae of traumatic brain injury. *Brain Injury*, 2, 273–290.

Haas, J. F., & Cope, D. N. (1985). Neuropharmacologic management of behavior sequelae in head injury: A case report. *Archives of Physical Medicine and Rehabilitation*, 66, 472–474.

Haig, A. J., & Ruess, J. M. (1990). Recovery from vegetative state of six months' duration associated with Sinemet (levodopa/carbidopa). *Archives of Physical Medicine and Rehabilitation*, 71, 1081–1083.

Hayes, R. L., Stonnington, H. H., Lyeth, B. G., Dixon, C. E., & Yamamoto, T. (1986). Metabolic and neurophysiologic sequelae of brain injury: A cholinergic hypothesis. *Central Nervous System Trauma*, 3, 163–173.

Jackson, R. D., Corrigan, J. D., & Arnett, J. A. (1985). Amitriptyline for agitation in head injury. *Archives of Physical Medicine and Rehabilitation*, 66, 180–181.

Lal, S., Merbtiz, C. P., & Grip, J. C. (1988). Modification of function in head-injured patients with Sinemet. *Brain Injury*, 2, 225–233.

Levin, H. S., Peters, B. H., Kalisky, Z., High, W. M., Jr., Von Laufen, A., Eisenberg, H. M., Morrison, D. P., & Gary, H. E., Jr. (1986). Effects of oral physostigmine and lecithin on memory and attention in closed head-injured patients. *Central Nervous System Trauma*, 3, 333–342.

Levine, A. M. (1988). Buspirone and agitation in head injury. *Brain Injury*, 2, 165–167.

Lewin, J., & Sumners, D. (1992). Successful treatment of episodic dyscontrol with carbamazepine. *British Journal of Psychiatry*, 161, 261–262.

Lipper, S., & Tuchman, M. M. (1976). Treatment of chronic post-traumatic organic brain syndrome with dextroamphetamine: First reported case. *Journal of Nervous and Mental Disease*, 162, 366–371.

McIntyre, F. L., & Gasquoine, P. (1990). Effect of clonidine on post-traumatic memory deficits. *Brain Injury*, 4, 209–211.

McLean, A., Jr., Cardenas, D. D., Burgess, D., & Gamzu, E. (1991). Placebo-controlled study of pramiracetam in young males with memory and cognitive problems resulting from head injury and anoxia. *Brain Injury*, 5, 375–380.

Michals, M. L., Crismon, M. L., Roberts, S., & Childs, A. (1993). Clozapine response and adverse effects in nine brain-injured patients. *Journal of Clinical Psychopharmacology*, 13, 198–203.

Mooney, G. F., & Haas, L. J. (1993). Effect of methylphenidate on brain injury-related anger. *Archives of Physical Medicine and Rehabilitation*, 74, 153–160.

Mysiw, W. J., Jackson, R. D., & Corrigan, J. D. (1988). Amitriptyline for post-traumatic agitation. *American Journal of Physical Medicine & Rehabilitation*, 67, 29–33.

Ommaya, A. K., & Gennarelli, T. A. (1974). Cerebral concussion and traumatic unconsciousness. *Brain*, 97, 633–654.

Pourcher, E., Filteau, M.-J., Bouchard, R. H., & Baruch, P. (1994). Efficacy of the combination of buspirone and carbamazepine in early posttraumatic delirium. *American Journal of Psychiatry*, 151, 150–151.

Ratey, J. J., Leveroni, C. L., Miller, A. C., Komry, V., & Gaffar, K. (1992). Low-dose buspirone to treat agitation and maladaptive behavior in brain-injured patients: Two case reports. *Journal of Clinical Psychopharmacology*, 12, 362–364.

Rupright, S. J., Cantrell, R. C., & Kidman, S. B. (1992). Atypical pharmacology management of agitation in traumatic brain injury. *Archives of Physical Medicine and Rehabilitation*, 73, 1007.

Sloan, R. L., Brown, K. W., & Pentland, B. (1992). Fluoxetine as a treatment for emotional lability after brain injury. *Brain Injury*, 6, 315–319.

Speech, T. J., Rao, S. M., Osmon, D. C., & Sperry, L. T. (1993). A double-blind controlled study of methylphenidate treatment in closed head injury. *Brain Injury, 7,* 333–338.

Starr, M., Zafonte, R. D., & Bond, R. (1992). Psychopharmacotherapy in a patient with prolonged post-traumatic unconsciousness. *Archives of Physical Medicine and Rehabilitation, 73,* 1007.

van Woerkom, T. C. A. M., Teelken, A. W., & Minderhoud, J. M. (1977). Difference in neurotransmitter metabolism in frontotemporal-lobe contusion and diffuse cerebral contusion. *Lancet, 1,* 812–813.

Vecht, C. J., van Woerkom, T. C. A. M., Teelken, A. W., & Minderhoud, J. M. (1975). Homovanillic acid and 5-hydroxyindoleacetic acid cerebrospinal fluid levels. *Archives of Neurology, 32,* 792–797.

Weinberg, R. M., Auerbach, S. H., & Moore, S. (1987). Pharmacologic treatment of cognitive deficits: A case study. *Brain Injury, 1,* 57–59.

Wroblewski, B., Glenn, M. B., Cornblatt, R., Joseph, A. B., & Suduikis, S. (1993). Protriptyline as an alternative stimulant medication in patients with brain injury: A series of case reports. *Brain Injury, 7,* 353–362.

Yassa, R., & Cvejic, J. (1994). Valproate in the treatment of posttraumatic bipolar disorder in a psychogeriatric patient. *Journal of Geriatric Psychiatry & Neurology, 7,* 55–57.

II

Clinical States

8

Neuropsychological Evaluation of Traumatic Brain Injury in the United States: A Critical Analysis

Brick Johnstone
Ty S. Callahan

As the need for psychological services in rehabilitation has grown (Frank, Gluck, Buckelew, 1990), neuropsychologists have established themselves as important members of interdisciplinary rehabilitation teams. In fact, Leung (1990) reported that 48% of psychologists who work in rehabilitation settings have advanced training in neuropsychology. Neuropsychology has enjoyed relative success in rehabilitation primarily due to the broad training neuropsychologists receive in the emotional, behavioral, and cognitive aspects of brain dysfunction. However, changes in the health care delivery system, based on health care reform, suggest that if neuropsychologists are to further secure their position in rehabilitation, it is necessary to critically evaluate the delivery of neuropsychological services in such settings.

For example, psychologists in rehabilitation settings are evaluating specific cognitive abilities using many tests that were originally developed to differentiate between individuals with and without brain dysfunction, with an emphasis on localization and lateralization of neuroanatomic lesions. Although a primary goal of neuropsychological rehabilitation is to improve functional abilities (or, at a minimum, to direct rehabilitation services), current evaluation practices are limited in terms of directly addressing TBI patients' functional needs. Although tests are used to predict functional outcomes, the ecological validity of most neuropsychological tests has not been adequately demonstrated. The assessment procedures are not necessarily deficient in and of themselves—they simply have not been developed or validated for functional purposes.

In addition, neuropsychologists need to better define their role in rehabilitation relative to other rehabilitation disciplines. Health care reform and managed care initiatives are forcing service providers to (a) justify the necessity of their services, (b) eliminate those services not directly linked to positive outcomes, and (c) reduce duplicity of services both within and between disciplines. Given the overlap between disciplines in rehabilitation (which is not unexpected given the interdisciplinary nature of rehabilitation), all disciplines need to better determine their "niche."

Thus, it can be argued that neuropsychologists need to focus on two critical areas to further the utility of neuropsychology in rehabilitation: (a) to empirically demonstrate the worth of neuropsychology in both predicting and impacting functional outcome, and (b) to establish a place for it in rehabilitation as it relates to other disciplines.

This chapter reviews the historical emphasis on neurological and diagnostic evaluation in the development of the field, examines current deficiencies in neuropsychological training, relates neuropsychology to other rehabilitation disciplines, justifies the need for a greater functional emphasis, and critically evaluates current neuropsychological procedures in the United States, all from a functional perspective. The focus of the chapter is cognitive dysfunction, although it is acknowledged that the emotional and behavioral sequelae of brain dysfunction are equally important to evaluate and treat following traumatic brain injury (TBI). It is also acknowledged that neuropsychology is a valuable and necessary component of rehabilitation. However, we hope to stimulate thought into how neuropsychologists can improve their services in rehabilitation settings.

HISTORICAL ORIGINS OF NEUROPSYCHOLOGY

To understand the limited functional (vs. diagnostic) utility of neuropsychological evaluations, it is necessary to review the origins of the field. Neuropsychology was initially developed to assist in the diagnosis of brain dysfunction, with an emphasis on the localization, lateralization, and detection of specific lesion sites (Hartman, 1988, 1991; Kreutzer, Leininger, & Harris, 1990; Loring, 1991). Prior to the advent of neuroradiological techniques, which allow for detailed structural and functional images of the brain (e.g., magnetic resonance imaging [MRI], computed tomography [CT], positron emission tomography [PET], and single photon emission computed tomography [SPECT]), neuropsychology was needed to make inferences regarding brain structure. This is no longer the case. However, in rehabilitation settings, neuropsychological procedures developed to speculate regarding structural abnormalities continue to be used, when in fact what is needed is evaluation of specific cognitive abilities that have direct relevance to everyday functions.

With advances in the diagnostic capabilities of neuroradiological techniques, there is less of a need for diagnostic neuropsychological evaluation. In rehabilitation, the need for diagnostic assessments for individuals with documented TBI is minimal because the localization of structural lesions has little direct functional utility. Determination of the nature and extent of cognitive deficits is of primary importance so that appropriate interventions can be initiated. There are no medical or psychological interventions specific to focal structural lesions, although there are interventions specific to cognitive dysfunctions (Sohlberg & Mateer, 1989; Wilson, 1987). For example, the identification of a possible right parietal lesion has no direct treatment implications. However, the elucidation of specific visuospatial deficits (regardless of their structural etiology) has important implications for the remediation of deficits as they pertain to functional abilities (e.g., driving, performing specific vocational or household responsibilities, etc.).

Several neuropsychological approaches have been utilized in rehabilitation, including normative-based batteries closely allied with the psychometric tradition (e.g., Halstead–Reitan Neuropsychological Battery [Reitan & Wolfson, 1985]), and approaches more closely related to the behavioral neurology tradition (e.g., Process Approach [Kaplan, 1988], variations of Luria-Nebraska Neuropsychological Battery [Golden, 1981]). The particular strengths and weaknesses of these approaches, from a functional perspective, have been discussed previously (Johnstone & Frank, 1995), and many rehabilitation professionals have found them to be useful in their own clinical experiences. However, from a scientist-practitioner perspective, the relationship between these neuropsychological measures/approaches and real-life functional outcomes needs to be empirically demonstrated.

NEUROPSYCHOLOGY TRAINING GUIDELINES

Functional applications of neuropsychological assessments are also limited due to existing training guidelines for neuropsychology. Related to the origins of the field, current training guidelines emphasize neurological, neuroanatomical, and diagnostic issues with minimal if any attention to training in rehabilitation, functional utility, and resources available for individuals with brain dysfunction (Reports of the INS-Division 40 Task Force on Education Accreditation and Credentialing, 1987). Furthermore, there are relatively few and nonspecific guidelines for training in interventions specific to brain dysfunction. It is evident that, as long as diagnostic training is emphasized, the use of neuropsychology for functional purposes will be slow to develop.

Review of American Psychological Association (APA) Division 22 (Rehabilitation Psychology) guidelines for postdoctoral fellowship training (Draft Guidelines for Post-Doctoral Training in Rehabilitation Psychology, 1992) illustrates weaknesses in Division 40 (Clinical Neuropsychology) training guidelines regarding functional issues. Division 22 guidelines are very specific regarding issues in rehabilitation; they call for specific training in cognitive retraining, vocational assessment, vocational rehabilitation, issues in independent living, and psychosocial adjustment models of disability and chronic illness. To maintain neuropsychology's position in rehabilitation, and to acknowledge the growing need for more functional neuropsychological evaluations, INS-Division 40 should consider providing additional training guidelines (Johnstone & Frank, 1995). This would ensure that all practicing neuropsychologists are aware of rehabilitation issues, and thus can provide better services to their consumers (i.e., patients and referral sources).

The heavy emphasis on the diagnostic utility of neuropsychology is also evident in the written examination for board certification in neuropsychology (American Board of Clinical Neuropsychology [ABCN]). It has five content areas that are proposed as essential core areas of knowledge: (a) neuropsychological assessment, (b) clinical neuropsychology, (c) basic and clinical neuroscience, (d) behavioral neurology, and (e) general clinical psychology. Obviously, it is important to know neurological etiologies of cognitive dysfunction, but it is equally important to know how to apply cognitive test results toward treatment considerations. Given the current training guidelines and board certification examination content areas, deficiencies in training regarding practical rehabilitation issues appear significant. Thus, neuropsychology risks falling behind other disciplines and psychology specialities as long as rehabilitation issues are minimized in training.

ISSUES IN THE FUNCTIONAL UTILITY
OF NEUROPSYCHOLOGY

Most neuropsychological measures and test batteries emphasize information that is important in the identification of deficits and diagnoses, but that has not been shown to be empirically related to functional abilities (i.e., daily living, vocational, educational, etc.). These problems regarding the ecological validity of neuropsychological tests and batteries have been frequently summarized, and the reader is referred to other articles for specific reviews (Johnstone & Frank, 1995; Robbins, 1989; Wilson, 1993). However, it is also important to address a less frequently discussed limitation of neuropsychological measures—namely, their construct validity. In general, it is often unclear which specific cognitive skills are measured by common neuropsychological tests. As a result, it is difficult to make predictions regarding unitary cognitive constructs, or to provide direction for the remediation of specific cognitive abilities. Test results are summarized by various constructs (e.g., attention, language, memory, executive functioning, etc.). However, these constructs are complex; to assume that commonly used tests are exhaustive or exclusive measures of these constructs is erroneous. In addition, variability in the language used to describe the skills measured by particular tests reflects considerable disagreement on assumed underlying constructs. For example, the fact that a single assessment procedure, such as the Trail Making Test (Reitan & Wolfson, 1985), is described by different sources as measuring sustained attention, psychomotor speed, or cognitive flexibility at the very least suggests lack of agreement in the constructs. Although many would agree that performance on Trails A and B is related to all these skills and more, it is inappropriate to state that the measure is a singular test of any one specific cognitive skill.

These problems in construct validity have direct relevance for the neuropsychologist working in rehabilitation. When research has not established a relationship between a particular test and a particular ability, which is often the case, extrapolation is made based on assumptions at the level of these constructs. Just as it is more convenient to describe test procedures as representing unitary neuropsychological skills, it is also easier to discuss a profile of neuropsychological skills as independent or, at best, hierarchical. The problem is that global functional abilities are most assuredly the result of complex interactions between various basic skills. As such, the need exists to focus on unitary cognitive abilities that can lead to basic functional recommendations. Other disciplines (e.g., occupational therapy, vocational evaluation, which evaluate more functionally relevant skills) may be more appropriate to evaluate how impairment in basic, unitary cognitive skills (and their interactions) impact more complex functional abilities that are specific to an individual's vocational, educational, or daily functioning. For example, although certain neuropsychological measures (e.g., Category Test [Halstead, 1947], Wisconsin Card Sorting Test [Heaton, 1981]) make inferences regarding reasoning abilities, they are limited in their ability to directly predict how a person will perform when he or she returns to work. In contrast, vocational evaluations can directly assess those skills a person needs for a specific vocation, and do not need to speculate about possible deficits. However, vocational evaluators can effectively combine their results with the results provided by neuropsychological evaluation to provide the most comprehensive treatment planning.

Neuropsychology is also limited in terms of functional utility secondary to the manner in which "outcome" is conceptualized in the neuro-psychological literature. Neuropsychological research typically defines outcome in terms of cognitive (i.e., an individual has a good or bad "outcome" based on neuropsychological test results). Several authors have noted problems in this manner of conceptualizing outcome (Johnston, Kirshblum, Zorowitz, & Shiflett, 1992; Johnstone & Frank, 1995. Rosenthal & Millis, 1992), stating the need to differentiate among impairment, disability, and handicap. A cognitive impairment (which neuro-psychological tests identify) may or may not result in a disability. For example, someone with a memory impairment may not have a vocational disability if he or she utilizes appropriate compensatory strategies. As such, neuropsychological research needs to focus on the effects of cognitive impairment on functional abilities (i.e., vocational, educational, daily living, etc.), rather than view "cognition" as an outcome area.

THE RELATIONSHIP BETWEEN NEUROPSYCHOLOGY AND OTHER REHABILITATION DISCIPLINES

As previously stated, neuropsychologists have established themselves as integral members of rehabilitation teams. The interdisciplinary nature of rehabilitation demands close collaboration among disciplines. However, neuropsychologists (and other rehabilitation professionals) must critically evaluate their place in rehabilitation, particularly related to duplicity of services. Given the overlap of services typically offered by neuropsychologists, speech pathologists, occupational therapists, vocational evaluators, and so on, it is necessary for all disciplines to better determine designated areas of practice. Although the interdisciplinary nature of a rehabilitation team is determined by the personal expertise of individual professionals at various settings, it is also important to consider this issue from a professional level (i.e., how to train students in neuropsychology, speech pathology, occupational therapy, etc., so as to enhance the interdisciplinary nature of rehabilitation).

It can be argued that neuropsychologists are better trained to integrate findings regarding TBI than other rehabilitation professionals, given their training in neurological, cognitive, emotional, and behavioral aspects of TBI. However, neuropsychologists must also acknowledge professional limitations. To illustrate this point, consider the overlap between services provided by neuropsychology and speech pathology. Many notable psychologists are nationally renowned language experts, as evidenced in their development of commonly used language measures. Their involvement in the evaluation and treatment of language disorders is appropriate. However, psychologists with such specialized language skills are the exception rather than the rule. INS-Division 40 guidelines in clinical neuropsychology do not have any guidelines for specific training in language disorders. As such, most neuropsychologists are generally not thoroughly trained in language dysfunction (and particularly interventions), and thus should allow speech pathologists to be primarily responsible for evaluating and treating language disorders. Conversely, it can be argued that the evaluation of cognitive abilities should be the primary responsibility of neuropsychologists, given the greater training they receive in this area.

Also consider the evaluation of *problem-solving* and *executive* skills in a rehabilitation setting. These terms are nonspecific and hard to define; as such, they are difficult to objectively evaluate. Neuropsychologists typically evaluate "executive" abilities by means of objective measures. However, the ecological validity of objective neuropsychological tests of executive functions has not been demonstrated, and some have argued that executive functions are difficult to evaluate from objective tests (Stuss, 1987; Johnstone & Frank, 1995). This is not a limitation in training or competency, but a limitation in the application of objective measures without demonstrated functional utility. Several authors (Johnstone & Frank, 1995; Stuss, 1987) have argued that executive functions cannot be effectively evaluated in a laboratory setting. In contrast, vocational counselors provide evaluations of vocational abilities with a minimal emphasis on specific cognitive abilities. Collaborative evaluations between neuropsychologists and vocational evaluators may provide the most comprehensive and useful information because the disciplines generally complement each other's weaknesses. Arguing this point, Lees-Haley (1989) suggested that "vocational" neuropsychology needs to focus on causal factors of vocational dysfunction, compared with "clinical" neuropsychology, which focuses on causal factors of brain dysfunction. It is important to note that Bigler (1991) called for the need to integrate neuropsychology with neuroradiology, although there have been minimal suggestions of coordinating evaluations between neuropsychology and other rehabilitation services. If it is important to coordinate these evaluations for diagnostic purposes, it is at least as important to integrate them for functional purposes.

CURRENT NEUROPSYCHOLOGICAL APPLICATIONS IN THE REHABILITATION OF TBI

There have been many descriptions of neuropsychological applications in rehabilitation. In general, most articles describe commonly used cognitive measures and test batteries, but do not critically evaluate the appropriateness of their use for functional purposes. Unfortunately, as

Erickson and Binder (1986) argued, the use and description of traditional neuropsychological measures are assumed to have meaning for individuals with cognitive dysfunction. However, it should not be assumed that reporting of cognitive test scores can adequately direct rehabilitation or vocational planning, especially because it is often unclear what most neuropsychological tests specifically measure. Given psychologists' expertise in research methodology, and that health care reform is necessitating demonstration of all rehabilitation services' efficacy, it is critical for the profession to empirically demonstrate the usefulness of neuropsychology in rehabilitation. In the future, it may be insufficient to claim that neuropsychology has functional utility based solely on clinical experience.

Articles regarding the use of neuropsychology in rehabilitation almost all focus on specific tests or test batteries; they give minimal attention to specific cognitive abilities and their relation to functional skills. For example, Blieberg and Kaplan (1992) discussed the use of the Halstead–Reitan Neuropsychological Test Battery (HRB) in rehabilitation for various populations including TBI, with an emphasis on the tests of the HRB. Similarly, Lynch (1990) described commonly used cognitive tests in the rehabilitation of TBI, with little discussion of the relationship between the tests listed and appropriate interventions. Minimal information specifically states how neuropsychological evaluations can be used to direct rehabilitation, most likely because this has never been adequately demonstrated. Several authors have called for more functional emphases of neuropsychological evaluation (Heinrichs, 1990; Johnstone & Frank, 1995; Kreutzer, Leininger, & Harris, 1990; Mapou, 1988), with a general consensus that neuropsychology needs to emphasize treatment planning as it relates to functional abilities.

FUNCTIONAL NEUROPSYCHOLOGICAL EVALUATION OF TBI

If neuropsychological evaluations are to have greater functional utility in the evaluation and treatment of TBI, it is necessary to critically evaluate neuropsychological assessment methods from a functional perspective. In general, it can be argued that previous assessment methods have focused on tests rather than cognitive abilities, as well as diagnostic rather than functional utility. However, for neuropsychology to have grater functional relevance, it must deemphasize tests and focus on those cognitive abilities associated with brain dysfunction. Utilizing a functional neuropsychological evaluation model, it is necessary to: (a) identify specific unitary cognitive abilities that have functional relevance and are testable in a laboratory setting; (b) report the test results based on functional descriptions, rather than just citing test indices; and (c) integrate neuropsychological results with other discipline findings. Conceptualizing neuropsychological evaluation in this manner calls for the use of any tests that have appropriate construct and ecological validity, as per Mapou (1988), regardless of their connection to a specific battery of tests or a neuropsychological approach (i.e., battery vs. process). Any test can be used to evaluate specific cognitive abilities if it has been shown to be an accurate measure of a specific cognitive ability, *and* if it has been shown to have ecological validity. Tests should not be used if it is unclear what they measure, or if they do not appear to have any functional relevance. Unfortunately, there are few measures that meet these criteria.

Different from previous diagnostic neuropsychological evaluations, the focus of a functionally oriented evaluation model is on relatively unitary cognitive constructs, with minimal focus on complex interactions between more basic cognitive skills. Drawing inferences regarding complex functional abilities from neuropsychological tests is not necessary when direct assessment of specific vocational/functional abilities can be better evaluated by others (i.e., vocational, educational professionals, etc.).

Following is a proposed model for the functional neuropsychological evaluation of TBI, emphasizing cognitive abilities shown to be commonly affected following TBI. We critically evaluate, from a functional perspective, those cognitive abilities (e.g., intelligence, academic skills, memory, attention, language, visuospatial, executive, emotional/behavioral) that are commonly evaluated in neuropsychological evaluations in rehabilitation settings. Although we focus on cognitive abilities, when appropriate we have critiqued certain tests based on their ability to measure relatively unitary cognitive constructs, or if they have demonstrated relationship to functional outcomes. However, it is acknowledged that many tests may be effectively used, depending on individual preference and training. It is our hope that this proposal can serve as a general guideline for functional evaluations, and hopefully initiate further interest in this area.

Intelligence

Although *intelligence* is vaguely defined, it is useful as an estimate of overall cognitive abilities. More functionally based evaluations should focus on global verbal and visuospatial abilities, rather than the description of individual subtests that have minimal functional utility. Determination of an individual's level of intelligence (e.g., superior vs.

borderline) can serve as a general predictor of ability to succeed in vocational and educational settings. Furthermore, IQ scores can serve as an "anchor" for estimating the degree of decline in other cognitive abilities. The Wechsler Adult Intelligence Scale–Revised (WAIS–R [Wechsler, 1981]) may be the best, or at least the most popular, measure of global intelligence, although other shorter IQ tests are gaining popularity.

Academic Abilities

For obvious reasons, it is important to evaluate specific academic abilities, including reading, reading comprehension, mathematical abilities, and written language skills. For individuals with TBI who are returning to academic settings, it is imperative to coordinate neuropsychological findings with appropriate educational interventions and programs. The Woodcock Johnson–Revised Tests of Achievement, (WJ–R [Woodcock & Mather, 1989]) may be one of the more appropriate academic measures to use, given that other commonly used tests, such as the Wide Range Achievement Test 3 (WRAT 3 [Wilkenson, 1993]), do not assess reading comprehension or written language skills.

Memory

It is important to investigate various memory abilities, rather than just cite memory scores from commonly used tests. Most often these index scores do not provide the functionally relevant information that is needed for rehabilitation. It can be argued that three basic memory functions need to be evaluated for functional purposes: registration, retention, and retrieval. In essence, does an individual have difficulties initially encoding material (registration), consolidating it into long-term memory (retention), or recalling it from memory (retrieval)? Differentiation of these specific abilities has important rehabilitation implications. Haut, Franzen, and Rogers (1992) provided recommendations regarding the adaptation of currently used tests, such as the Wechsler Memory Scale–Revised (WMS–R, [Wechsler, 1987]) for more functional purposes.

Attention

Attention deficits are frequently reported following TBI, with specific remediation strategies used to improve them (Sohlberg & Mateer, 1989). Although attention interventions are commonly utilized and have been shown to improve attention (Sohlberg & Mateer, 1989), several limitations regarding the evaluation and treatment of attention deficits must be noted. Barkley (1994) and Johnstone and Frank (1995) suggested it may not be appropriate to evaluate "attention" by objective tests. In addition, several studies (e.g., Schmidt, Trueblood, Merwin, & Durham, 1994; Shum, McFarland, & Bain, 1990) have questioned the construct validity of various attentional processes (e.g., divided, sustained, focused, etc.). These findings question which aspects of attention should be measured and whether attention measures (not attention as a construct) have valid real-world applications. Although the measurement of attention deficits is considered an integral part of cognitive rehabilitation, the need exists to be more specific in the evaluation, labeling, and treatment of specific attention processes.

Language

As previously stated, several prominent psychologists have established themselves as experts in language functioning, and are appropriate to evaluate and treat language disorders. However, individuals who follow specific INS-Division 40 guidelines do not receive training in language evaluation. Although language tests are commonly administered by psychologists, it may be most appropriate for functional language evaluations to be performed by speech pathologists. Psychologists can report relative performance on measures of picture naming, verbal fluency, and so on, but are not traditionally trained in interventions for language deficits. Furthermore, given that neuropsychology and speech pathology are both integral rehabilitation disciplines, the need exists to determine relative practice boundaries from a professional standpoint. If psychologists actively evaluate language deficits, they should ensure that they seek out and receive adequate training in this area.

Visuospatial Abilities

The term *visuospatial* is relatively nonspecific, and thus it is difficult to evaluate specific visuospatial abilities per se. As such, it may be best to evaluate relatively basic visuospatial abilities that have functional relevance, including visuospatial perception (ability to accurately perceive/ estimate visuospatial relations) and perceptual-motor skills (ability to copy/ draw). Also, as previously argued, it is most appropriate for neuropsychologists to integrate their findings with different disciplines to improve the description and prediction of functional skills (e.g., occupational evaluation of driving abilities, cooking skills, specific vocational skills, etc.).

Executive Functions

It has been argued that "executive" functions are difficult to describe and quantify, and therefore cannot be adequately evaluated in a laboratory setting (Mattson & Levin, 1990). Vocational and daily living skills are frequently too complex to predict from nonspecific tests of "executive" functions. For example, problem-solving skills are frequently reported in neuropsychological reports, with commonly used problem-solving measures, such as the Category Test, (Halstead, 1947), the Wisconsin Card Sorting Test, (Heaton, 1981), and the Tactual Performance Test (Halstead, 1947). However, each one of these tests measures different abilities, and the relationship of these tests to more functional abilities is questionable (Johnstone & Frank, 1995). As such, neuropsychological evaluations should focus on the delineation of specific unitary cognitive abilities that may be basic components of more complex executive skills. These basic executive skills may be best termed *information-processing abilities*, and may be most appropriately conceptualized to include cognitive speed, sequencing, and flexibility. Thus, inferences can be made regarding relatively simplistic cognitive abilities, including how fast a person thinks, if he or she can follow logical sequences of information, and if he or she can process more than one stream of information at a time. In addition, it may be appropriate to differentiate between general verbal versus visual information-processing abilities based on global results (i.e., memory, intelligence, etc.). These findings can then be integrated with appropriate vocational evaluations of specific job skills.

SUMMARY

Neuropsychological evaluation is a standard part of rehabilitation. However, neuropsychological services have demonstrated limited functional utility due to issues of training, origins of the field, and lack of critical examination of neuropsychology's application in rehabilitation settings. Functionally oriented evaluations that emphasize abilities rather than tests are needed, and the assessment of relatively unitary cognitive abilities rather than complex interactions of cognitive abilities is mandatory. Evaluation of these specific unitary cognitive constructs can be used to direct remediation of specific cognitive abilities (Sohlberg & Mateer, 1989; Wilson, 1987). Neuropsychologists can help guarantee the success they have enjoyed in rehabilitation by empirically demonstrating the effectiveness of standard services and working closely with other rehabilitation disciplines to reduce duplicity of services.

REFERENCES

Barkley, R. A. (1994). Can neuropsychological tests help diagnose ADD/ADHD? *ADHD Report, 2,* 1–3.

Bigler, E. D. (1991). Neuropsychological assessment, neuroimaging, and clinical neuropsychology: A synthesis. *Archives of Clinical Neuropsychology, 6,* 113–132.

Blieberg, J., & Kaplan, D. (1992). Evolution of neuropsychology using the Halstead–Reitan Neuropsychological Test Battery. In S. Hanson & D. M. Tucker (Eds.), *Physical medicine and rehabilitation: State of the art review. Neuropsychological assessment.* (pp. 415–432). Philadelphia: Hanley & Belfus, Inc.

Draft guidelines for post-doctoral training in Rehabilitation Psychology (1992). *Division 22 Newsletter, 19,* 7–13.

Erickson, R. C., & Binder, L. M. (1986). Cognitive deficts among functionally psychotic patients: A rehabilitative perspective. *Journal of Clinical and Experimental Neuropsychology, 8,* 257–274.

Frank, R. G., Gluck, J. P., & Buckelew, S. P. (1990). Rehabilitation: Psychology's greatest opportunity? *American Psychologist, 45,* 757–761.

Golden, C. J. (1981). A standardized version of Luria's neuropsychological tests: A quantitative and qualitative approach to neuropsychological assessment. In S. Filskov & T. Boll (Eds.), *Handbook of Clinical Neuropsychology.* New York: Wiley.

Halstead, W. C. (1947). *Brain and Intelligence.* Chicago: University of Chicago Press.

Hartman, D. E. (1988). Review of R. E. Tartar, D. H. Van Thiel, & K. L. Edwards, Medical neuropsychology: The impact of disease on behavior. *Archives of Clinical Neuropsychology, 3,* 299–301.

Hartman, D. E. (1991). Reply to Reitan: Unexamined premises and the evolution of clinical neuropsychology. *Archives of Clinical Neuropsychology, 6,* 147–165.

Haut, M. W., Franzen, M. D., & Rogers, M. J. C. (1992). Assessment of memory. In S. Hanson & D. M. Tucker (Eds.), *State of the art review: Physical medicine and rehabilitation. Neuropsychological assessment* (pp. 451–466). Philadelphia: Hanley and Belfus, Inc.

Heaton, R. K. (1981). *Wisconsin Card Sorting Test Manual.* Odessa, FL: Psychological Assessment Resources.

Heinrichs, W. R. (1990). Current and emergent applications of neuropsychological assessment: Problems of validity and utility. *Professional Psychology: Research and Practice, 21,* 171–176.

Johnston, M. V., Kirshblum, S., Zorowitz, R., & Shiflett, S. C. (1992). Prediction of outcomes following rehabilitation of stroke patients. *Neurorehabilitation, 2,* 72–97.

Johnstone, B., & Frank, R. G. (1995). Neuropsychological assessment in rehabilitation: Current limitations and applications. In B. Johnstone & R. G. Frank (Eds.), *Neurorehabilitation: Functional assessment in rehabilitation* (pp. 75–86). New York: Elsevier.

Kaplan, E. (1988). A process approach to neuropsychological assessment. In T. Boll and B. K. Bryant (Eds.), *Clinical neuropsychology and brain function.* (pp. 125–167). Washington, DC: American Psychological Association.

Kreutzer, J. S., Leininger, B. E., & Harris, J. A. (1990). The evolving role of neuropsychology in community integration. In J. S. Kreutzer & P. Wehman (Eds.), *Community integration following traumatic brain injury* (pp. 49–66). Baltimore: Paul H. Brookes.

Lees-Haley, P. R. (1989). Vocational neuropsychology: A rehabilitation perspective. *Journal of Private Sector Rehabilitation, 4,* 123–129.

Leung, P. (1990). Position openings in rehabilitation psychology: A ten-year survey. *Rehabilitation Psychology, 35,* 157–160.

Loring, D. W. (1991). A counterpoint to Reitan's note on the history of clinical neuropsychology. *Journal of Clinical and Experimental Neuropsychology, 6,* 167–171.

Lynch, W. J. (1990). Neuropsychological assessment. In M. Rosenthal, E. R. Griffith, M. R. Bond, & J. D. Miller (Eds.), *Rehabilitation of the adult and child with traumatic brain injury* (2nd ed., pp. 310–326). Philadelphia: F. A. Davis.

Mapou, R. L. (1988). Testing to detect brain damage: An alternative to what may no longer be useful. *Journal of Clinical and Experimental Neuropsychology, 10,* 271–278.

Mattson, A. J., & Levin, H. S. (1990). Frontal lobe dysfunction following closed head injury: A review of the literature. *Journal of Nervous and Mental Disease, 178,* 282–291.

Prigatano, G., Fordyce, D. J., Zeiner, H. K. (1986). *Neuropsychological rehabilitation after brain injury.* Baltimore: Johns Hopkins University Press.

Reitan, R. M., & Wolfson, D. (1985). *The Halstead-Reitan Neuropsychological Test Battery.* Tucson, AZ: Neuropsychology Press.

Reports of the INS-Division 40 Task Force on education accreditation, and credentialing. (1987). *The Clinical Neuropsychologist, 1,* 29–34.

Robbins, D. E. (1989). The Halstead–Reitan Neuropsychological Battery. In M. D. Franzen (Ed.), *Reliability and validity in neuropsychological assessment* (pp. 91–107). New York: Plenum.

Rosenthal, M., & Millis, S. (1992). Relating neuropsychological indicators to psychosocial outcome after traumatic brain injury. *Neurorehabilitation, 2,* 1–8.

Schmidt, M., Trueblood, W., Merwin, M., & Durham, R. L. (1994). How much do "attention" test tell us? *Archives of Clinical Neuropsychology, 9,* 383–394.

Shum, D. H. K., McFarland, K. A., & Bain, J. D. (1990). Construct validity of eight tests of attention: Comparison of normal and closed head injured samples. *The Clinical Neuropsychologist, 4,* 151–162.

Stuss, D. T. (1987). Contribution of frontal lobe injury to cognitive impairment after closed head injury: Methods of assessment and recent findings. In H. S. Levin, J. Grafman, & H. M. Eisenberg (Eds.), *Neurobehavioral recovery from head injury.* New York: Oxford University Press.

Sohlberg, M. M., & Mateer, C. A. (1989). *Introduction to cognitive rehabilitation: Theory and practice.* New York: Guilford.

Wechsler, D. (1981). *Manual for the Wechsler Adult Intelligence Scale-Revised.* New York: Psychological Corporation.

Wechsler, D. (1987). *Manual for the Wechsler Memory Scale-Revised.* New York: Psychological Corporation.

Wilkenson, G. S. (1993). WRAT 3: *Wide Range Achievement Test administration manual (3rd edition).* Wilmington, DE: Wide Range, Inc.

Wilson, B. A. (1987). *Rehabilitation of memory.* New York: Guilford.

Wilson, B. A. (1993). Ecological validity of neuropsychological assessment: Do neuropsychological indexes predict performance in everyday activities? *Applied and Preventive Psychology, 2,* 209–215.

Woodcock, R. W., & Mather, N. (1989). *Woodcock-Johnson Tests of Achievement.* Allen, TX: DLM Teaching Resources.

9

Assessment of Agitation During the Acute Phase of Recovery

John D. Corrigan

Denny-Brown (1945) first observed that the presence of excitability and restlessness in patients who had experienced closed head injuries was predictive of delayed recovery and prolonged disability, including return to work. Levin and Grossman (1978) found that agitated patients on a neurosurgery unit were more likely to experience anxiety, depression, and thought disturbance after the resolution of the agitation and upon 3-month follow-up. Reyes, Bhattacharyya, and Heller (1981) found that restless and agitated patients demonstrated poorer long-term psychological adjustment; those with marked early agitation were more likely to require later institutionalization for behavioral disturbance. Despite the consistency of these findings, systematic research on the causes, correlates, and effects of agitation has been largely lacking. Most of the published literature has focused on interventions, particularly pharmacological interventions, for managing agitation during the acute phase of recovery. To some degree, clinical and other research efforts have been limited by two factors: (a) lack of agreement as to the definition of the construct, and (b) lack of an objective means of measuring it. A brief review of the existing literature in which agitation after traumatic brain injury (TBI) has been defined, as well as differences in presumed incidence arising from differences in definitions, are provided before addressing problems in measurement.

DEFINITION OF THE CONSTRUCT

Denny-Brown (1945) never actually used the word *agitation*. He described patients as restless and excitable, as well as demonstrating emotional outbursts. He studied 200 consecutive admissions to the Boston

City Hospital immediately following head injury (ages 15–55 years, with "vagrants" and "chronic alcoholic addicts" excluded), and found that 6% was excited or restless, and another 9% demonstrated emotional outbursts. The Denny-Brown study, like most that followed, used the observations of experienced professionals to make a presence–absence determination of the existence of these behaviors.

Levin and Grossman (1978) used the word *agitation* to describe "combativeness, thrashing, truncal rocking, screaming and signs of sympathetic activation" observed in some patients during coma and later stages of the early recovery (p. 725). Their prospective sample of patients hospitalized on a neurosurgical unit following nonpenetrating TBI found that 34% exhibited agitation. Again, a presence–absence determination was made by experienced professionals.

Reyes et al. (1981) reported the first of two studies, in which the researchers made a distinction between restlessness and agitation. In this study, *restlessness* was defined as constant activity that the patient was capable of briefly inhibiting, and *agitation* was defined as constant, uninhibited movement. This distinction suggested that excessive activity was present in both instances, with qualitative differentiation based on the patient's ability to inhibit this behavior. These authors studied consecutive admissions to an acute rehabilitation unit, and found that 37% was restless and an additional 14% was agitated. *Restlessness* and *agitation* were two categories on a five-category rating of activity; the other three categories were *coma, sluggish*, and *appropriately active*. On admission to the rehabilitation unit, patients were assigned to one of the five categories based on the observation of an experienced professional. Thus, like previous studies, agitation was treated as a presence–absence determination, although, in this case, restlessness was also distinguished as present or absent.

A fourth and final study examining a prospective group of patients for the presence of agitation was that reported by Brooke, Questad, Patterson, and Bashak (1992). These authors also made a distinction between restlessness and agitation, although their definitions were considerably more complex than those used by Reyes and colleagues. *Restlessness* was defined as behavior that interferes with care, therapy, or safety; does not meet severity criteria for agitation; and is continuous. *Agitation* was defined as episodic motor or verbal behavior severe enough to be rated on the Overt Aggression Scale (Yudofsky, Silver, Jackson, Endicott, & Williams, 1986), require physical or chemical restraints, or disrupt patient care. Like Reyes and colleagues, this definition also suggested that restlessness may be a less severe form of agitation. In a prospective study of trauma center admits with at least a 1-week stay, they found 35% was restless and 11% was agitated. These results are similar to those found by Reyes and colleagues. Brooke and colleagues felt that restlessness was a significantly different phenomenon than agitation, and that, without making the distinction, agitation is overdiagnosed and treated too aggressively. Despite mention of the Overt Aggression Scale, these authors also used a presence–absence approach to their observation of the construct.

Work on agitation at The Ohio State University began in the mid-1980s, and the problems with defining the construct evident today were apparent then as well. Our work has implicitly or explicitly made the following assumptions regarding the nature of agitation. First, although component behaviors of agitation may have specific clinical and heuristic value, the key concept is an excess of behavior, regardless of its type. Excessive movement, emotional display, or orienting behavior resulting in short attention span are all manifestations of agitation. Second, restlessness is a degree of agitation, not an independent construct. Like Reyes and colleagues, for purposes of measurement we have attempted to operationalize the degree to which the excessive behavior can be inhibited. In contrast, we have used a three-way partition. We have not ascribed the term *restlessness* to the less excessive levels because we feel this would obscure the continuous nature of the actual construct. Brooke and colleagues appropriately observed that the degree of agitation needs to be taken into account in determining the aggressiveness of the intervention. However, this does not mean that restlessness is a different phenomenon than agitation. Finally, related to both assumptions, we believe aggressive behavior is an important component of agitation, but agitation is not limited to aggressive behaviors.

From these assumptions, we recently proposed the following definition of *agitation:* an excess of one or more behaviors occurring during an altered state of consciousness. This definition is consistent with our presumption that excess is the defining characteristic, rather than the component behaviors. Furthermore, by limiting the construct to excesses that occur during altered states of consciousness, we presume a neurophysiological substrate as opposed to a psychological substrate. Agitated behavior has been studied in Alzheimer's disease, psychotic patients, and persons with moderate and severe mental retardation. Whether the neurophysiological substrate is the same in each case is not known. It would appear important, as a starting point, to differentiate agitation in association with cerebral compromise from behavioral disorders occurring in the absence of the same.

MEASURING AGITATION

As the previous review revealed, the study of agitation has lacked a valid and reliable method of objective measurement. Although simple presence–absence determinations can be made reliably, the construct cannot actually be measured. Most clinical use and more in-depth research questions require the ability to make subtle distinctions in the presence of agitation. The most needed clinical use is for serial monitoring, rather than diagnosis. From a research point of view, the least studied questions concern the course of agitation. Both of these purposes would be greatly advanced by a measuring instrument. It was with this intent that the development of the Agitated Behavior Scale (ABS; Corrigan, 1989) was initiated at The Ohio State University.

Because agitation lacked definition, the initial development of the ABS gave significant emphasis to content validity. To ensure that there was no aspect of the construct ignored, item-generation procedures sought an exhaustive list of descriptors of agitation to establish the initial item pool. All available published works, whether research or clinical, were reviewed, and terms or phrases used to describe agitated behavior were extracted. Independently, an experienced, interdisciplinary group of rehabilitation professionals were asked to generate descriptors in two ways. On one occasion, they were asked to list all of the behaviors they considered to represent agitated behaviors. On another occasion, Kelly's (1955) construct *elicitation technique* was used to "tease out" any other subtleties of their individual concepts of agitation that may not have been elicited by direct request. After removal of duplications, descriptors from all three methods resulted in an initial 39-item pool, describing the component behaviors of agitation.

Because it was our view that it was not the behavior alone, but the excess of the behavior that was the key aspect of agitation, a two-dimensional rating system was developed for use in the second stage of item selection. Raters were asked to categorize each behavior along two 4-point scales: one scale denoting levels of frequency of occurrence of the behavior, the other denoting levels of severity. Over a 2-month period, registered nurses on the Traumatic Head Injury Unit at The Ohio State University rated patients 1 day each week at the end of the day shift. Nurses were asked to only rate patients they considered to be agitated. Because two nurses worked each shift, further item selection could be based on both reliability of observation and relatedness of the item to the overall construct. On completing the rating form, each nurse made two general assessments as to the degree to which the patient was agitated. Using these observations, the original 39-item pool was reduced to 14 items based on the reliability of observation, relatedness to the overall construct, minimal occurrence, and retention of unique component behaviors. The initial study also showed that some descriptors could be combined. The interested reader can refer to Corrigan (1989) for a detailed treatment of this second step in item selection. The resulting 14 items that constitute the ABS are shown in Fig. 9.1.

AGITATED BEHAVIOR SCALE

Patient _____   Period of Observation:
                                       a.m.
Observ. Environ._____   From:_____p.m._____/_____/_____
                                       a.m.
Rater/Disc._____   To:_____p.m._____/_____/_____

At the end of the observation period indicate whether the behavior described in
each item was present and, if so, to what degree: slight, moderate or extreme.
Use the following numerical values and criteria for your ratings.

   1 = **absent:** the behavior is not present.
   2 = **present to a slight degree:** the behavior is present but does not prevent
        the conduct of other, contextually appropriate behavior. (The individual
        may redirect spontaneously, or the continuation of the agitated behavior
        does not disrupt appropriate behavior.)
   3 = **present to a moderate degree:** the individual needs to be redirected from
        an agitated to an appropriate behavior, but benefits from such cueing.
   4 = **present to an extreme degree:** the individual is not able to engage in
        appropriate behavior due to the interference of the agitated behavior,
        even when external cueing or redirection is provided.

DO NOT LEAVE BLANKS.

_____   1. Short attention span, easy distractibility, inability to concentrate.
_____   2. Impulsive, impatient, low tolerance for pain or frustration.
_____   3. Uncooperative, resistant to care, demanding.
_____   4. Violent and or threatening violence toward people or property.
_____   5. Explosive and/or unpredictable anger.
_____   6. Rocking, rubbing, moaning or other self-stimulating behavior.
_____   7. Pulling at tubes, restraints, etc.
_____   8. Wandering from treatment areas.
_____   9. Restlessness, pacing, excessive movement.
_____ 10. Repetitive behaviors, motor and/or verbal.
_____ 11. Rapid, loud or excessive talking.
_____ 12. Sudden changes of mood.
_____ 13. Easily initiated or excessive crying and/or laughter.
_____ 14. Self-abusiveness, physical and/or verbal.

_____   Total Score

FIG. 9.1.   The Agitated Behavior Scale (ABS).

The initial validation study also revealed a marked distinction in the
utility of duration versus severity ratings. Uniformly, the nurses' overall
perceptions of the extent of agitation were correlated with their perceptions of the severity, rather than the duration, of the behavior. Thus, the
duration dimension was eliminated from the final 14-item scale, and the
4-point severity rating remained:

1 = absent
2 = present to a slight degree
3 = present to a moderate degree
4 = present to an extreme degree

In use of the ABS, we have further refined this dimension by describing for each level the extent to which a person is able to inhibit the behavior and/or the extent to which the inability to inhibit it is functionally limiting. These further definitions are as follows:

Slight—the behavior is present, but does not prevent the conduct of other contextually appropriate behavior. Patients may redirect themselves spontaneously, or the continuation of the agitated behavior does not preclude the conduct of the appropriate behavior.
Moderate—indicates the individual may need to be redirected from an agitated behavior to an appropriate one, but is able to benefit from such cueing.
Extreme—indicates that the individual is not able to engage in appropriate behavior due to interference by the agitated behavior, even when external cueing or redirection is provided.

Although professional staff who are not familiar with TBI may find these distinctions difficult, staff who have had even minimal exposure to agitated patients appear able to grasp these distinctions quite readily. It should be noted that this delineation of the extent of inhibition is made at the item level. As is discussed later, all people do not uniformly show the same excesses in all behaviors at all times. This observation led us to ask what behaviors appear to show related amounts of agitation; in other words, is there an underlying factor structure?

FACTOR STRUCTURE OF THE ABS

Corrigan and Bogner (1994) provided a detailed report of the systematic investigation of the ABS's factor structure. Principal components factor analysis had been conducted in the original validation study to ensure that no items eliminated represented a unique component of agitated behaviors. That analysis afforded some a priori ideas about underlying factor structure. However, subsequent clinical experience with the instrument stimulated additional hypotheses. Corrigan and Bogner (1994) used confirmatory factor analysis to test whether and which hypothesized underlying structure best fit actual data.

Four models were tested: one-factor, two-factor, three-factor, and four-factor models. The one-factor model presumed that there were no underlying factors, and that component behaviors did not relate to each other in systematic ways, except as part of the overall construct of agitation. The two-factor model was based on the factor structure observed in the validation study, and distinguished between directed and nondirected agitation. The former included behaviors that seemed to involve some intent, regardless of the cogency. The latter included behaviors that seemed to represent a heightened state of activity without an apparent purpose. The three-factor model included one factor that narrowed the concept of directed agitation to aggressive behaviors. A second factor included behaviors that seemed to be characterized by disinhibition. A third factor, lability, included excessive emotional display. Our work with patients who had brain injury marked by anoxia suggested that this third factor may have some unique importance in some subpopulations. The four-factor model was the same as the three-factor model, except that the disinhibition factor was further partitioned into behaviors that were highly repetitive and self-stimulating in nature.

Confirmatory factor analysis suggested that the three- and four-factor models fit the observed data significantly better than the one- and two-factor models. These results suggest that there was an underlying factor structure that could have some heuristic value, and that the disinhibition, aggression, and lability distinctions were the most parsimonious description of that structure. The four-factor model did not increase goodness of fit with the data, thus the three-factor model was adopted. Inspection of factor analyses that forced even more factors suggested that little was gained in increased variance. As with the four-factor model, the additional factors further partitioned the disinhibition factor.

Each of the models allowed factors to be correlated, and in each case factors were highly related. For the three-factor model, Aggression and Disinhibition shared 36% of variance ($r = .600$); Disinhibition and Lability shared 73% of variance ($r = .852$); and Aggression and Lability shared 63% of variance ($r = .793$). These high innercorrelations suggest that the factors are part of an overall construct that is largely homogeneous, but for which factors can be identified. Thus, in clinical use, the total agitation score should still be considered the most sensitive indicator of agitation. However, the use of subscale scores may provide additional information about unique characteristics of individuals or subpopulations, and/or unique effects of interventions. Subscale scores can be calculated by adding the ratings from the component items as follows:

- Disinhibition is the sum of Items 1, 2, 3, 6, 7, 8, 9, and 10;
- Aggression is the sum of Items 3, 4, 5, and 14;
- Lability is the sum of Items 11, 12, and 13.

It is not an error that Item 3 is included in both the Disinhibition and Aggression subscales; this behavior was hypothesized to be part of both.

MEASUREMENT CHARACTERISTICS OF THE ABS

Corrigan and Bogner (1995) recently published a summary of the measurement characteristics of the ABS. Its validation, and thus the majority of its use, has been with brain-injured persons in an acute phase of recovery. Tabloski, McKinnon-Howe, and Remington (1995) reported its use with nursing home residents experiencing dementia, primarily of the Alzheimer's type. Based on the validation studies, the ABS can be used by nursing staff, physical therapists, and occupational therapists. At The Ohio State University, the ABS is completed by the primary nurse at the end of each shift. Novack and Penrod (1993) reported that, in their facility, the ABS is used by the therapists at the end of each session. Again, the validation work used therapists' 30-minute observations from treatment sessions, as well as primary nurses' observations from 8-hour shifts.

Based on a prospective sample of persons with acquired brain injury during the acute phase of recovery, mean agitation scores can be expected to cluster around 21. These samples were of all patients, not just those deemed agitated. Similarly, we found that a standard deviation of approximately 7 is relatively consistent. Zielinski, Theroux-Fichera, Tremont, and Mittenberg (1994) found similar results for a prospective sample of persons with TBI admitted to a trauma service. For these patients, the mean ABS score was 18.73, and the standard deviation was 6.19. These slightly lower scores may have been due to selection bias inherent in trauma service versus rehabilitation samples. It was notable that their highest score was 37, which, in our experience, is low for a sample of rehabilitation patients.

For clinical use, we partition the total and subscale scores into levels of severity. Any score 21 or below is considered within normal limits for the population; scores from 22 to 28 (i.e., one standard deviation above the mean) imply mild agitation; scores from 29 to 35 (i.e., two standard deviations above the mean) imply moderate agitation; and scores greater than 35 are considered severe. This convention assists in graphing results, as well as discussing patient change.

The original validation studies found that all of the items included in the ABS met minimum criteria for interrater reliability. Different staff rating the same patient on the same day showed that all total score interrater correlations exceeded $r = .70$ (Corrigan, 1989). Internal consistencies using Cronbach's alpha ranged from .83 to .92 in the original validation study (Corrigan, 1989). Corrigan and Bogner (1994) found Cronbach's alphas exceeding .88 in their recent samples.

In terms of validity, the steps taken to ensure content validity were described earlier. The original validation studies (Corrigan, 1989) also

136

demonstrated concurrent validity with staff perceptions of the extent of agitation. Studies since then have provided preliminary support for construct validity, including: (a) the demonstration of predictable relationship with cognitive status (Corrigan & Mysiw, 1988), (b) differentiation from confusion and inattention (Corrigan, Mysiw, Gribble, & Chock, 1992), (c) differentiation of orthopedic and head-injured patients treated on a trauma unit (Zielinski et al., 1994), and (d) identification of an interpretable underlying factor structure (Corrigan & Bogner, 1994).

CONCLUSIONS

Agitation ". . . is often observed, usually treated, but rarely measured" (Corrigan & Bogner, 1994, p. 368). As many as one third of patients with acquired brain injuries treated in acute hospital settings are likely to experience agitation. As many as one half of those admitted to acute rehabilitation will demonstrate this behavior. When agitation is severe, as described in Rancho Level IV (Malkmus, Booth, & Kodimer, 1980), it must be treated by behavioral, environmental, or pharmacological means. The potential prognostic value of identifying agitation has been observed in every study in which the question has been asked (Denny-Brown, 1945; Levin & Grossman, 1978; Reyes et al., 1981).

Although the construct of agitation is important, advancements in understanding have been limited by both a lack of consensus regarding definition and lack of a measurement tool. This chapter described the underpinnings of one definition of agitation (i.e., excesses of behavior occurring during altered states of consciousness), as well as the development of an instrument to measure it. Regardless of whether this definition is broadly accepted, clearly researchers and clinicians must better define their use of this term. Regardless of whether the ABS is found to be a useful measurement tool, researchers and clinicians must address the reliability and validity of the measurement devices they are using. Although findings based on a broader sampling of patients from other institutions are needed to evaluate the utility of the ABS, at this juncture it appears to be both a reliable and valid measure of agitation.

REFERENCES

Brooke, M., Questad, K., Patterson, D., & Bashak, K. (1992). Agitation and restlessness after closed head injury: A prospective study of 100 consecutive admissions. *Archives of Physical Medicine and Rehabilitation, 73,* 320–323.
Corrigan, J. D. (1989). Development of a scale for assessment of agitation following traumatic brain injury. *Journal of Clinical and Experimental Neuropsychology, 11,* 261–277.

Corrigan, J. D., & Bogner, J. A. (1994). Factor structure of the Agitated Behavior Scale. *Journal of Clinical and Experimental Neuropsychology, 16*, 386–392.

Corrigan, J. D., & Bogner, J. A. (1995). Assessment of agitation following brain injury. *Neurorehabilitation, 5*, 205–210.

Corrigan, J. D., & Mysiw, W. J. (1988). Agitation following traumatic head injury: Equivocal evidence for a discrete stage of cognitive recovery. *Archives of Physical Medicine and Rehabilitation, 69*, 487–492.

Corrigan, J. D., Mysiw, W. J., Gribble, M., & Chock, S. (1992). Agitation, cognition and attention during post-traumatic amnesia. *Brain Injury, 6*, 155–160.

Denny-Brown, D. (1945). Disability arising from closed head injury. *Journal of the American Medical Association, 127*, 429–436.

Kelly, G. A. (1955). *The psychology of personal constructs* (Vol. 1). New York: Norton.

Levin, H. S., & Grossman, R. G. (1978). Behavioral sequelae of closed head injury. *Archives of Neurology, 35*, 720–727.

Malkmus, D., Booth, B. J., & Kodimer, C. (1980). *Rehabilitation of the head injured adult: Comprehensive cognitive management.* Downey, CA: Professional Staff Association of Ranchos Los Amigos Hospital, Inc.

Novack, T. A., & Penrod, L. (1993). Using the Agitated Behavior Scale to evaluate restlessness/agitation following traumatic brain injury. *Neurorehabilitation, 3*, 79–82.

Reyes, R. L., Bhattacharyya, A. K., & Heller, D. (1981). Traumatic head injury: Restlessness and agitation as prognosticators of physical and psychological improvement in patients. *Archives of Physical Medicine and Rehabilitation, 62*, 20–23.

Tabloski, P. A., McKinnon-Howe, L., & Remington, R. (1995) Effects of calming music on the level of agitation in cognitively impaired nursing home residents. *American Journal of Alzheimer's Care and Related Disorders, 10*(1), 10–15.

Yudofsky, S. C., Silver, J. M., Jackson, W., Endicott, J., & Williams, D. (1986). The Overt Aggression Scale for the objective rating of verbal and physical aggression. *American Journal of Psychiatry, 143*, 35–39.

Zielinski, R., Theroux-Fichera, S., Tremont, G., & Mittenberg, W. (1994). Normative data for the Agitated Behavior Scale. Poster presented at the 102nd Annual APA convention, Los Angeles, CA.

10

The Incidence and Impact of Substance Abuse Following Traumatic Brain Injury

John D. Corrigan

The fourth edition of the American psychiatric Association's *Diagnostic and Statistical Manual* (*DSM–IV*; American Psychiatric Association, 1994) defines *substance abuse* as ". . . a maladaptive pattern of substance use leading to clinically significant impairment or distress" (p. 182). "Clinically significant impairment or distress" is considered present when one of the following consequences of use occurs recurrently within a 12-month period: (a) failure to fulfill major obligations at home, work, or school; (b) engaging in potentially hazardous behavior (e.g., drinking and driving); (c) legal problems; or (d) social or interpersonal problems (e.g., arguments with spouse, getting in physical fights). A diagnosis of substance dependence is a more serious disorder and, when present, takes precedence over a diagnosis of substance abuse. Substance abuse and substance dependence are substance-use disorders; intoxication is a substance-induced disorder. In brain-injury rehabilitation, considerable attention has been given to the relationship between intoxication and traumatic brain injury (TBI). However, substance abuse and substance dependence have not been adequately addressed in this population. In this chapter, a brief overview of recent studies examining both intoxication and substance abuse as they effect outcomes from TBI is provided. This discussion is followed by a brief review of what is known about use and abuse in patients undergoing rehabilitation after brain injury. The chapter concludes with a discussion of the implications for brain-injury rehabilitation. For convenience, the term *substance abuse* is used to refer to all substance-use disorders (i.e., abuse and dependence).

EFFECTS ON OUTCOME

Corrigan (1995) recently reviewed North American studies in which the presence or mediating effects of either intoxication or a history of substance abuse were examined in adolescents and adults who had experienced TBI. Extrapolation from these studies suggests that between one third and one half of adolescents and adults who incur TBI will be intoxicated at the time of their injury. The additional proportion who are intoxicated by other drug use is not known. Those intoxicated will tend to be younger, male, and more likely to have been injured in a moving vehicle accident or an assault. Those intoxicated at time of injury will also be more likely to have a history of substance abuse preceding the injury. This latter relationship makes it difficult to distinguish between the mediating effects of intoxication versus those arising from a history of substance abuse. Studies that have examined the co-occurrence of intoxication and substance abuse have found very high rates (Brooks et al., 1989; Ruff et al., 1990; Sparadeo & Gill, 1989). For example, Brooks and colleagues found that 80% of subjects identified as alcoholic were reported to have been intoxicated at time of injury, and 100% had at least some alcohol present in their bodies. Sparadeo and Gill found that 95% of their subjects with a history of alcohol abuse had positive blood alcohol levels (although they were not necessarily intoxicated).

With these apparently high rates of co-occurrence, studies that seek to examine the effect of either intoxication or substance abuse, without accounting for the mediating effect of the other, risk overestimating the extent of the relationship. Only one study of a sample of persons with TBI accounted for both variables—the Ruff et al. examination of the effects on outcome based on the National Traumatic Coma Data Bank. These researchers found that a history of excessive alcohol use (the highest use category in their method) significantly increased the likelihood of mortality and mass lesions, and significantly decreased the likelihood of a "good" Glasgow Outcome Scale (GOS) rating at discharge. When the effects of a history of abuse were accounted for, there was no independent relationship between intoxication and either mortality or morbidity. Jurkovich et al. (1993) found remarkably similar findings based on a large, prospective study of trauma center admissions, although the proportion of their sample who had incurred TBI was not reported.

Few studies have provided insight into the effects of substance abuse on long-term recovery from brain injury. Dikmen, Donovan, Loberg, Machamer, & Temkin, (1993) performed neuropsychological assessments on a prospective sample of trauma center admissions, 1 month and 1 year following TBI. Their subjects represented the full range of brain-injury severity. Results were compared with friend and family controls who were assessed at the same intervals. Dikmen and colleagues found that substance abusers were more likely to be male and have a lower education. Those with more severe histories of abuse had lower incomes and were more likely to have preexisting psychiatric conditions. They found main effects for both TBI and substance abuse on neuropsychological performance, but no interaction. The effect of substance abuse was less when age, education, and gender differences were taken into account. They further concluded that the effect could be attributed to subjects who appeared to have more chronic histories of abuse.

Dunlop et al. (1991) conducted an archival study from Social Security disability files of persons who experienced TBI and showed deterioration in neurobehavioral functioning 6 months to 1 year following injury. From 193 files of persons with TBI, 34 such cases of deterioration were identified. These 34 cases were then matched with 34 cases of individuals with TBI who showed the same level of functioning at 6 months postinjury. Those who deteriorated were twice as likely to have a history of alcohol abuse than those who did not. This study was not able to identify causal factors, although resumption of use would appear to be one viable working hypothesis.

Corrigan's (1995) review included studies of samples drawn from rehabilitation settings. These findings suggest that almost two thirds of persons treated in brain-injury rehabilitation programs will have a history of alcohol or other drug use that is abusive at least. Those with histories will be: (a) more likely to be males over the age of 30, (b) have had less education, (c) have a lower socioeconomic status (SES), and (d) have been intoxicated at time of injury. Individuals with histories of abuse will be approximately twice as likely to have had other TBIs than the one precipitating current treatment. This group will have greater functional limitations by virtue of their substance use, their most recent brain injury, or previous brain injuries. However, it would be risky to presume that substance abuse is less prevalent in younger persons who experience TBI. The methods of detection used in most studies more easily identify individuals who have been abusing substances over a longer period of time and have accumulated more substance-abusing "events" (e.g., previous injuries, moving vehicle violations, family or work consequences). Late adolescents and adults in their early 20s may have similar patterns of use, but have not had the time to accumulate these more visible indications of a history of abuse.

Taken together, these results suggest that practitioners of brain-injury rehabilitation need to be cognizant of substance abuse in the population they treat. Although there are only a minimum number of studies avail-

able, the existing literature suggests that it may be conservative to estimate that two thirds of adolescents and adults in brain-injury rehabilitation programs can be diagnosed as substance abusing. Those with a
history will be vulnerable to poorer outcomes for a variety of reasons.
Among a group with more chronic histories of abuse, level of functioning is likely to be lower prior to injury and, presumably, after as well.
The presence of a history of abuse, if not intoxication, may interact with
the brain injury to increase the resulting impairment. Persons with a
history of abuse, particularly those who are more chronic abusers, may
have fewer resources, including social supports, for facilitating their
continued recovery following discharge from inpatient rehabilitation.
Finally, it would be reasonable to expect that those who resume use will
experience less recovery, if not deteriorate. In the next section, the nature and extent of substance use is described in persons who are attempting community integration following brain injury.

PATTERNS OF USE

Kreutzer and colleagues at the Medical College of Virginia published
some of the first research findings regarding the scope of the problem of
substance abuse in rehabilitation populations. Kreutzer, Doherty, Harris, and Zasler, (1990) described alcohol use among adolescents and
adults evaluated in an outpatient medical rehabilitation clinic. The average age of their sample exceeded 31 years, and the sample averaged
approximately 4 years postinjury. Based on responses to the General
Health and History Questionnaire (Kreutzer, Leininger, Doherty, &
Waaland, 1987), approximately 25% of the sample indicated they did not
consume alcohol prior to their injury, whereas 72% indicated they ab-
stained subsequent to their injury. Approximately 12% indicated they
had a drinking problem prior to their injury, whereas 8% indicated they
had such a problem after. From the Quantity–Frequency–Variability Index (QFVI; Cahalan & Cisin, 1968), 58% of respondents were classified
as moderate or heavy drinkers prior to injury, whereas 20% reported this
extent of consumption after. Results from the brief Michigan Alcohol
Screening Test (Brief MAST; Pokorney, Miller, & Kaplan, 1972) indicate
approximately 14% of the sample could be classified as problem drinkers. These authors concluded that this population's preinjury consumption of alcohol was significantly higher than same-age peers. However,
their postinjury consumption was consistent with the consumption of
peers. They estimated that between 8% and 14% could be classified as
having a substance-abuse problem related to alcohol, and that approximately 20% were moderate- or high-volume drinkers.

Kreutzer, Wehman, Harris, Burns, and Young (1991) described the patterns of alcohol and other drug use among a sample of adults with TBI referred to a supported employment program. The average age of this sample was 31 years, and they averaged more than 6 years postinjury. Approximately two thirds of this group were moderate or heavy drinkers preinjury, based on responses to the QFVI (in most cases, completed by a significant other). Postinjury, 28% were moderate or heavy consumers of alcohol, and 23% were classified as problem drinkers based on Brief MAST scores. In this study, the use of other drugs was assessed, indicating that 36% used illicit drugs prior to injury and 4% did so after. Marijuana was the most frequent other drug used, followed by cocaine. Again, this study revealed that this sample of persons with TBI tended to have higher levels of substance use prior to injury when compared with same-age peers but lower levels after. This study also found that there were higher levels of criminal arrests among individuals who reported alcohol or other drug use.

Corrigan, Rust, and Lamb-Hart (1995) recently described the nature and extent of substance abuse among persons with TBI referred to a program for treatment of substance abuse after brain injury. Not surprisingly, between 80% and 95%, depending on the screening instrument, had substance-abuse problems. Sixty percent of this sample had incurred injuries that were substance-abuse related. Moving vehicle accidents, assaults, and falls were all disproportionately substance-use related. The demographic characteristics of their sample were not significantly different from the general population of persons with TBI, specifically those followed in the TBI Model Systems database (Gordon, Mann, & Willer, 1993). Corrigan and colleagues found alcohol was the preferred drug for 83% of their sample, and almost three quarters of those who preferred alcohol indicated that beer was their drink of choice. For the entire sample, 98% reported some alcohol use. Marijuana was the secondary drug of choice, with 54% of respondents indicating use of this substance. For the entire sample, 17% reported cocaine use, whereas another 9% reported crack use.

Corrigan, Rust, and Lamb-Hart (1995) found that alcohol was the overwhelming drug of choice, followed by marijuana—an observation also made by Kreutzer et al. (1991). However, Corrigan and colleagues cautioned that the pattern of preferred drug use may be different in samples drawn predominantly from urban populations. Like Kreutzer and colleagues, Corrigan et al. (1995) used the QFVI to measure the extent of alcohol consumption. Similar to Kreutzer and colleagues' findings, prior to injury their sample consumed significantly more alcohol than same-age peers, and approximately comparable amounts after. Corrigan and colleagues questioned whether it is acceptable that consumption equaled that of peers, given that 42% of males ages 21–29 are medium- and high-volume alcohol users. Given the likely interaction between alcohol use and recovery of function and community integration, the advisability of drinking the same as peers would appear questionable.

Corrigan et al. (1995) observed two additional alarming findings regarding patterns of use. First, approximately 20% of persons in their sample who were abstainers or light drinkers preinjury became high-volume users after injury. Another 36% who were low-volume users became medium- or high-volume users after injury. These data suggest that the problems of substance abuse after injury may not be restricted to those with a prior history. These authors also found that the amount of consumption increased as time postinjury increased. Their sample was an average of 3.5 years postinjury. Among individuals less than 2 years postinjury, just over 25% consumed medium and high volumes of alcohol. For those 2–6 years postinjury, this percentage increased to 40%, reaching 50% for those more than 6 years postinjury.

Similar to the Kreutzer et al. (1991) observation that criminal arrests appeared related to substance use, Corrigan et al. (1995) found that half of those more than 2 years postinjury had at least one arrest, and that 32 arrests had occurred among 21 clients who were at least this far postinjury. The study also detailed other ways in which this population presented significant costs to society. A high percentage of accidents were substance-use related, including three quarters of the accidents incurred by individuals who were medium- and high-volume users. The sample showed high use of medical services, including an average of .5 hospital admissions per year for those more than 12 months postinjury. The same group averaged .5 emergency room visits per year. Whereas 90% of the group was working or in school prior to injury, only 36% were so engaged at time of referral. Forty-one percent had their primary income from government supports, and another 22% relied on family or relatives for their primary source of income. Brain-injury rehabilitation professionals have long been aware of the significant cost to society of those individuals who must be sustained in nursing homes or other long-term-care facilities. However, these data indicate that there can be significant costs to society among those living in the community as well.

IMPLICATIONS FOR REHABILITATION

Given the current emphasis on outcomes to justify health care expenditures, it seems risky in brain-injury rehabilitation to ignore the problems of substance abuse. The majority of our clients had or could have diagnosable substance-use disorders. With the potential for substance abuse to limit the positive outcomes of rehabilitation, it would seem prudent for rehabilitation professionals to more aggressively address this problem. It is likely that awareness of substance-abuse problems among rehabilitation professionals is significantly better today than it was in 1988, when the National Head Injury Foundation (NHIF) Task Force on Substance Abuse published their white paper. However, personal observations suggest that rehabilitation professionals are not comfortable with the issues of substance abuse, and are not sure what they should be doing about it.

Langley, Lindsay, Lam, and Priddy (1990) proposed a scheme for level of intervention during brain-injury rehabilitation based on clients' relative risks. Corrigan (1995) made similar recommendations, including proposing that it is reasonable to expect that every individual admitted for acute brain-injury rehabilitation is at least at risk for substance-abuse problems. Therefore, both patient and family education should include systematic attempts to describe how alcohol and other drug use could affect recovery from TBI. The Ohio Valley Center for Head Injury Prevention and Rehabilitation (1994) published *A User's Manual for Faster More Reliable Operation of a Brain after Head Injury*. It presents eight issues that individuals and their families should consider when making choices about their substance use following brain injury. Presentation of similar information in discussion settings with families and patients would appear to be a minimal step toward secondary prevention. Supporting this effort should be institutional policies prohibiting use during acute rehabilitation, as well as systematic education of staff so that they (a) are comfortable with discussion of the subject with their patients, and (b) reinforce positive choices that their patients may be considering.

A second level of intervention should be to identify and provide additional treatment to those individuals who have a substance-abuse history. As a prerequisite, every brain-injury rehabilitation team should have the expertise within it to conduct sensitive substance-abuse assessments with both families and patients. *Sensitive* is used here to mean both the ability to detect and the skill to do it collaboratively with the patient and family. Although research methods have used paper-and-pencil screening devices, at this juncture there appears to be no substitute for well-informed professionals, attuned to the nuances and stigma of substance abuse, conducting an interview with the patient and significant others. The basis for recommending screening interviews instead of screening instruments is beyond the scope of this chapter. However, substance abuse is often marked by the individual's and, in some cases, the family's minimization of consequences. Furthermore, it is not difficult to understand why individuals and families may be reluctant to volunteer negative information during acute rehabilitation, when their primary goal is to enlist the maximum assistance available from the brain-injury rehabilitation team. A sensitive method of substance-abuse detection allows the provision of additional education and support to patients and families during the acute stay, which in turn serves to increase the probability of making a successful referral for ongoing intervention following discharge. Clearly, issues as complex as substance abuse will not be resolved during inpatient rehabilitation. However, added attention and discussion of this issue and its relationship to recovery will increase the success of subsequent referrals.

Following inpatient rehabilitation, there must be better capability for initiating and sustaining treatment, particularly for brain-injured persons who have cognitive and/or physical impairments that make them unusual cases in existing substance-abuse treatment programs. Corrigan, Lamb-Hart, and Rust (1995) described a program of intervention for substance abuse following brain injury. It uses a resource and service coordination model to make linkages with existing substance-abuse providers, and sustains those linkages over the prolonged course of community integration. This model of treatment is relatively inexpensive, can be made available in rural and urban communities, and could be an important adjunct to outpatient rehabilitation services. The model was developed as an alternative to specialized, residential programs for persons with substance abuse and TBI. Although it would be premature to assert that a specialized, facility-based program is never needed, the 5-year history of this project suggests that existing substance-abuse facilities and programs can be assisted to adapt their services to meet the needs of this population. Indeed, substance-abuse facilities are already treating a surprisingly high proportion of individuals who have experienced brain injuries, although these individuals often have poorer outcomes and are a source of staff frustration. The project at The Ohio State University uses a case consultation model to: (a) assist substance-abuse program staff to understand individuals' unique strengths and weaknesses, (b) adapt services and treatment plans to individuals' abilities, (c) troubleshoot problems as they arise, and (d) assist in "wrapping around" other resources and services that individuals require to stabilize their health, financial, social, and vocational status. Preliminary outcome data from this program indicate that alcohol and other drug use reduction is at least as successful as substance-abuse programs in general. Similarly, return-to-work rates are equivalent to those for a general population of persons with disability.

Although few brain-injury rehabilitation programs have the three tiers of addressing substance abuse described earlier, widespread implementation of such programming would be a significant step in addressing this important problem among persons with TBI. Our clients who have or will abuse alcohol or other drugs cannot afford to ignore the additional consequences that a recent brain injury introduces. As a field, we cannot afford to have the effectiveness of rehabilitation efforts underestimated because of the mediating effects on outcome of substance-use disorders.

ACKNOWLEDGMENT

Preparation of this chapter was supported, in part, by Grant H235L20001 from the U.S. Department of Education, Rehabilitation Services Administration, to the Ohio Valley Center for Head Injury Prevention and Rehabilitation.

REFERENCES

American Psychiatric Association. (1994). *Diagnostic and Statistical Manual IV*. Washington, DC: American Psychiatric Association.

Brooks, N., Symington, C., Beattie, A., Campsie, L., Bryden, J., & McKinlay, W. (1989). Alcohol and other predictors of cognitive recovery after severe head injury. *Brain Injury, 3*(3), 235–246.

Cahalan, D., & Cisin, I. H. (1968). American drinking practices: Summary of findings from a national probability sample: I. Extent of drinking by population subgroup. *Quarterly Journal of Studies on Alcohol, 29*, 130–151.

Corrigan, J. D. (1995). Substance abuse as a mediating factor in outcome from traumatic brain injury. *Archives of Physical Medicine and Rehabilitation, 76*, 302–309.

Corrigan, J. D., Lamb-Hart, G. L., Rust, E. (1995). A program of intervention for substance abuse following traumatic brain injury. *Brain Injury, 9*, 221–236.

Corrigan, J. D., Rust, E., Lamb-Hart, G. L. (1995). The nature and extent of substance abuse problems among persons with traumatic brain injuries. *Journal of Head Trauma Rehabilitation, 10*(3), 29–45.

Dikmen, S. S., Donovan, D. M., Loberg, T., Machamer, J. E., & Temkin, N. R. (1993). Alcohol use and its effects on neuropsychological outcome in head injury. *Neuropsychology, 7*(3), 296–305.

Dunlop, T. W., Udvarhelyi, G. B., Stedem, A. F., O'Connor, J. M., Isaacs, M. L., Puig, J. G., & Mather, J. H. (1991). Comparison of patients with and without emotional/behavioral deterioration during the first year after traumatic brain injury. *Journal of Neuropsychiatry and Clinical Neurosciences, 3*, 150–156.

Gordon, W. A., Mann, N., & Willer, B. (1993). Demographic and social characteristics of the traumatic brain injury model system database. *Journal of Head Trauma Rehabilitation, 8,*(2), 26–33.

Jurkovich, G. J., Rivara, F. P., Gurney, J. G., Fligner, C., Riles, R., Mueller, B. A., & Copass, M. (1993). The effect of acute alcohol intoxication and chronic alcohol abuse on outcome from trauma. *Journal of the American Medical Association, 270*(1), 51–56.

Kreutzer, J. S., Doherty, K. R., Harris, J. A., & Zasler, N. D. (1990). Alcohol use among persons with traumatic brain injury. *Journal of Head Trauma Rehabilitation, 5*(3), 9–20.

Kreutzer, J. S., Leininger, B., Doherty, K., & Waaland, P. (1987). *The General Health and History Questionnaire*. Richmond, VA: Rehabilitation Research and Training Center on Severe Traumatic Brain Injury, Medical College of Virginia.

Kreutzer, J. S., Wehman, P. H., Harris, J. A., Burns, C. T., & Young, H. F. (1991). Substance abuse and crime patterns among persons with traumatic brain injury referred for supported employment. *Brain Injury, 5*(2), 177–187.

Langley, M. J., Lindsay, W. P., Lam, C. S., & Priddy, D. A. (1990). A comprehensive alcohol abuse treatment programme for persons with traumatic brain injury. *Brain Injury, 4*(1), 77–86.

National Head Injury Foundation. (1988). *Substance Abuse Task Force: White Paper*. Southborough, MA: Author.

Ohio Valley Center for Head Injury Prevention and Rehabilitation. (1994). *A user's manual for faster more reliable operation of a brain after head injury*. Columbus, OH: Author.

Pokorney, A. D., Miller, B. A., & Kaplan, H. B. (1972). The Brief MAST: A shortened version of the Michigan Alcoholism Screening Test. *American Journal of Psychiatry, 129*, 342–345.

Ruff, R. M., Marshall, L. F., Klauber, M. R., Blunt, B. A., Grant, I., Foulkes, M. A., Eisenberg, H., Jane, J., & Marmarou, A. (1990). Alcohol abuse and neurological outcome of the severely head injured. *Journal of Head Trauma Rehabilitation, 5*(3), 21–31.

Sparadeo, F. R., & Gill, D. (1989). Effects of prior alcohol use on head injury recovery. *Journal of Head Trauma Rehabilitation, 4*(1), 75–82.

11

Florid Confabulation Following Brain Injury

Zvi Kalisky
B. P. Uzzell

Confabulation, according to Berlyne (1972), is a falsification of memory occurring in clear consciousness in association with an organically derived amnesia. The neuropsychological mechanism of confabulation is not known. Factors such as suggestibility (Pick, 1905; cited in Berlyne, 1972), improper sense of chronological order (Van der Horst, 1932; cited in Berlyne, 1972), vivid daydreaming and difficulty distinguishing fantasy from reality (Whitty & Lewin, 1957), filling amnestic gaps (Barbizet, 1963), and abnormal psychological reaction (Weinstein & Lyerly, 1968) have been implicated in the production of confabulations.

It has been suggested that there are two types of confabulation: (a) florid, fantastic, or spontaneous, unprovoked fabrications, sometimes elaborate and bizarre; or (b) momentary or provoked, filling in of memory gaps (Berlyne, 1972; Kapur & Coughlan, 1980; Kopelman, 1987). Several investigators have pointed to a strong association between confabulation and frontal lobe dysfunction (DeLuca & Cicerone 1991; Kapur & Coughlan, 1980; Luria, 1980; Stuss, Alexander, Lieberman, & Levine, 1978). Confabulation was found to be strongly related to an inability to withhold answers, monitor responses, and provide verbal self-regulation (Mercer, Wapner, Gardner, & Benson, 1977), all of which are characteristic of frontal lobe dysfunction. It has been hypothesized that spontaneous confabulation is related to a greater degree of frontal dysfunction than is momentary confabulation (Kapur & Coughlan, 1980; Kopelman, 1987). However, this hypothesis does not explain satisfactorily the large variation in content and form of florid confabulation—specifically, why some patients show delusional elements in their confabulations and others do not. The fact that confabulation is often associated with reduplicative and misidentification syndromes was noted by Weinstein and Lyerly (1968).

Indeed, a close look at described case reports reveals that, in addition to an intrusional component consisting of an unchecked flow of thoughts, memories, and fantasies, a delusional element was frequently present. This included grandiose ideas (Berlyne, 1972; Damasio, Graff-Radford, Eslinger, Damasio, & Kassell, 1985), misidentification delusion of persons (Capgras' syndrome; Alexander, Stuss, & Benson, 1979), misidentification delusion of places (reduplicative paramnesia; Benson, Gardner, & Meadows, 1976; Ruff & Volpe, 1981), and dreamy state with false sense of familiarity (déjà vu; Staton, Brumback, & Wilson, 1982).

Because organic delusions and dreamy states have frequently been associated with temporal lobe disease (Freeman, 1980), it appears natural to question whether temporal lobes play a role in the production of confabulation. To answer this question, a retrospective study of five patients with florid confabulation was undertaken.

METHODS

Four patients with traumatic brain injury (TBI) and, for comparison, one patient with anterior communicating artery aneurysm (who exhibited highly florid and bizarre confabulation) were chosen for a retrospective study from 350 neurological patients consecutively admitted to Del Oro Institute for Rehabilitation in the years 1990–1994. Patients with histories of dementia or active psychiatric illness were excluded. The history; content of the confabulation; and findings in the computed tomography (CT) scan, magnetic resonance imaging (MRI), or single photon emission computed tomography (SPECT) were reviewed. The case of anterior communicating artery aneurysm was included because of the striking similarity of the neurobehavioral manifestations to head injury, and the relatively defined anatomical involvement seen in this type of lesion (Damasio et al., 1985).

RESULTS

The five patients selected for the study were males, aged 24–60. In addition to florid confabulation, all exhibited profound anterograde amnesia, varying degree of disinhibited behavior, and poor insight into their deficits. The following are summaries of the case reports.

Case 1

A 34-year-old male sustained depressed right frontal skull fracture and right eye injury secondary to a pipe explosion. He underwent elevation of the skull fracture and right eye enucleation. He was transferred to the rehabilitation unit about 1 week after the injury. On admission, he was disoriented to time and place and only partially oriented to person. He showed severe impairment of recent memory, as well as some retrograde amnesia. Initial hospital course was marked by uncooperative behavior, denial of deficits, and confabulation. The patient stated that he was pregnant and carrying the child for his wife, who had not been able to become pregnant because of complications. He also stated that he had undergone Caesarean section in the past. (His wife reported to have a previous difficult pregnancy and labor.) He also stated that he was a retired Air Force pilot who flew combat missions during the Gulf War. He described in detail the instrument and technique of flying, which he later admitted to have learned from flight simulator games. Several episodes occurred when he looked outside and insisted that the scenery viewed represented his hometown in Michigan, not in Houston. He exhibited confabulation, at times elaborate, in response to questions about activities on the rehabilitation unit, or when asked to repeat a story. Neuropsychological testing revealed severe memory deficits, disorientation, agitation, expressive language deficit, poor planning, poor insight, and decreased initiation. An MRI of the brain showed a large area of gliosis or encephalomalacia in the right frontal region and a smaller lesion in the left frontal lobe (see fig. 11.1). A SPECT study revealed significant decrease in activity in the anterior and orbital frontal regions, with milder decreased activity in the right superior temporal and parietal regions.

The patient showed steady cognitive recovery, and the confabulation disappeared within about 6 weeks. He was discharged to the outpatient clinic, completed the program successfully, and returned to a modified job situation. About 2 months after discharge from the program, he experienced a brief episode of visual hallucinations and leg weakness. Two months later, he was admitted after a grand mal seizure. Electroencephalography (EEG) showed focal slowing in the right frontal temporal region. Subsequently, seizures have been well controlled with carbamazepine. He has ultimately shown an excellent recovery.

Case 2

A 24-year-old male who suffered head injury when his 18-wheeler truck collided with a parked vehicle was admitted to an acute hospital unconscious, responding to pain only. A CT scan of his brain revealed bitemporal hemorrhagic contusions and cerebral edema. An intracranial pressure monitor was inserted, and he was treated medically. He improved steadily, regaining consciousness and gradually talking and walking. However, he remained confused, disoriented, and restless, and wandered in the halls. He was transferred to the rehabilitation unit 3 weeks

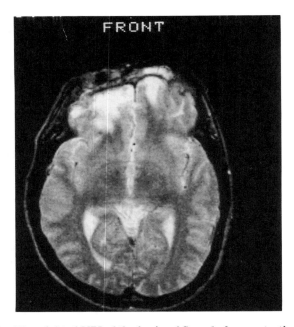

FIG. 11.1.   T2-weighted MRI of the brain of Case 1, demonstrating extensive bifrontal gliosis and encephalomalacia, with an accompanying depressed frontal bone fracture.

after injury. On admission, he was found to be disoriented, with paraphasia, hyperfluency, and confabulation. He had severe anterograde amnesia; was restless, disinhibited, and at times agitated; and in complete denial of deficits. When questioned about the accident, he stated that he was driving a truck carrying a tank for an embarkation port for Desert Shield Operation, and that the truck collided with another vehicle carrying a howitzer gun. He boasted constantly about his military career, stating that he was a commando expert in U.S. Special Forces, and had participated in numerous secret missions behind enemy lines. (Actually he had been involved in maintaining electronic equipment during military service.) He soon insisted that the hospital was a secret installation of the U.S. Special Forces disguised as a hospital to conceal its true identity. He also became suspicious of his wife, claiming that she had an affair with another man. Neuropsychological testing revealed disorientation and the presence of retrograde amnesia, poor insight, decreased cognitive flexibility, perseverations of thoughts, and poor problem solving. An MRI of the brain showed small bilateral frontal subdural hygromas.

The patient was discharged 2 months after admission to the outpatient clinic. His confabulation diminished, but he continued to exhibit disinhibited behavior and agitation. Paranoid ideation regarding his wife intensified, and he was transferred to a neurobehavioral unit. He eventually showed good recovery and resumed work as a truck driver.

Case 3

A 31-year-old male, a Vietnam veteran with history of war injury, was struck in the right temporal region by a rock thrown from a lawn mower. He had a 5-minute loss of consciousness, a right temporal depressed skull fracture, blood in both external ear canals, and right periorbital ecchymosis. Initially he was lethargic and verbalized inappropriately, but was able to move all extremities. A skull x-ray showed significant depression of the right temporal squamous bone; a CT scan showed significant depression of the right temporal bone, with right to left shift and right temporal lobe edema. He underwent elevation of the depressed skull fracture and repair of two dural tears. Contamination of the brain with the patient's hair was noted during surgery. Postoperatively, he initially was unable to verbalize and had weakness on the left side. Postoperative CT scan showed white matter edema involving the right temporal lobe and frontal regions and shift of midline structures. He was confused and stated that the hospital was not in the United States, but in Vietnam, and that it was wartime. He insisted on sleeping under the bed in his hospital room at night, stating that it was perfectly acceptable because of the threat of enemy attack during war. He later changed the location of the hospital, insisting that it was the Walter Reed Hospital in Washington, DC. He also insisted that he could not sleep at night because his roommate was talking, although he did not have a roommate. Neuropsychological testing 18 days postinjury revealed both general and verbal abilities in the average range. Performance abilities were in the borderline range. These values were below the level of a lawyer (patient's occupation). A second neuropsychological evaluation 50 days postinjury showed both general and verbal abilities in the high average range. Performance abilities were in the average range. A third neuropsychological evaluation 2½ years later showed general and verbal abilities in the superior range and performance abilities in the high average range.

Case 3 had a grand mal seizure 15 months postinjury, as well as a Jacksonian seizure. By this time he had returned to his law practice full time, and denied any difficulties. However, his wife reported personality changes, lack of assertiveness, and marital problems, for which the patient was undergoing counseling.

Case 4

A 34-year-old male suffered severe closed head injury as a result of a high-speed motor vehicle accident. His initial Glasgow Coma Scale score was eight, and a CT scan of the brain revealed diffuse swelling. He underwent ventriculostomy and remained in coma for 6 days. An MRI revealed bifrontal hygromas and posterior subdural hematoma. He was transferred to the rehabilitation unit about a month after the injury, and was severely confused, restless, impulsive, and, at times, agitated. He had severe anterograde amnesia and profuse confabulation. He stated he was injured in a plane crash, which he described at length. He stated he was at work (or sometimes in school), describing in detail imaginary trips, business meetings, and dinners with customers. He became irate and defensive when confronted with the implausibility of his stories, insisting that they actually happened. Florid confabulation was also noted during story repetition. The confabulation subsided gradually over the next 2 months, and he showed overall cognitive improvement. Spontaneous confabulation disappeared when he came out of the post-traumatic amnesia but provoked confabulation persisted for a while longer. Neuropsychological testing performed about 2 months postinjury revealed disorientation to time and severe deficits in rote learning and executive functioning. Intelligence was in the average range. A follow-up CT scan of the brain revealed residual bifrontal subdural hygroma. The patient eventually showed good recovery, and returned to his former job as a salesman.

Case 5

A 60-year-old male, an art dealer, was admitted to the hospital with acute headache and confusion. A CT scan of the brain revealed hematoma in the low medial left frontal lobe, and angiography showed anterior communicating artery aneurysm requiring a craniotomy and clipping. He subsequently developed hydrocephalus, and a right ventriculoperitoneal shunt was surgically inserted. He was transferred to the rehabilitation unit about 1 month after the acute onset. On admission, he was found to be confused and disoriented in all spheres. He was restless and irritable, and showed no insight into deficits or concern regarding personal appearance. He had severe anterograde and retrograde amnesia spanning approximately 7 years. He exhibited highly florid and, at times, bizarre confabulation about autobiographical or semantic information. For example, when asked about his job, he stated that his responsibilities included negotiating with foreign governments to buy their national treasures. He cited the governments of Egypt, France, Greece, and Cyprus as his negotiating partners. He insisted that one of his therapists and several of his friends were not real persons, but impostors. On several occasions, he reported an unusual sense of familiarity with certain parts of the hospital, as if he had lived there all his life. He stated that at times he felt that he was living in a dream. He frequently misidentified the rehabilitation unit as a psychiatric unit in another state, in which he had actually been hospitalized 30 years previous for treatment of depression. He also misidentified the hospital cafeteria as a dining room of a club in another state, where he had been a member. He claimed that a certain building near the hospital was being used for sinister purposes. He later admitted that his interpretation of the building was due to a spy movie seen some 40 years ago, which flashed back whenever he looked at the building. This memory was highly vivid and real. Neuropsychological testing revealed severe impairment of auditory and visual memory, rote learning psychomotor speed, and auditory processing speed. Response style was marked by perseveration, confabulation, and disinhibition. His verbal intelligence was in the superior range and performance ability in the average range. A CT scan of the brain revealed an area of gliosis in the left medial frontal lobe (see Fig. 11.2A). A SPECT study revealed large areas of decrease in tracer activity in the right orbitofrontal region and in the right anterior temporal lobe (see Fig. 11.2B). Mild decrease in activity was noted in the left parietal lobe. Steady improvement in memory and behavior occurred. Follow-up about 5 months after the onset showed that confabulation had diminished, but had not disappeared completely.

DISCUSSION

The findings of severe amnesia and significant frontal lobe dysfunction in all patients are in agreement with the current notion held by many researchers—that the two crucial factors involved in confabulation are amnesia and frontal lobe damage (DeLuca & Cicerone, 1991; Kapur & Coughlan, 1980; Stuss et al., 1978). All five patients exhibited a marked intrusional component in their confabulation. However, a delusional element was present in the four patients who had temporal lobe lesions, in addition to the frontal involvement (Case 1, right superior temporal-parietal region; Case 2, both temporal lobes; Case 3, right temporal region; Case 5, large lesion involving the right anterior temporal lobe). These findings are compatible with other studies showing association between various types of delusions and temporal lobe disease. Highly bizarre somatic delusions were present in Case 1, and episodes of déjà vu and feeling of living in a dream were seen in Case 5. Both of these manifestations are known to be part of dreamy states of temporal lope

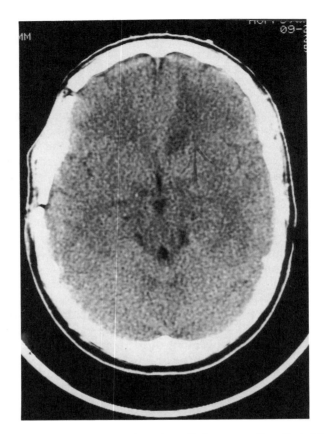

FIG. 11.2A.   CT scan of the brain of Case 5, demonstrating diminished density in the left medial frontal white matter, consistent with cerebral infarction.

epilepsy (Bancaud, Brunet-Bourgin, Chauvel, & Halgren, 1994; Mullan & Penfield, 1959; Penfield, 1955). Grandiose delusions were observed in Cases 1 and 2. Organic mania with grandiose behavior has been associated with left and right temporal lobe lesion (Cohen & Niska, 1980; Jampala & Abrams, 1983; Rosenbaum & Barry, 1975). Reduplicative paramnesia was seen in Cases 1 and 5, who had, in addition to right temporal lesions, right and left small parietal changes, respectively. Reduplicative paramnesia has been reported to be associated with abnormalities of various cerebral areas in the right hemisphere (Benson et al., 1976; Kapur, Turner, & King, 1988; Ruff & Volpe, 1981; Staton, Brumback, & Wilson, 1982). Case 5 exhibited Capgras' syndrome, believing that certain persons were not themselves but their impostors. Capgras' syndrome, although occurring primarily in the context of functional psychoses, has been reported to be associated with temporal lobe abnormalities (Christodoulou, 1977; Lewis, 1987).

Case 5, who had bleeding from an anterior communicating artery aneurysm, had more extensive delusional findings in comparison with the head-injured patients. These manifestations included Capgras' syndrome, déjà vu, reduplicative paramnesia, and persecutory delusions. The reason for this is unknown. It is quite possible that it is related to the large size of the right temporal lesion seen in this case (the cause of which remains undetermined).

The findings in Cases 1 and 5—of temporal lobe lesions on the SPECT, with no such findings present in the CT scan or MRI—have been observed by other investigators, who have pointed out the superior sensitivity of brain perfusion SPECT compared with CT scan or MRI in the detection of lesions after TBI (Ichise et al., 1994; Newton et al., 1992; Tikofsley, 1994; Wilson & Wyper, 1992). Furthermore, positron emission tomography (PET) and SPECT studies in patients with an anterior communicating artery aneurysm revealed diminished activity in the medial temporal regions, suggesting that damage to the basal forebrain may result in diminished metabolic activity in the medial temporal lobes (Damasio et al., 1985; Volpe, Herscovitch, & Raichle, 1984).

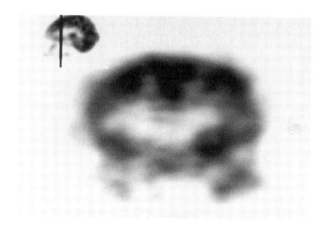

FIG. 11.2B.   SPECT study of the brain of Case 5, showing a coronal image (two slices thick), and demonstrating diminished activity in the right orbital frontal and right anterior temporal regions.

Because our study was limited due to small number of patients, the observed association between delusional component of confabulation and temporal lobe lesions warrants further investigation. Unlike the delusional component, the intrusional element was present in all cases. It consisted of free flow of thoughts, memories, and fantasies into the patients' consciousness. It was usually provoked by conversation, and encompassed both autobiographical and semantic information (such as story repetition). A distinct feature of these intrusions was that patients frequently expressed firm belief in their validity and became quite irritated when the truthfulness of their stories was questioned. It appears as if these intrusive thoughts became a new reality for the patients.

The causes of inability to differentiate thoughts or fantasies from reality are unknown. However, it appears that the medial frontal lobes may play a major role in this matter. This is supported by findings in patients who underwent bilateral anterior cingulectomy, but had other frontal regions left intact (Whitty & Lewin, 1957, 1961). These patients experienced a transient confusional state, in which they noted difficulty, although not complete inability, distinguishing between their thoughts and events of the external world. In response to questions, the patients fabricated elaborate stories and admitted, on further questioning, that their response had been a thought or dream that was indistinguishable from reality. These patients also exhibited limited disorientation to time, and their speech tended to be somewhat disinhibited both in content and format (Whitty & Lewin, 1957).

The previous observations indicate that controlled lesions limited to the cingulate gyri in the medial frontal lobes produced a near confabulatory state, combined with mild memory impairment for time and verbal disinhibition. Based on these findings, it may be speculated that more extensive damage in these areas could cause amnesia and frontal lobe dysfunction to be more pronounced, and could result in a full-scale confabulatory state.

The mechanism that allows people to control the flow of their thoughts, memories, or fantasies, and enables them to distinguish these from reality, remains unknown. However, an interesting explanation may be found in the concept of reality monitoring (Johnson, 1991). *Reality monitoring* is the process by which people discriminate between memories derived from perception and those reflectively generated via thought, imagination, dreams, and fantasy (Johnson & Raye, 1981). This process is the consequence of the coordinated activity of a number of processes embedded in a complex memory system. It involves two types of judgment processes: (a) nondeliberate evaluation of information such as the type and amount of perceptual detail, and (b) deliberate evaluation of the meaningful content of the information in light of other memories and knowledge. Reality monitoring is a frontal lobe function. Disruption of the "reality monitor" may lead to an inability to distinguish between what belongs to the realm of thoughts or memory and what belongs to the outside world; or it may lead to the inability to judge whether a certain thought is plausible or nonsensical (Johnson, 1991).

Reality monitoring may be part of a larger mechanism by which the frontal lobe controls and modulates the limbic system. The fronto-limbic association is established by a fairly compact fiber bundle that follows the white matter of the cingulate gyrus caudally, issuing fibers to the overlying cortex and the hippocampal gyrus (Nauta, 1971). The cingulate gyrus has rich afferent and efferent connection with the prefrontal region, which suggests prefrontal participation in a regulatory process. Further support for the involvement of prefrontal and anterior cingulate cortices in memory-retrieval process is given by recent studies using PET on normal subjects. These studies showed increased blood flow in these regions during retrieval from episodic memory in auditory sentence-recognition tasks (Tulving, Kapur, Craik, Moscovitch, & Houle, 1994). The left and right prefrontal regions are part of an extensive neuronal network that subserves episodic remembering. The left prefrontal cortex is associated with retrieval of information from semantic memory, and with simultaneously encoding novel aspects of the retrieved information into episodic memory. The right prefrontal cortex is more involved with episodic memory retrieval (Tulving, Kapur, Markowitsch, Craik, Habib, & Houle, 1994). It is possible that reality monitoring is one of the functions performed by the prefrontal and anterior cingulate cortices during the memory-retrieval process.

CONCLUSION

The substate of confabulation appears to be a disruption of the fronto-limbic association, which results in the breakdown of the control and modulation exerted by the frontal lobes on the limbic system, producing malfunctioning of the reality testing and feedback. When the frontal lobe damage is mild and the fronto-limbic association not severely disrupted, the patient may exhibit only provoked confabulation. When the frontal lobe's damage is extensive and the disruption of the association severe, florid confabulation is likely to be seen. In addition to this, if there is temporal lobe damage, the confabulation may include delusional elements, especially if the right temporal lobe is involved.

ACKNOWLEDGMENTS

The authors wish to thank Dr. Bruce J. Barron, Department of Nuclear Medicine, University of Texas Health Science Center, and Dr. Jeffrey C.

London, Department of Radiology, Columbia HCA Medical Center Hospital, Houston, Texas, for assisting in neuroimaging interpretation.

REFERENCES

Alexander, M. P., Stuss, D. T., & Benson, D. F. (1979). Capgras' syndrome: A reduplicative phenomenon. *Neurology, 29*, 334–339.

Bancaud, J., Brunet-Bourgin, F., Chauvel, P., & Halgren, E. (1994). Anatomical origin of déjà vu and vivid "memories" in human temporal lobe epilepsy. *Brain, 117*, 71–90.

Barbizet, J. (1963). Defect of memorizing of hippocampalmammillary origin. *Journal of Neurology, Neurosurgery and Psychiatry, 26*, 27–135.

Benson, F. D., Gardner, H., & Meadows, J. C. (1976). Reduplicative paramnesia. *Neurology, 26*, 147–151.

Berlyne, N. (1972). Confabulation. *British Journal of Psychiatry, 120*, 31–39.

Christodoulou, G. N. (1977). The syndrome of Capgras'. *British Journal of Psychiatry, 130*, 556–564.

Cohen, M. R., & Niska, R. W. (1980). Localized right cerebral hemisphere dysfunction and recurrent mania. *American Journal of Psychiatry, 137*, 847–848.

Damasio, A. R., Graff Radford, N. R., Eslinger, B. J., Damasio, H., & Kassell, N. (1985). Amnesia following basal forebrain lesions. *Archives of Neurology, 42*, 263–271.

DeLuca, J., & Cicerone, K. D. (1991). Confabulation following aneurysm of the anterior communication artery. *Cortex, 27*, 417–423.

Freeman, A. M. (1980). Delusions, depersonalization and unusual psychopathological symptoms. In R. C. W. Hall (Ed.), *Psychiatric presentations of medical illness: Somatopsychic disorders* (pp. 75–89). New York: SP Medical & Scientific Books.

Ichise, M., Chung, D. G., Wang, P., Wortzman, G., Gray, B. G., & Franks, W. (1994). Technetium-99m-HMPAO SPECT, CT and MRI in the evaluation of patients with chronic traumatic brain injury: A correlation with neuropsychological performance. *Journal of Nuclear Medicine, 35*, 217–226.

Jampala, V. C., & Abrams, R. (1983). Mania secondary to left and right hemisphere damage. *American Journal of psychiatry, 140*, 1197–1199.

Johnson, M. K. (1991). Reality monitoring: Evidence from confabulation in organic brain disease patients. In G. P. Prigatano & D. L. Schacter (Eds.), *Awareness of deficit after brain injury: Clinical and theoretical issues* (pp. 176–197). New York: Oxford University Press.

Johnson, M. K., & Raye, C. L. (1981). Reality monitoring. *Psychological Reviews, 88*, 67–85.

Kapur, N., & Coughlan, A. K. (1980). Confabulation and frontal lobe dysfunction. *Journal of Neurology, Neurosurgery and Psychiatry, 43*, 461–463.

Kapur, N., Turner, A., & King, C. (1988). Reduplicative paramnesia. Possible anatomical and neuropsychological mechanisms. *Journal of Neurology, Neurosurgery and Psychiatry, 51*, 579–581.

Kopelman, M. D. (1987). Two types of confabulation. *Journal of Neurology, Neurosurgery and Psychiatry, 50*, 1482–1487.

Lewis, S. W. (1987). Brain imaging in a case of Capgras' syndrome. *British Journal of Psychiatry, 150*, 117–121.

Luria, A. R. (1980). *Higher cortical functions in man* (2nd ed.). New York: Basic Books.

Mercer, B., Wapner, W., Gardner, H., & Benson, F. (1977). A study of confabulation. *Archives of Neurology, 34*, 429–433.

Mullan, S., & Penfield, W. (1959). Illusions of comparative interpretation and emotion. *Archives of Neurology and Psychiatry, 81*, 269–284.

Nauta, W. J. H. (1971). The problem of the frontal lobe: A reinterpretation. *Journal of Psychiatric Research, 8*, 167–187.

Newton, M. R., Greenwood, R. J., Britton, K. E., Charlesworth, M., Nimmon, C. C., Carrol, M. J., & Dolke, G. (1992). A study comparing SPECT with CT and MRI after closed head injury. *Journal of Neurology, Neurosurgery and Psychiatry, 55*, 92–94.

Penfield, W. (1955). The role of the temporal cortex in certain psychical phenomena. *Journal of Mental Sciences, 101*, 451–465.

Rosenbaum, A. H., & Barry, M. J. (1975). Positive therapeutic response to lithium in hypomania secondary to organic brain syndrome. *American Journal of Psychiatry, 132*, 1072–1073.

Ruff, R. L., & Volpe, B. T. (1981). Environmental reduplication associated with right frontal and parietal lobe injury. *Journal of Neurology, Neurosurgery and Psychiatry, 44*, 382–386.

Staton, R. D., Brumback, R. A., & Wilson, H. (1982). Reduplicative paramnesia: A disconnection syndrome of memory. *Cortex, 18*, 23–36.

Stuss, D. T., Alexander, M. P., Lieberman, A., & Levine, H. (1978). An extraordinary form of confabulation. *Neurology, 28*, 1166–1172.

Tikofsley, R. S. (1994). Predicting outcome in traumatic brain injury. What role for rCBF/SPECT. *Journal of Nuclear Medicine, 35*, 947–948.

Tulving, E., Kapur, S., Craik, F. I. M., Moscovitch, M., & Houle, S. (1994). Hemispheric encoding/retrieval asymmetry in episodic memory: Positron emission tomography findings. *Proceedings of the National Academy of Science, USA, 91*, 2016–2020.

Tulving, E., Kapur, S., Markowitsch, H. J., Craik, F. I. M., Habib, R., & Houle, S. (1994). Neuroanatomical correlates of retrieval in episodic memory: Auditory sentence recognition. *Proceedings of the National Academy of Science, USA, 91* 2012–2015.

Weinstein, E. A., & Lyerly, O. G. (1968). Confabulation following brain injury. *Archives of General Psychiatry, 18*, 348–354.

Whitty, C. W. M., & Lewin, W. (1957). Vivid day dreaming: An unusual form of confusion following anterior cingulectomy. *Brain, 80*, 72–76.

Whitty, C. W. M., & Lewin, W. (1961). A Korsakoff syndrome in the post cingulectomy confusional state. *Brain, 83*, 648–653.

Wilson, J. T. L., & Wyper, D. (1992). Neuroimaging and neuropsychological functioning following closed head injury: CT, MRI, and SPECT. *Journal of Head Trauma Rehabilitation, 7*, 29–39.

Volpe, B. T., Herscovitch, P., & Raichle, M. E. (1984). Positron emission tomography defines metabolic abnormality in mesial temporal lobes of two patients with amnesia after rupture and repair of anterior communicating artery aneurysm. *Neurology, 34* (Suppl. 1), 188.

12

Physiological Rehabilitation of Disordered Speech Following Closed Head Injury

Bruce E. Murdoch

Dysarthria has been reported to be one of the most persistent sequelae of severe closed head injury (CHI), often remaining beyond the resolution of any concomitant language disorder (Najenson, Sazbon, Fiselzon, Becker, & Schecter, 1985; Sarno & Levin, 1985). In recent years, improved posttrauma medical care has resulted in a greater number of survivors following severe CHI, thereby increasing the need for development of specialist CHI rehabilitation programs. To date, however, little attention has been paid to the development of programs for the rehabilitation of the communication deficits, including dysarthria, exhibited by persons following severe CHI (Ylvisaker & Urbanczyk, 1990). The majority of severe CHI cases is found in either adolescents or young adults, and the presence of a persistent motor speech impairment can significantly inhibit a return to normal work, as well as social and community activities. Hence, the need for an effective program for the rehabilitation of dysarthria subsequent to severe CHI is urgent.

Traditional therapeutic approaches to the rehabilitation of dysarthric speech in CHI, as in the case of dysarthrias associated with other neurological conditions (e.g., Parkinson's disease, cerebrovascular accident, etc.), are based primarily on subjective, perceptual techniques, and consequently lack the objectivity and specificity required to ensure the most effective rehabilitation. In fact, as stated by Gentil (1993), many clinicians believe that current speech treatments for dysarthrics are of questionable benefit. What is needed is a more objective, physiological approach to dysarthria therapy—one that is based on a comprehensive instrumental assessment of the functioning of the speech production apparatus' components. Such an approach, referred to as the *physiologi-*

cal approach, has been advocated by Hardy (1967) and Netsell and colleagues (Netsell, 1984, 1986; Netsell & Daniel, 1979; Netsell, Lotz, & Barlow, 1989).

The physiological or multiple speech-component approach to dysarthria rehabilitation is based on a neurobiological view of human speech. It evolved from the following concept: assessment of the individual motor subsystems of the speech mechanism (i.e., respiratory, laryngeal, velopharyngeal, and articulatory subsystems) is crucial in defining the underlying speech motor pathophysiology necessary for the development of optimal treatment programs (Abbs & De Paul, 1989; Netsell, 1986). Therefore, in this approach the initial step is to undertake a comprehensive physiological assessment of the various components of the speech-production mechanism of the dysarthric speaker to determine: (a) those components that are malfunctioning, and (b) the physiological nature and severity of the malfunction. Essentially, the goal of the multiple speech-component assessment is to evaluate the integrity of the speech components (e.g., lips, tongue, jaw, velopharynx, larynx, etc.) and systems (e.g., articulation, phonation, respiration, etc.) that generate or valve the expiratory airstream, and subsequently relate this information to the perceived dysarthric symptom (Kearns & Simmons, 1990). Subsequent to the physiological assessment, treatment procedures are selected, taking into account the physiological nature of the malfunction as well as the interaction of any coexisting linguistic or cognitive deficits with the motor impairment. This requires the clinician to determine the relative contributions of the underlying neuromuscular impairments to the patient's deviant perceptual speech features. A hierarchy of factors for treatment intervention are then listed, with treatment initially being directed at those parts of the speech mechanism primarily responsible for the speech deficit.

Several reports in the literature have confirmed that the physiological approach to the rehabilitation of dysarthria can be a more objective and effective method of speech rehabilitation than traditional perceptual-based therapy (Bellaire, Yorkston, & Beukelman, 1986; Netsell & Daniel, 1979; Netsell & Hixon, 1992; Workinger & Netsell, 1992). In recent years, colleagues and I at the Motor Speech Research Unit, The University of Queensland, have adopted the physiological approach to develop more effective programs specifically for the treatment of dysarthria following CHI. In line with the components of the physiological approach outlined earlier, our research has included two major steps. The first step involved the development of a profile of the physiological functioning of the various components of the speech-production apparatus in a group of speech-disordered CHI subjects. Based on the outcome of the physiological assessment, the second step involved the development and application of appropriate instrumental treatment methods based on biofeedback techniques. The aim of the present chapter is to demonstrate the principles of the physiological approach to rehabilitation of disordered speech by reference to the assessment and treatment strategies used in two CHI patients with persistent speech disorder subsequent to motor vehicle accidents.

PHYSIOLOGICAL EVALUATION OF THE SPEECH MECHANISM

As outlined previously, the aim of the physiological evaluation of the speech mechanism is to determine the severity and physiological nature of the malfunctions. To be of value in deciding treatment priorities, the physiological assessment should be comprehensive, covering as many components of the speech-production apparatus as possible. An example of a comprehensive speech physiology examination for dysarthric patients is that described by Netsell et al. (1989). Ideally, the assessment should evaluate the physiological functioning of the respiratory system (including the rib cage and abdomen/diaphragm musculature), the larynx, the velopharynx, as well as the articulators (e.g., tongue, lips, etc.). A variety of instruments are currently available for assessing the functioning of these various components. However, a discussion of these procedures is beyond the scope of this chapter (see Baken, 1987, for a detailed review of instruments available for assessing the speech-production mechanism). Techniques described here are restricted to those used in my laboratory to date for the assessment of CHI subjects. These instruments, together with the relevant parameters measured by each, are listed in Table 12.1.

Multiple Component Evaluation

Evaluation of Respiration. Subjects undergo a standard clinical spirometric assessment of respiratory function, yielding measures of respiration rate, tidal volume, vital capacity, forced expiratory volume, expiratory reserve volume, and inspiratory reserve volume. These values are compared with predicted values, taking into account the patient's age, gender, and height. In addition to these nonspeech respiratory tasks, lung volume changes during selected speech tasks are also recorded. Speech tasks for respiratory evaluation consist of the subject engaging in several minutes of spontaneous conversation with the investigator, and reading the Grandfather Passage (Darley, Aronson, & Brown, 1975). Each subject also performs a syllable-repetition

TABLE 12.1
Physiological Examination of the Speech Mechanism

Speech Component	Instrumentation	Parameter Measured
Respiratory system	Spirometer	• Vital capacity
		• Forced expiratory volume
	Strain-gauge belt pneumograph or Respitrace	• Lung volume changes
		• Relative contribution of the rib cage and abdomen to lung volume changes
		• Configuration of the chest wall during speech
	Aerophone II	• Subglottal pressure
Larynx	Indirect:	
	Electroglottography	• Duty cycle, closing time, Fo
	Aerophone II	• Aerodynamic measures (e.g., glottal resistance, phonatory flow rate)
	Direct:	
	Videostroboscopy	• Vocal-fold movements
Velopharynx	Accelerometry	• Oral/nasal coupling index
	Nasometer	• Nasalance
	Videofluoroscopy	• Soft palate movements
Oro-facial system		
Tongue	Rubber bulb pressure transducer	• Tongue strength and endurance
	Electropalatograph	• Tongue placement on hard palate
Lip	Semiconductor strain-gauge transducer	• Lip pressure

task, calling for intermittent, rapid, discrete increments in vocal stress in a pattern repeated several times on a single expiration, as well as a series of vowel prolongations. In addition to lung volume changes, the reading task allows calculation of the mean syllables per breath and speaking rate (syllables/minute).

Recording of the respiratory system's performance during speech production is carried out using the computerized strain-gauge belt pneumograph system developed by Murdoch, Chenery, Bowler, and Ingram (1989). Briefly, this system involves simultaneous, but independent, recording of circumferential-size changes of the rib cage and abdomen. The rib cage and abdominal components of the respiratory system must be coordinated in their respective movements (i.e., they each contribute simultaneously to changes in total lung volume and production of subglottal air pressures during speech). Knowledge of how lung volume changes are partitioned between the various components of the respiratory apparatus (i.e., rib cage and abdomen) is of fundamental importance to understanding the physiological bases of both normal and disordered speech production.

As an alternative to the strain-gauge belt pneumograph system, speech breathing can also be monitored by respiratory-inductive plethysmography (Respitrace). This system is currently used in many speech laboratories and clinical settings. As in the case of the strain-gauge system, Respitrace transduces circumferential changes in the rib cage and abdomen during breathing. Instead of the movement being detected by strain gauges, however, changes in chest wall size are detected by alterations in the inductance of two wire loops passed around the torso: one at the level of the rib cage and the other around the abdomen.

One other important indicator of respiratory function for speech production is the ability of the patient to generate subglottal air pressure during speech (Netsell et al., 1989). Subglottal air pressure is estimated using an Aerophone II (Kay Elemetrics) airflow measurement system. The Aerophone II consists of a hand-held transducer module, together with a powerful data acquisition and processing software program that runs on a 486DX IBM-compatible computer. The transducer module consists of miniaturized transducers capable of recording airflow, air pressure, and acoustic signals during speech. A face mask, through which a thin flexible tube of silicon rubber is inserted to record intra-oral pressure, is attached to the hand-held transducer module. To estimate subglottal pressure, the patient is asked to repeat /ipipipi/ into the face mask, with the rubber tube located in the oral cavity, for several seconds. The point of maximum intra-oral pressure during the pronunciation of the voiceless stop /p/ is calculated automatically over six repetitions, and is used as the estimate of subglottal air pressure.

Evaluation of Laryngeal Function. Physiological evaluation of laryngeal function is carried out using both indirect and direct techniques. The indirect methods include electroglottography (electrolaryngography) and aerodynamic examination. Electroglottography is an electrical impedance method of estimating vocal-fold contact during phonation, which is designed to allow investigation of laryngeal microfunction (cycle-by-cycle periodicity and contact). The electroglottographic assessment is conducted using a Fourcin laryngograph interfaced with a Waveform Display System (Kay Elemetrics Model 6091), running on a 486DX IBM-compatible computer. The system records the degree of vocal-fold contact and the vocal-fold vibratory patterns during phonation; these features are then displayed in the form of an Lx waveform. The Waveform Display System allows for acquisition and real-time viewing of the Lx waveform on the computer monitor, as well as storage and analysis of waveform segments. Although some caution must be used in interpreting electroglottographic results, a number of authors have acknowledged that this procedure provides a useful estimate of vocal-fold contact during the glottal cycle and gives some insight into the regulation, maintenance, and quality of phonation (Childers & Krishnamurthy, 1985; Hanson, Gerratt, Karin, & Berke, 1988; Motta, Cesari, Iengo, & Motta, 1990).

Aerodynamic measures allow examination of the macrofunctions of the larynx, such as laryngeal airflow, glottal resistance, glottal power, and glottal resistance. Estimates of these parameters are obtained by way of an Aerophone II Airflow Measurement System (described earlier).

Videostroboscopy is a fiberoptic procedure that enables the researcher to directly examine laryngeal function and vocal-fold movement. The procedure involves the use of an endoscope connected to a video camera and a strobe light source. Stroboscopy involves the rapid sampling of vocal-fold position at particular time intervals, producing a composite moving image of different cycles. This technique allows important components of the glottal cycle (e.g., mucosal wave, symmetry and amplitude of vibration, glottal shape at closure, and timing relationships) to be observed.

Evaluation of Velopharyngeal Function. Velopharyngeal function is assessed using a modified version of the nasal accelerometric technique proposed by Horii (1980). The technique involves the use of two miniature accelerometers (Knowles Electronics Model BU-1771), as recommended by Lippmann (1981), to detect nasal and throat vibrations during speech. One miniature accelerometer is attached to the upper side of the nose over the lateral nasal cartilage just in front of the nasal bone; the other is attached to the side of the neck over the lamina of the thyroid cartilage. The output signals from each accelerometer are amplified by a DC amplifier, and the amplified signals are then relayed to a computerized physiological data acquisition system composed of a 486DX IBM-compatible computer equipped with a 16-channel analog/digital converter. The software used for data acquisition is ASYSTANT PLUS (MacMillan Software Company). The system yields an index of oral/nasal coupling (The Horii Oral-Nasal Coupling Index) during production of a range of nasal and non-nasal sounds, words, and sentences.

Another instrument available for assessment of nasality is the Nasometer (Kay Elemetrics Model 6200-2). The Nasometer is a computer-assisted instrument that measures nasality derived from the ratio of acoustic energy output from the nasal and oral cavities during speech. Acoustic energy is detected by two-directional microphones (one placed in front of the nares and the other in front of the mouth) separated by a sound separator plate. The instrument yields a "nasalence" score consisting of a ratio of nasal to oral, plus nasal acoustic energy calculated as a percentage.

Although not a routine part of the test battery used in my laboratory, another useful technique for assessing velopharyngeal function is videofluoroscopy. This is an x-ray procedure requiring the services of a radiologist. It is currently used in my laboratory to assess a restricted number of dysarthric subjects.

Evaluation of the Oro-Facial System.   The strength, range, and speed of movement of the lip and tongue muscles are assessed by a variety of force-transduction systems. To date, the principal transducer for assessing lip strength and endurance has been similar to that described by Abbs, Barlow, and Netsell (1978). This transducer is composed of a flexible, stainless steel ring that is open in one section to form two levers, which can be placed between the lips. Attached to the surface of the ring are two etched linear foil strain-gauge transducers; these set up a signal when the two levers are pressed toward each other by the lips. Because of its mechanical properties, the above-lip transducer is limited to assessment of lip strength and endurance during performance of nonspeech tasks. Consequently, it is currently being replaced by a new miniaturized lip transducer similar to that described by Hinton and Luschei (1992). The new transducer is based on semiconductor strain-gauge technology. Because of its small size, it is capable of generating interlabial pressure measurements during speech production without interfering with normal articulatory movements.

The tongue force transducer system in current use is similar to that described by Robin, Somodi, and Luschei (1991). It is composed of an air-filled soft rubber bulb connected to a pressure transducer. The transducer estimates tongue strength and endurance during performance of nonspeech tasks only. Dynamic measurements of tongue behavior are obtained by way of an electropalatogram (Miligrant-Wells EPG-3). This technique involves the use of a false palate fitted with an array of electrodes, enabling the examiner to estimate tongue placement during production of a range of sounds. This technique is used with a restricted number of cases only because a false palate must be constructed for each patient.

Case Reports

As described earlier, according to the physiological approach to the rehabilitation of dysarthria following CHI, the first step is to define treatment
priorities on the basis of a comprehensive physiological assessment of
the speech-production mechanism. The two cases presented next are
examples of CHI patients' performance on the instrumental battery described in the previous section. In the following section, the outcome of
treatments—selected on the basis of the physiological assessments, and
applied to these same two CHI cases—is evaluated. Thus, the principles
of the physiological approach to rehabilitation of dysarthria following
CHI are demonstrated.

Case 1.   Subject 1 was a 21-year-old male who had suffered a CHI as
a result of a motor vehicle accident $2^{1}/_{2}$ years prior to assessment. At the
time of hospital admission, he was given a Glasgow Coma Scale (GCS)
score of 4, and was therefore classified as severely head injured. The
findings of a computed tomography (CT) scan taken shortly after admission indicated the presence of a subarachnoid hemorrhage and contusion to the right side of the cerebellum, close to the vicinity of a skull
fracture extending toward the foramen magnum. On the basis of a perceptual assessment conducted immediately prior to the instrumental
evaluation, Subject 1 was diagnosed as having a mild–moderate spastic-
ataxic dysarthria, with ataxic perceptual speech characteristics such as
excess and equal stress, prolonged intervals, reduced loudness variation, and reduced rate of speech predominating in his verbal output.
Therefore, the perceptual deficits identified in Subject 1's speech were
generally consistent with the neuroradiological finding of cerebellar
damage.

Instrumental assessment of respiratory function revealed that Subject
1 had reduced lung volumes and capacities. In particular, both his vital
capacity and forced expiratory volume were more than 20% below predicted levels for a person of his age, gender, and height. In addition,
kinematic assessment revealed that Subject 1 exhibited impaired two-
part coordination of the chest wall during the expiratory phase of speech
breathing. Further, both his speaking rate (syllables/minute) and mean
number of syllables/breath were markedly reduced compared with non-
neurologically impaired controls.

The physiological evaluation of laryngeal activity indicated a hyperfunctional pattern of laryngeal activity, both aerodynamically and at the
level of vocal-fold vibration. In particular, the results revealed a short
closing time, a reduced phonatory flow rate, elevated subglottal pressure, and high-glottal resistance compared with non-neurologically im-

paired control subjects. Fundamental frequency, duty cycle, average phonatory sound pressure level, and ad/abduction rate of the vocal folds were found to be within the normal range. The instrumental assessments provided no evidence of abnormal velopharyngeal activity. Likewise, measures of strength, endurance, and rate of repetitive movements were normal for both the lips and tongue.

Overall, the instrumental findings suggest that treatment of Subject 1's dysarthric speech should focus initially on the remediation of respiratory and laryngeal dysfunction. Specifically, therapy should be directed toward improving the control of expiratory airflow during speech by improving the two-part coordination of the chest wall (i.e., by improving the coordinated action of the rib cage and abdomen/diaphragm). In addition, the marked degree of hyperfunctional laryngeal activity recorded for this subject would appear to require specific therapy to reduce laryngeal hypertension. Specific therapy aimed at the treatment of velopharyngeal dysfunction would appear unwarranted. Likewise, no immediate need was identified to improve lip or tongue strength.

Case 2. Subject 2 was a 55-year-old male who had suffered a severe CHI (GCS score of 4) as a result of a motor vehicle accident 2 years prior to assessment. A CT scan taken soon after hospital admission revealed the presence of a small brain stem hematoma and a small hematoma/contusion of the right temporal lobe. Skull fractures in the left superior parietal vault and ethmoid bone were also indicated. On the basis of a perceptual speech analysis carried out prior to the instrumental evaluation, Subject 2 was classified as a moderate spastic-flaccid dysarthric speaker. His major deviant speech dimensions included: reduced pitch and loudness variation, reduced pitch level, loudness decay, shortened phrases, decreased speech rate, rate decay, excess stress, reduced breath support for speech, hypernasality, harshness, strained-strangled vocal quality, intermittent breathiness, hoarseness, glottal fry, imprecision of consonants and vowels, prolonged phonemes, prolonged intervals, forced inspiration and expiration, and audible inspiration.

The instrumental assessment of respiratory function identified the presence of reduced lung volumes and capacities, as well as problems with the two-part coordination of the chest wall during speech. The values recorded for both vital capacity and forced expiratory volume were found to be more than 20% below the values predicted based on Subject 2's age, gender, and height. Respiratory dysfunction was also indicated, by below normal values for speaking rate (syllables/minute) and mean number of syllables per breath when reading.

Hyperfunctional laryngeal activity was identified as the primary mode of laryngeal function for Subject 2 based on vocal-fold vibratory patterns and aerodynamic measures. Subject 2 exhibited a high fundamental frequency, a fast closing time, a very high subglottal pressure, and an elevated sound pressure level compared with non-neurologically impaired control subjects. Phonatory flow rate, glottal resistance, and ad/abduction rate of the vocal folds were found to be within the normal range.

A marked degree of velopharyngeal dysfunction was indicated by the finding of oral/nasal coupling indices on non-nasal sounds of more than twice that recorded from normal controls. However, instrumental assessment of lip strength failed to show impairment of lip strength or endurance. Both tongue strength and endurance were below normal. Although Subject 2 could achieve a normal rate of repetitive tongue movements, this appeared to be achieved by a reduction in the degree of tongue pressure on each repetition.

Both the perceptual and instrumental findings for Subject 2 suggested that therapeutic intervention was required in the respiratory, laryngeal, velopharyngeal, and oro-facial subsystems of his speech-production mechanism. Specifically, with regard to respiration, therapy should be directed primarily toward improving the coordination of the rib cage and abdomen during the expiratory phase of speech breathing. The instrumental laryngeal findings suggest that therapy for the laryngeal subsystem should focus on reducing laryngeal tension and developing a less forceful pattern of voice production. Resonance therapy, required for the velopharyngeal dysfunction identified in Subject 2, would need to address the problem of maintaining adequate palatal function during speech to achieve a greater degree of oral resonance. Based on the instrumental results available, specific articulation therapy should focus on improving the tongue's strength and endurance.

PHYSIOLOGICAL REHABILITATION OF DISORDERED SPEECH BREATHING FOLLOWING CLOSED HEAD INJURY

Subsequent to a comprehensive physiological evaluation of the speech mechanism, the second step in the physiological approach to the rehabilitation of dysarthria is determining which components of the speech-production apparatus are to be treated first and what methods of treatment are to be applied. As mentioned previously, the principle is to establish a hierarchy of components for treatment, with intervention being directed at those parts of the speech mechanism determined to be the major contributors to the overall speech deficit. With regard to the two CHI cases described in the previous section, it was noted that impaired speech breathing was a major factor contributing to overall speech disturbance. Ideally therapy should target several components of the speech mechanism simultaneously for subjects with multiple dysarthric symptoms. However, according to Rosenbek and La Pointe (1985), if a speech-breathing deficit is present, this often requires remediation before other areas of speech can be targeted. Consequently, therapy aimed at improving their speech breathing was seen as the primary target for rehabilitation in each case.

Treatment of dysarthria can involve either traditional or instrumental methods. Although the majority of dysarthria treatment continues to involve traditional treatment based on behavioral methodology, an increasing body of evidence indicates that instrument-based therapy is more efficacious. In particular, there is increasing support for the use of instruments capable of providing biofeedback (Carman & Ryan, 1989; Daniel & Guitar, 1978; Nemec & Cohen, 1984; Netsell & Cleeland, 1973). For the two CHI cases reported here, both traditional and biofeedback therapy were used to improve speech breathing.

Procedure

To study the efficacy of the traditional versus the physiological therapy techniques, an A-B-A-B single-subject experimental design was employed, involving baseline assessments (A_1), a period of traditional therapy (B_1), a withdrawal phase (A_2), and biofeedback therapy (B_2). Both CHI subjects participated in all four stages of the study. In all stages, speech breathing was assessed using both perceptual measures (including rating scales of intelligibility and respiratory support for speech) and instrumental measures (including both kinematic and spirometric assessments).

The two CHI subjects were required to read a standard passage, "The Grandfather Passage" (Darley et al., 1975), to obtain a sample of their speech for perceptual analysis. The speech was recorded onto audiotape using a high-quality tape recorder and microphone. It was then independently rated by two judges, both qualified and experienced speech/language pathologists, on the dimensions of respiratory support for speech and intelligibility using the scales developed by FitzGerald, Murdoch, and Chenery (1987).

The procedure and instrumentation for the kinematic assessment of speech breathing followed that of Murdoch et al. (1989). This technique has been described in detail elsewhere (see Manifold & Murdoch, 1993), and therefore is only described briefly here. The system uses a pair of strain-gauge belt pneumographs to sense circumferential changes in the rib cage and abdomen. The transducer for recording circumferential change in the rib cage was wrapped around the torso midway between the sternal notch and xiphoid process, whereas that for sensing circumferential change in the abdomen was fitted around the torso at the umbilicus. Signals from the abdominal and rib cage transducers were amplified by a DC amplifier and passed simultaneously to two separate recording and storage instruments. Outputs from both transducers were then displayed on a computer fitted with a physiological data acquisition system to yield a relative volume chart on the computer monitor. This chart takes the form of an x–y plot, with rib cage circumference displayed on the y axis (circumference increasing upward) and abdominal circumference displayed on the x axis (circumference increasing to the right). The relative volume chart displayed as an x–y plot was used to provide visual biofeedback to the subjects during the biofeedback therapy stage (B_2). The outputs from the rib cage and abdominal transducers were also independently recorded on one channel of a four-channel oscillographic recorder. Recordings are made during performance of two types of activities: respiratory maneuvers (nonspeech tasks), which are necessary for calibration of the system, and utterances (speech tasks). Speech tasks for kinematic evaluation included sustained vowel productions, syllable repetitions, counting, and reading a declarative passage. Parameters determined included: (a) lung volume changes, (b) relative contributions of the rib cage and abdomen to lung volume changes (percent rib cage contribution), (c) configuration of the chest wall during speech production, (d) frequency of slope changes in the expiratory limbs, and (e) incidence of rib cage and abdominal paradoxing. The spirometric assessment was conducted using a Mijnhardt Vicatest-P1 Spirometer.

Baseline Assessment.   Six baseline assessments were carried out over 2 weeks for each subject. At each assessment, the various parameters of speech breathing were measured, and an audiotaped speech sample was recorded for perceptual analysis.

Traditional Therapy.   Following the baseline stage, both subjects received 2 weeks of intensive traditional therapy for speech breathing, involving daily 45-minute sessions for 10 days. A common session plan was used for both subjects. Each session began with instruction in good posture for optimal breathing patterns, as well as exercises for relaxation of the head, neck, and shoulders. To target controlled exhalation, the subject and therapist used tactile, kinesthetic, and visual feedback during quiet breathing.

A U-tube manometer was used—in the way described by Rosenbek and La Pointe (1985)—to increase the amount of air pressure generated by each subject and for greater periods of time. The duration and air pressure were recorded for 5–10 trials per session. Each subject was then timed, using a stopwatch, on his or her ability to sustain the fricatives /s/ and /ʃ/ and vowels /a/ and /i/. The aim was to increase the time that the sounds could be sustained without compromising the vocal quality, pitch, or loudness. Serial speech tasks were also included in each session, in which the subjects were required to recite the alphabet or count in one breath. Appropriate phrasing was taught, using sentence and paragraph material, to enable the subjects to monitor their breathing patterns while reading. Speech breathing and perceptual assessments were carried out following the first, third, fifth, seventh, and tenth treatment sessions.

Withdrawal Phase. During the next 12 weeks, subjects received no therapy. Speech-breathing and perceptual speech assessments were conducted at 2, 5, 6, 7, and 8 weeks following the end of traditional therapy.

Biofeedback Therapy. During the final stage, both subjects received further speech breathing therapy, this time using a visual biofeedback approach. Therapy sessions were conducted daily for 10 days, with each session lasting for a maximum of 40 minutes, or less if the subject tired before that time.

All sessions commenced with a reminder of good posture for breathing, as well as relaxation of the head, neck, and shoulders. The subjects were then allowed as much time as necessary to familiarize themselves with the strain-gauge belt pneumograph. They were also instructed on how to manipulate the visual feedback by altering the relative contributions of the rib cage and abdomen during exhalation. Initially subjects focused on one strain-gauge belt pneumograph at a time. This allowed them to master the control of the rib cage and abdomen separately before attempting to coordinate the two. Subjects were then required to match a target relative volume chart, comprising a 45 degree straight line overlaid on a computer screen, during performance of a variety of speech and nonspeech tasks. A hierarchy of tasks was devised. Subjects progressed through each level once a consistent approximation of the target could be achieved. These tasks included: quiet breathing, production of sustained vowels, syllable repetitions, serial speech, reading, and spontaneous conversation. Throughout each session, the visual feedback was fully explained, and the subjects were prompted where necessary to make necessary adjustments to their breathing pattern. Occasionally the visual feedback was removed to allow the subjects practice in monitoring their own exhalation. During the period of biofeedback therapy, speech-breathing and perceptual speech assessments were conducted on Days 1, 3, 5, 7, and 10.

Results

Subject 1.   Consistent with his initial diagnosis of cerebellar damage and ataxic dysarthria, the primary speech-breathing deficits exhibited by Subject 1 during the baseline assessments included: incoordination of the respiratory musculature, manifested as slope changes and paradoxical movements in the relative volume charts recorded during his performance of the various speech tasks (i.e., vowel prolongations, syllable repetition, counting, and reading), and inconsistency of the relative contribution of the rib cage (% RC) during production of the various speech tasks. Figure 12.1 shows a relative volume chart typical of those produced by Subject 1 during the baseline period.

The aim of the traditional therapy was to improve respiratory support for speech and coordination of the chest wall during speech breathing. During the traditional therapy stage, Subject 1 continued to evidence incoordination of the respiratory musculature and inconsistency of the relative contribution of the rib cage (% RC) across the majority of the speech tasks. However, a consistent increase in % RC was noted during reading (see Fig. 12.2). An increase in the average number of slope changes and paradoxical movements was also noted to accompany the traditional therapy stage across all speech tasks (see Fig. 12.3).

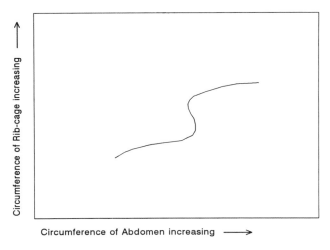

FIG. 12.1.   Relative volume chart recorded from Subject 1 during vowel prolongation in the baseline stage.

As was expected, relative volume charts recorded during the withdrawal stage were similar to baseline traces, characterized by variable % RC values and incoordination. As in the case of the traditional therapy, based on the outcome of the baseline assessments of speech breathing, the biofeedback therapy targeted the incoordination of the respiratory musculature and inconsistent patterns of rib cage contribution during breathing. To achieve these goals, Subject 1 was expected to match a target expiratory trace in a hierarchy of expiratory tasks using visual feedback. In the first week of biofeedback therapy, Subject 1, who evidenced some high-level cognitive-language deficits following the CHI, was unable to build on the skills taught in previous sessions. To account for this problem, each biofeedback session began with the most basic task of the hierarchy described earlier. Also due to his cognitive deficits, the subject initially had difficulty understanding the relationship between the visual biofeedback and his breathing pattern. To simplify this relationship, early biofeedback sessions were spent focusing on one component of the respiratory mechanism at a time. Initially, only one strain-gauge belt pneumograph was fitted. The subject experimented with this, trying to manipulate the visual biofeedback during nonspeech and speech tasks. This was helpful in familiarizing the subject with the instrumentation. It also served as a foundation for the more difficult tasks involving coordination of both components of the respiratory mechanism.

During the early sessions of biofeedback therapy, Subject 1 had some difficulty matching the target trace, the number of slope changes, and paradoxical movements actually increasing. The increased frequency of

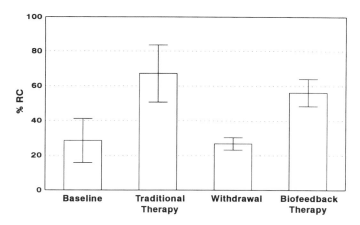

FIG. 12.2. Mean percentage of rib cage contribution (% RC) to expiration recorded from Subject 1 during reading.

A

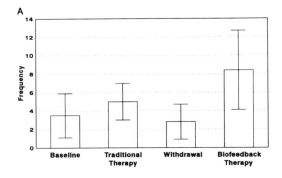

B

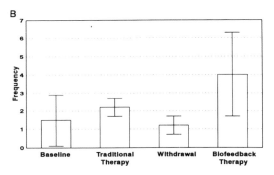

FIG. 12.3. Mean frequency of (a) slope changes and (b) para-doxical movements recorded from Subject 1 during vowel prolongation.

these features, however, may have resulted from Subject 1's increased ability to self-monitor his breathing pattern. The occurrence of slope changes may have represented adjustments in the two-part coordination of the chest wall in an effort to match the target trace. This is suggested by the fact that, although more frequent, the slope changes in the early sessions of biofeedback therapy were smaller in amplitude and duration than slope changes noted in the previous three stages, including the baseline stage. Toward the end of the biofeedback stage, however, Subject 1 was more able to minimize the occurrence of slope changes and paradoxical movements in his expiratory traces, initially only with the aid of visual biofeedback. Examples of relative volume charts recorded toward the end of the biofeedback stage are shown in Fig. 12.4. These changes in speech breathing during the biofeedback stage also corresponded to an increase in % RC during reading (see Fig. 12.2) and an improvement in the perceptual rating given to Subject 1 by two qualified speech pathologists with regard to perceived respiratory support for speech.

Subject 2. Baseline assessments showed a consistent pattern of speech breathing in Subject 2. It was composed of a predominance of

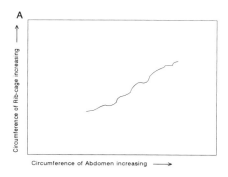

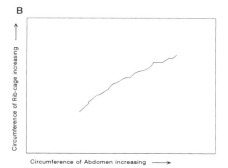

FIG. 12.4. Relative volume chart recorded from Subject 1 during (a) vowel prolongation and (b) deep breathing in the biofeedback stage.

abdominal contribution in the initial half of exhalation, followed by a predominance of rib cage contribution in the latter half of exhalation, which coincided with a degree of abdominal paradoxing caused by relaxation of the abdominal muscles at the end of expiration. An example of a relative volume chart, typical of those recorded by Subject 2 in the baseline phase, is shown in Fig. 12.5.

Traditional therapy had a positive effect on speech breathing during reading, with a consistent increase in the rib cage contribution (% RC) to exhalation during reading of a standard passage being noted (see Fig. 12.6). For the other speech tasks (e.g., vowel prolongations), however, the pattern of speech breathing was less consistent across the traditional therapy stage, with some relative volume charts showing a predominance of rib cage activity and others a predominance of abdominal contribution to the exhalation. In addition, the frequency of occurrence of slope changes and paradoxical movements in the relative volume charts also increased during the traditional therapy stage. These latter increases possibly reflect an increase in Subject 2's ability to self-monitor his speech breathing patterns as a result of training provided as part of traditional therapy.

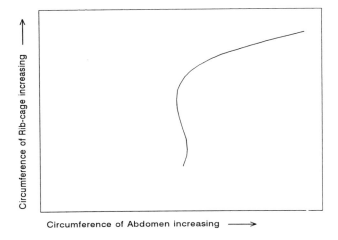

FIG. 12.5.   Relative volume chart recorded from Subject 2 during vowel prolongation in the baseline stage.

During the withdrawal stage, the % RC values recorded during performance of the various speech tasks, including reading (see Fig. 12.6), returned to near baseline levels. The frequency of occurrence of slope changes and paradoxical movements in the majority of expiratory traces remained high, possibly reflecting Subject 2's maintenance of the self-monitoring learned in traditional therapy.

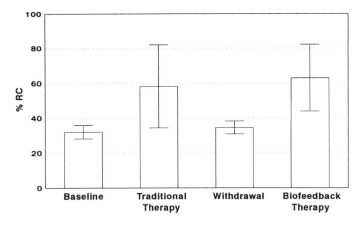

FIG. 12.6.   Mean percentage of rib cage contribution (% RC) to expiration recorded from Subject 2 during reading.

Subject 2 showed marked improvement in the relative contribution of the rib cage (% RC) to lung volume reduction during all speech tasks as a result of biofeedback therapy. He had a high level of motivation and task commitment, both of which aided rapid achievement of biofeedback therapy goals. Subject 2 had minimal cognitive impairment, and understood the requirements of the biofeedback task well. By the end of the biofeedback stage, he was able to closely match the target trace (see Fig. 12.7).

The expiratory traces recorded during the biofeedback therapy stage showed an increase in the occurrence of slope changes, and, to a lesser extent, in the number of paradoxical movements. Like the previous subject, however, the slope changes and paradoxical movements were consistently of small amplitude and short duration, and probably represented minor adjustments of respiratory control throughout the exhalation. When visual feedback was provided, Subject 2 was able to minimize the frequency of slope changes, although this ability did not generalize to situations where visual biofeedback was not allowed.

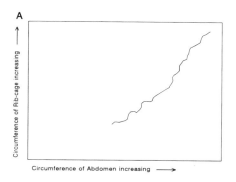

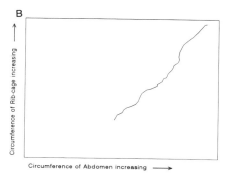

FIG. 12.7. Relative volume chart recorded from Subject 2 during (a) vowel prolongation and (b) deep breathing in the biofeedback stage.

As with Subject 1, the alterations in the speech-breathing pattern as a result of biofeedback therapy corresponded to an improvement in the perceptual rating given by two qualified speech pathologists with regard to Subject 2's respiratory support for speech.

DISCUSSION AND CONCLUSIONS

The results showed that both traditional and biofeedback therapy were able to effect positive changes in the speech-breathing patterns of both subjects. Biofeedback therapy, however, was more consistent in producing the desired physiological changes in speech breathing than traditional therapy alone. In particular, assessments made toward the end of the biofeedback phase revealed that both subjects had learned to self-monitor their breathing patterns so as to produce more control exhalations during speech production. Overall, the preliminary results presented are supportive of the physiological approach to rehabilitation of disordered speech following CHI. For both subjects, however, the remediation of speech breathing, as outlined, is only the first step in the overall program needed for the treatment of their speech disorder. Although in both cases the improvements in the pattern of speech breathing were mirrored by improvements in their perceived level of respiratory support for speech, in neither case did the changes in speech breathing significantly alter the intelligibility of speech. The results of the multicomponent physiological analysis showed that, in both subjects, in addition to problems with speech breathing, dysfunction at other levels of the speech-production apparatus was present (e.g., laryngeal dysfunction was present in each case). In addition to speech-breathing problems, dysfunction in these other components would influence speech intelligibility. Consequently, following treatment for speech-breathing problems, therapy would need also to be aimed at other levels of the speech mechanism. Ultimately, having directed individual therapy at components named major contributors to the speech disorder, treatment should be focused on all dysfunctional components of the speech mechanism simultaneously. Only then could general improvement of the speech disorder be expected with a corresponding improvement in speech intelligibility.

In conclusion, the aim of the present chapter was to outline the steps involved in a multicomponent or physiological approach to rehabilitation of dysarthria following CHI. Based on the preliminary findings of a study where this approach was applied to two CHI subjects, it is concluded that the physiological approach is potentially an effective method for the treatment of dysarthria caused by CHI.

REFERENCES

Abbs, J. H., Barlow, S. M., & Netsell, R. (1978). *Lip closing force: Normative data and some clinical observations*. Unpublished manuscript, Speech Motor Control Laboratories, Waisman Centre, Madison, Wisconsin.

Abbs, J. H., & De Paul, R. (1989). Assessment of dysarthria: The critical prerequisite to treatment. In M. M. Leahy (Ed.), *Disorders of communication: The science of intervention* (pp. 206–227). London: Taylor & Francis.

Baken, R. J. (1987). *Clinical measurement of speech and voice*. Boston: College-Hill Press.

Bellaire, K., Yorkston, K. M., & Beukelman, D. R. (1986). Modification of breath patterning to increase naturalness of a mildly dysarthric speaker. *Journal of Communication Disorders, 19,* 271–280.

Carman, B. G., & Ryan, G. (1989). EMG biofeedback and the treatment of communication disorders. In J. V. Basmajian (Ed.), *Biofeedback—Principles of practice for clinicians* (3rd ed., pp. 287–295). Baltimore: Williams & Wilkins.

Childers, D. G., & Krishnamurthy, A. K. (1985). A critical review of electroglottography. *CRC Critical Reviews in Biomedical Engineering, 12,* 131–161.

Daniel, B., & Guitar, B. (1978). EMG biofeedback and recovery of facial and speech gestures following neural anastomosis. *Journal of Speech and Hearing Disorders, 43,* 9–20.

Darley, F. L., Aronson, A. E., & Brown, J. R. (1975). *Motor speech disorders*. Philadelphia: W. B. Saunders.

FitzGerald, F. J., Murdoch, B. E., & Chenery, H. J. (1987). Multiple sclerosis: Associated speech and language disorders. *Australian Journal of Human Communication Disorders, 15,* 15–33.

Gentil, M. (1993). Speech rehabilitation in dysarthria. *Folia Phoniatrica, 45,* 31–35.

Hanson, D. G., Gerratt, B. R., Karin, R. R., & Berke, G. S. (1988). Glottographic measures of vocal fold vibration: An examination of laryngeal paralysis. *Laryngoscope, 98,* 541–548.

Hardy, J. C. (1967). Suggestions for physiological research in dysarthria. *Cortex, 3,* 128–156.

Hinton, V. A., & Luschei, E. S. (1992). Validation of a modern miniature transducer for measurement of interlabial contact pressure during speech. *Journal of Speech and Hearing Research, 35,* 245–251.

Horii, Y. (1980). An accelerometric approach to nasality measurement: A preliminary report. *Cleft Palate Journal, 17,* 254–261.

Kearns, K. P., & Simmons, N. N. (1990). The efficacy of speech-language pathology intervention: Motor speech disorders. *Seminars in Speech and Language, 11,* 273–295.

Lippmann, R. P. (1981). Detecting nasalization using a low-cost miniature accelerometer. *Journal of Speech and Hearing Research, 24,* 314–317.

Manifold, J. A. Y., & Murdoch, B. E. (1993). Speech breathing in young adults: Effect of body type. *Journal of Speech and Hearing Research, 36,* 657–671.

Motta, G., Cesari, U., Iengo, M., & Motta, G. (1990). Clinical application of electroglottography. *Folia Phoniatrica, 42,* 111–117.

Murdoch, B. E., Chenery, H. J., Bowler, S., & Ingram, J. C. L. (1989). Respiratory function in Parkinson's patients exhibiting a perceptible speech deficit: A kinematic and spirometric analysis. *Journal of Speech and Hearing Disorders, 54,* 610–626.

Najenson, T., Sazbon, L., Fiselzon, J., Becker, E., & Schecter, I. (1978). Recovery of communicative functions after prolonged traumatic coma. *Scandinavian Journal of Rehabilitation Medicine, 10,* 15–21.

Nemec, R. E., & Cohen, K. (1984). EMG biofeedback in the modification of hypertonia in spastic dysarthria: Case report. *Archives of Physical Medicine and Rehabilitation, 65,* 103–104.

Netsell, R. (1984). Physiological studies of dysarthria and their relevance to treatment. *Seminars in Speech and Language, 5,* 279–291.

Netsell, R. (1986). *A neurobiological view of speech production and the dysarthrias.* San Diego: College-Hill Press.

Netsell, R., & Cleeland, C. S. (1973). Modification of lip hypertonia in dysarthria using EMG feedback. *Journal of Speech and Hearing Disorders, 38,* 131–140.

Netsell, R., & Daniel, B. (1979). Dysarthria in adults: Physiologic approach in rehabilitation. *Archives of Physical Medicine and Rehabilitation, 60,* 502–508.

Netsell, R., & Hixon, T. J. (1992). Inspiratory checking in therapy for individuals with speech breathing dysfunction. *American Speech and Hearing Association, 34,* 152.

Netsell, R., Lotz, W. K., & Barlow, S. M. (1989). A speech physiology examination for individuals with dysarthria. In K. M. Yorkston & D. R. Beukelman (Eds.), *Recent advances in clinical dysarthria* (pp. 4–37). Boston: College-Hill Press.

Robin, D. A., Somodi, L. B., & Luschei, E. S. (1991). Measurement of strength and endurance in normal and articulation disordered subjects. In C. A. Moore, K. Yorkston, & D. R. Beukelman (Eds.), *Dysarthria and apraxia of speech: Perspectives on management* (pp. 173–184). Baltimore: Brookes.

Rosenbek, J. D., & La Pointe, L. L. (1985). The dysarthrias: Description, diagnosis and treatment. In D. F. Johns (Ed.), *Clinical management of neurogenic communicative disorders* (2nd ed., pp. 251–310). Boston: Little, Brown.

Sarno, M. T., & Levin, H. S. (1985). Speech and language disorders after closed head injury. In J. K. Darby (Ed.), *Speech evaluation in neurology: Adult disorders* (pp. 323–339). New York: Grune & Stratton.

Workinger, M., & Netsell, R. (1992). Restoration of intelligible speech 13 years post-head injury. *Brain Injury, 6,* 183–187.

Ylvisaker, M. S., & Urbanczyk, B. (1990). The efficacy of speech-language pathology intervention: Traumatic brain injury. *Seminars in Speech and Language, 11*(4), 215–224.

13

Vegetative State: Challenges, Controversies, and Caveats A Physiatric Perspective

Nathan D. Zasler

The rehabilitation community has raised its voice in response to recent publications and implied statements by specialists in neurology and neurosurgery that may directly impact the diagnosis and treatment of patients who are minimally responsive following severe traumatic brain injury (TBI). A recent publication, authored by a multisociety task force sans rehabilitation specialists, entitled "Medical Aspects of the Persistent Vegetative State" appeared in the *New England Journal of Medicine*, triggering a strong response from those in clinical rehabilitation (Multi-Society Task Force on PVS, 1994b). Specifically, we were concerned with the differences in opinion on nomenclature issues, accuracy of diagnosis of the vegetative state, implications regarding quality of life relative to level of functional disability, and concerns regarding potential use of recent literature to make clinical decisions that may adversely and inappropriately impact on clinical and research decisions. A transcultural, multination, transdisciplinary consensus panel convened in England in early 1995, providing a foundation for future discourse and resolution of some of the rehabilitation community's aforementioned concerns. More recent cross-disciplinary developments, supported and facilitated to a great extent, by the Brain Injury Association (formerly National Head Injury Foundation) in the United States have resulted in an ongoing dialogue and effort to continue work on formation of guidelines for diagnosis and treatment of vegetative, as well as, minimally responsive states.

OVERVIEW OF NOMENCLATURE
AND ASSESSMENT ISSUES

One of the major problems faced by clinicians in the field of neuro-trauma care has been the lack of a consistent nomenclature germane to low-level neurological states following severe brain injury, both traumatic and non-traumatic (Zasler, Kreutzer, & Taylor, 1991). Another major issue has been the relative lack of understanding of the existing nomenclature and a tendency toward inappropriate diagnoses and subsequently incorrect conclusions regarding neurological and functional prognoses, as well as, necessary treatment. Ultimately, clinicians must universally agree on a nomenclature and understand the clinical implications of such a system relative to diagnosis, prognosis, and treatment.

Although the recent neurological and neurosurgical multisociety task force document clarified some of these issues, there are still significant concerns regarding some of the conclusions and recommendations made in the aforementioned document. Historically, nomenclature systems for minimally responsive patients with brain injury have been behaviorally based. Yet, within the context of prior paradigms, insufficient emphasis has been placed on neurobehavioral assessment. Clinicians must take adequate time to behaviorally assess patients at the bedside if any nomenclature system dependent on neurobehavioral criteria is to be used in an accurate and responsible fashion.

The assessment of the minimally responsive patient is further complicated by the need for a thorough understanding of the limitations of a brief bedside assessment in an otherwise severely disabled patient, given the normally expected fluctuations in levels of arousal and awareness. Additionally, the examiner must understand what clinical findings are consistent with cortical versus subcortical neurobehavioral responses, as well as, what factors, both neurologic and medical, may confound the neurobehavioral assessment.

DIAGNOSTIC NOMENCLATURE
IN SEVERE BRAIN INJURY

The major diagnostic neurobehavioral terms that are germane to a discussion of nomenclature in persons with severe alterations in consciousness are coma, vegetative state, minimally responsive state (akinetic mutism being a subcategory of this larger group), and locked-in syndrome. These terms describe the scope of neurobehavioral presentations for persons who typically present at Rancho Los Amigos Cognitive Behavioral Levels of I–III based on apparent outward "neurobehavioral appearance" following severe brain injury. To the clinician who has become sensitized to appropriate neurobehavioral assessment, there are significant differences between these different populations. For readers interested in a more comprehensive document presenting the rehabilitation perspective on recommended nomenclature in patients with severe alterations in consciousness, please see Giacino, Zasler, Whyte, Katz, Glenn, and Andary (1995).

Coma

Coma is a state of unarousable neurobehavioral unresponsiveness. Neurobehaviorally, patients in coma typically (a) present with eyes closed without evidence of opening either spontaneously or to external stimulation, (b) do not follow commands, (c) do not demonstrate goal directed/volitional behavior, (d) do not verbalize or mouth words, and (e) cannot sustain visual pursuit movements beyond a 45 degree arc. One must, of course, exclude neurobehavioral signs and symptoms of coma secondary to pharmacological treatment with agents such as paralytic or sedative drugs.

Vegetative State

Vegetative state (VS) patients demonstrate arousal without concurrent awareness. Neurobehaviorally, patients in a vegetative state (a) have periods of eye opening, either spontaneously or following stimulation, (b) may demonstrate subcortical physiological responses to external stimulation including generalized physiological responses to pain, such as posturing, tachycardia, and diaphoresis, as well as subcortical motor responses, such as a grasp reflex, (c) demonstrate return of so-called vegetative (autonomic) functions, including sleep–wake cycles, and normalization of respiratory and digestive system functions, and (d) may show roving eye movements without concomitant visual tracking ability.

   The presence of subcortical responses should not be considered as pathognomonic of VS because these findings may also be seen in minimally responsive patients. Additionally, there is no way that we are aware of to clinically assess internal awareness in a patient otherwise unable to express awareness relative to external environmental stimuli. Thus, it is theoretically possible that some patients who are indeed conscious at some level are incorrectly labeled as being in a VS. Practitioners should also understand that there is no neurodiagnostic or laboratory test that allows the clinician to diagnose VS. The diagnosis of VS is *only* made by serial neurobehavioral assessment.

   Patients in persistent or permanent vegetative state (PVS) meet all the neurobehavioral criteria that patients in vegetative state do. Note that the acronym PVS is now even more confusing due to the inability to determine which modifier is being referred to . . . persistent or permanent. There continues to be some controversy with regard to the use of modifiers such as persistent or permanent vegetative state (Giacino et al., 1995). Many practitioners, including the originator of the phrase "persistent vegetative state", Dr. Bryan Jennett, now believe that the modifier "persistent" should be abandoned as it is poorly understood by clinicians, families, and payors and it adds nothing to clinical management (Jennett, personal communication, 1995). Some practitioners believe that there is insufficient methodologically sound research to label any VS patient as permanently vegetative, thereby implying no potential for further neurologic improvement. Unfortunately, the multisociety task force has recommended that the term permanent be utilized in any patient 1 year after trauma or 3 months after hypoxic-ischemic insult (MSTF on PVS, 1994a/1994b). Smallpox, tuberculosis, bubonic plague, and spinal cord injury were all once thought to be permanent. Such nomenclature has the strong potential to create a self-prophesizing environment, which surely does not encourage clinicians and scientists to pursue treatments that may ameliorate the condition and potentially improve quality of life. Such pejorative labels also have the unfortunate tendency to negatively affect the manner in which clinicians broach patient care. One often observes clinicians becoming much more cavalier in their treatment aggressiveness and more relaxed in their commitment to the ongoing efforts of friends and family. It must also be realized that little methodologically sound prospective data exists regarding the natural history of patients in vegetative state beyond 1 year following trauma. So the question of whether we really know what happens to this group of patients is still up in the air. Lastly, clinicians must be aware of the fact that life expectancy determinations for a particular patient cannot accurately be made simply by looking at life expectancy averages for the vegetative population at large.

In general, it has been my philosophy to endorse a time frame of 1 year for traumatic and 3 months for hypoxic-ischemic brain injury for prognostic purposes relative to determining that emergence from vegetative state is statistically highly unlikely. Such a determination should only occur after an adequate period of extended patient observation and sufficient neuromedical assessment to rule-out treatable conditions potentially affecting ongoing neural and functional recovery. Any cases of late emergence, that is more than one year following trauma or 3 months following hypoxic-ischemic insult, from vegetative state should without a doubt be reported in peer-reviewed scientific literature.

Minimally Responsive State

Minimally responsive (MR) patients are no longer in a coma or VS but demonstrate low-level neurobehavioral response consistent with severe neurological impairment and disability. Patients who are MR are able to demonstrate, albeit intermittently and possibly incompletely, some level of awareness to environmental stimulation consistent with the presence of cognitive function. The examining clinician must take into consideration both the frequency and the context of the behavioral response to interpret the meaningfulness and/or purposefulness of a given behavior. This group of brain injury patients has been recognized only recently as a subcategory of its own. As a result, there is no formal prospective data per se of any significance regarding the natural history of recovery and/or morbidity in this group of patients. There is however experiential evidence that patients who are minimally responsive may continue to make improvements neurologically and functionally for many years postinsult, particularly when the initial event was traumatic as opposed to hypoxic-ischemic.

Unfortunately, the media in the United States often inaccurately represents information regarding late "miracle" recoveries following brain injury even when provided with contrary information and/or professional input suggesting alternative explanations. This is not uncommon in minimally responsive patients who are claimed to have been comatose or vegetative for extended periods of time. All too often, inadequate information is provided regarding prior neuromedical findings and work-up, present medications, and injury history. This type of media hype only serves to promulgate unfortunate misconceptions among less sophisticated health care providers and the lay community at large.

Akinetic Mutism

Akinetic mutism (AM) is a neurobehavioral condition marked by severe disturbances in behavioral drive. In actuality, it is a neurobehavioral subset of the MR subgroup. Generally, a minimal degree of movement (kinesis) and speech is elicitable. As opposed to most other low-level neurobehavioral disorders, AM is associated with damage to dopaminergic pathways, including the mesoceruleal, diencephalospinal, and/or mesocorticolimbic (Nemeth, Hegedus, & Monar, 1986). Patients with frontal AM tend to be more vigilant than those with midbrain AM, and the former group may even demonstrate episodic agitation. Patients with AM typically demonstrate eye opening with visual tracking, little-to-no spontaneous speech, and infrequent as well as minimal command following. This subgroup of MR patients may respond particularly well to treatment with dopaminergic agonist administration with agents such as amantadine, sinemet, and bromocriptine.

Locked-in Syndrome

Locked-in syndrome (LIS) is a relatively rare, albeit important, neuro-behavioral condition associated with lesions of the ventral pons. Clinically, patients with LIS present with anarthria and quadriplegia in the "complete form" of the condition. Disruption of corticospinal and cortico bulbar pathways at the level of the pons results in preservation of rostral and dorsal pontine function, thereby, implying intact cognitive function and arousal. Vertical eye movements and blinking are preserved, yet there is typically significant lower cranial nerve and sleep–wake cycle dysfunction. It is of utmost importance for clinicians to be aware of the differences in this patient population from VS and MR, relative not only to level of cognitive function but also long term neurologic prognosis.

LIMITATIONS OF ASSESSMENT AND PROGNOSIS

It is my belief that no medical specialty is particularly adept, based on either training or experience, with regard to differential diagnosis of patients who are in low-level neurologic states following severe TBI. That is, even the experts will often have trouble agreeing as to the state of consciousness that a particular patient has at a particular time, as was apparent in claimed persistent VS cases in the media such as that of Karen Quinlan. Such lack of agreement simply suggests that current assessment methodologies are lacking and have a limited degree of both specificity and sensitivity.

One can never be 100% sure that a patient is vegetative, never mind persistently or permanently vegetative. We can never determine with total accuracy whether there is any degree of cognitive awareness of either internal or external environment. A patient may be so motorically and communication impaired that it is impossible to get a "readable" behavioral response consistent with such awareness. This margin of error must be accounted for in both clinical and ethical arenas.

NATURAL HISTORY OF THE VEGETATIVE STATE

It is becoming evident that there are more and more case studies of *isolated* exceptions to the rule that "once vegetative, always vegetative," particularly beyond the 1 year threshold following traumatic insults

(Arts, Hof-Van Duin Van, & Lammens, 1985; Childs & Mercer, 1996; Horiguchi, Inami, & Shoda, 1990; May & Kaelbling, 1968; Rosenberg, Johnson, & Brenner, 1977; Snyder, Cranford, & Rubens, 1983; Stewart & Gonzalez-Rothi, 1990; Tanhehco & Kaplan, 1982). One cannot accurately compare, however, pure hypoxic-ixchemic brain injury outcomes with those of TBI, where there may or may not be associated hypoxic insult. Additionally, many reported cases of late recovery from prolonged post-traumatic VS (after 1 year) are at best anecdotal, often with poor documentation that the patient was truly in a VS. Consequentially, all patients should receive ongoing monitoring for *any* change in neurological or functional status before *and* after the 1 year mark (Choi, Barnes, Bullock, Germanson, Marmarou, & Young, 1994; Levin, Saydjari, Eisenberg, Foulkes, Marshall, & Ruff (1991).

From the available outcome data examining the evolution of VS, it is apparent that there is approximately a 3% incidence rate of VS at 1 year postinjury (Bartowski & Lovely, 1986; Braakman, Jennett, & Minderhoud, 1988). This obviously has significant implications for the thousands of individuals left in this condition annually in terms of appropriate resource utilization, as well as provision of adequate maintenance care. It is generally believed that patients who have previously received adequate neuromedical care and can confidently be said to be in VS 1 year after trauma do not belong in rehabilitation programs but rather in skilled nursing home facilities or, if appropriate and logistically possible, at home with family. Certainly, there are also implications for cost-shifting even before 1 year following trauma in a patient who remains vegetative, but the exact manner by which to do this is still being debated.

ROLE OF REHABILITATION IN LOW-LEVEL NEUROLOGIC STATES

One of the criticisms of the multisociety document was the lack of discussion, if not exclusion, of information regarding the role of rehabilitation outside of a cursory review of "coma stimulation" literature and a brief mention of possible pharmacotherapeutic interventions (Zasler, Giacino, & Sandel, 1994). Interdisciplinary rehabilitative management of this patient population involves preventing potential morbidity issues as well as providing appropriate neuromedical and rehabilitative interventions to maximize potential neurologic and functional outcome. Rational neuromedical and rehabilitation management of this patient population has been delineated in several articles (Giacino & Zasler, 1995; Horn, 1989; Sandel & Ellis, 1990; Whyte & Glenn, 1986).

A full neuromedical work-up must be performed prior to labeling a patient as vegetative. Adequate understanding of the "late" neuromedical sequelae of traumatic brain injury is essential in the care and treatment of this population. Medical conditions such as posttraumatic epilepsy, particularly of the nonconvulsive type, posttraumatic hydrocephalus, neuroendocrine dysfunction, occult infection, late subdural hematomas, and iatrogenically induced problems related to inappropriate use of pharmacological agents may all cause an individual to "look" vegetative when indeed they are not (Horn, 1989). Appropriate care should emphasize minimizing morbidity and treating any underlying condition(s) potentially suppressing neural recovery potential, good nursing care with a emphasis on skin, respiratory, and bowel/bladder care, and appropriate and timely prescription of adaptive equipment including seating and orthotics (Giacino & Zasler, 1995; Sandel & Ellis, 1990). Family involvement, education, and counseling should also be an integral part of *any* early recovery management program (ERMP).

The issue of whether so-called structured sensory stimulation (SSS) can in any way be a negative factor in recovery has only recently been theorized. Such issues of how stimulation may cause over-arousal and increase fatigue, decrease seizure threshold, and/or increase maladaptive plasticity including spasticity definitely need to be looked at more critically. Nonetheless, the literature supporting a utility for such structured stimulation programs is lacking and most clinicians in the field would acknowledge that SSS probably has no effect on either rate or eventual plateau of neural recovery (Zasler, Kreutzer, & Taylor, 1991). If sensory stimulation is offered, it should be done in a cost-efficient, ethical, and responsible fashion, not as the major component of the total program. The exact role of other, more controversial interventions, such as neural stimulation and pharmacotherapy for promoting recovery from VS, remains unanswered but definitely warrants further research in a controlled, blinded fashion to establish their efficacy (Giacino & Zasler, 1995).

As a community of health care providers, rehabilitation clinicians have sufficient experiential consensus as well as a growing base of prospective data regarding the efficacy of early and intensive rehabilitative treatment to minimize short- and long-term morbidity, decrease health care costs, and optimize long-term functional outcomes.

QUALITY OF LIFE ISSUES

Issues regarding quality of outcome must also be broached, particularly given the statements made in the multisociety document implying that "severe disability", presumptively as defined by the Glasgow Outcome

Scale (GOS), was as bad a functional outcome as vegetative state. Those of us who have worked with enough patients with severe disabilities know that there is a wide range of functional capabilities within the severe disability category (by GOS or any other grading system). It is important to acknowledge that severe disability occurs along a continuum of severity. It could be purely and/or mainly physical, or range from patients who are noncommunicative and totally dependent for care but aware, at least to some extent of their environment, to those who are communicative to some degree and able to assist with life tasks. Quality of life issues must be seen first from the standpoint of the patient and second from the standpoint of the family. Clinician opinions should rank tertiary, with payor opinions last. Severe disability may seem like a poor quality of life to one person but may seem quite acceptable to another given the potential options including VS and/or death.

CONCLUSIONS

Professionals and families dealing with individuals in prolonged VS following severe brain injury are faced with many issues, including but not limited to, withdrawal and withholding of care, as well as ethicolegal aspects of long-term care (Council on Scientific Affairs and Council on Ethical and Judicial Affairs, 1990; Sandel & Ellis, 1990). We can only broach these issues if we have a full and collective understanding of the issues at hand, including a commitment to continue efforts at researching better ways to manage such patients and developing methodologies to explore novel treatment approaches to facilitate emergence from VS.

The field of rehabilitation has clearly made critical contributions to the care of this special population including development of neurobehavioral assessment measures, formulation of interventions to decrease morbidity, and coordination of life care planning. The rehabilitation community strongly encourages all clinicians to advocate for consensus regarding guidelines for diagnosis, prognosis, and treatment of patients in coma, VS, and MR. Without involvement of all relevant parties in the process of guideline development, one runs the risk of adversely affecting the quality of health care service provided to this sector of patients. Multidisciplinary research efforts sponsored and endorsed by the major medical organizations (AAPM&R, ANA, AANS) should be encouraged. Ultimately, society's best interests would be served through more intensive collaborative efforts directed at promoting our understanding of the pathophysiology, diagnosis, and treatment of vegetative state, regardless of its duration.

REFERENCES

Arts, W. F. M., Dongen Van, H. R., Hof-Van Duin Van, J., & Lammens, E. (1985). Unexpected improvement after prolonged postraumatic vegetative state. *Journal of Neurology, Neurosurgery and Psychiatry, 48,* 1300–1303.

Bartowski, H. M., & Lovely, M. P. (1986). Prognosis in coma and the persistent vegetative state. *Journal of Head Trauma Rehabilitation, 1,* 1–6.

Braakman, R., Jennett, W. B., & Minderhoud, J. M. (1988). Prognosis of the posttraumatic vegetative state. *Acta Neurochirurchica, 95,* 49–52.

Childs, N. L., & Mercer, W. N. (1996). Brief report: Late improvement in consciousness after post-traumatic vegetative state. *New England Journal of Medicine, 1*(334), 24–25.

Choi, S. C., Barnes, T. Y., Bullock, R., Germanson, T. A., Marmarou, A., & Young, H. F. (1994). Temporal profile of outcomes in severe head injury. *Journal of Neurosurgery, 81,* 169–173.

Council on Scientific Affairs and Council on Ethical and Judicial Affairs. (1990). Persistent vegetative state and the decision to withdraw or withhold life support. *Journal of the American Medical Association, 263,* 426–430.

Giacino, J. T., & Zasler, N. D. (1995). Outcome following severe brain injury: The comatose, vegetative and minimally responsive patient. *Journal of Head Trauma Rehabilitation, 10*(1), 40–56.

Giacino, J. T., Zasler, N. D., Whyte, J., Katz, D. I., Glenn, M., & Andary, M. (1995). Recommendations for use of uniform nomenclature pertinent to patients with severe alterations in consciousness. *Archives of Physical Medicine and Rehabilitation, 76,* 205–209.

Horn, L. J. (1989, June). Rational management of the vegetative patient. Workshop on coma stimulation. *The Postgraduate Course on Rehabilitation of the Brain Injured Adult and Child.* Williamsburg, Virginia.

Levin, H. S., Saydjari, C., Eisenberg, H. M., Foulkes, M., Marshall, L. F., & Ruff, R. M. (1991). Vegetative state after closed head injury. *Archives of Neurology, 48,* 580–585.

May, P. G., & Kaelbling, R. (1968). Coma of over a year's duration with favorable outcome. *Diseases of the Nervous System, 29,* 837–840.

Multi-Society Task Force on PVS. (1994a). Medical aspects of the persistent vegetative state (first of two parts). *New England Journal of Medicine, 330*(21), 1499–1508.

Multi-Society Task Force on PVS. (1994b). Medical aspects of the persistent vegetative state (second of two parts). *New England Journal of Medicine, 330*(22), 1572–1579.

Nemeth, G., Hegedus, K., & Monar, L. (1986). Akinetic mutism and lock-in syndrome: The functional-anatomical basis for their differentiation. *Functional Neurology, 1*(2), 128–139.

Rosenberg, G. A., Johnson, S. F., & Brenner, R. P. (1977). Recovery of cognition after prolonged vegetative state. *Annals of Neurology, 2,* 167–168.

Sandel, M. E., & Ellis, D. W. (Eds.). (1990). *The coma-emerging patient.* Philadelphia, PA: Hanley & Belfus, Inc.

Snyder, B. D., Cranford, R. E., Rubens, A. B. (1983). Delayed recovery from postanoxic persistent vegetative state. *Annals of Neurology, 14,* 152.

Stewart, J. T., & Gonzalez-Rothi, L. J. (1990). Treatment of a case of akinetic mutism with bromocriptine. *Journal of Neuropsychiatry, 2,* 462–463.

Tanhehco, J., & Kaplan, P. E. (1982). Physical and surgical rehabilitation of patient after 6-year coma. *Archives of Physical Medicine and Rehabilitation, 63,* 36–38.

Whyte, J., & Glenn, M. B. (1986). The care and rehabilitation of the patient in a persistent vegetative state. *Journal of Head Trauma Rehabilitation, 1*, 39–53.

Zasler, N. D., Giacino, J., Sandel, M. E. (1994). Letter to the editor. *New England Journal of Medicine, 331*(20), 1381.

Zasler, N. D., Kreutzer, J. S., & Taylor, D. (1991). Coma recovery and coma stimulation: A critical review. *Neuro-Rehabilitation: An Interdisciplinary Journal, 1*(3), 33–40.

Timing and Outcomes

Brain Plasticity and Behavior During Development

Bryan Kolb

There is general agreement that injury to the brain in infancy has different consequences than similar injury in adulthood. In fact, this difference was noted as long ago as 1965 by Broca. However, no uniform agreement exists on how or why the consequences are different in infancy and adulthood. One of the most common views on the effects of early brain injury has come to be known as the Kennard Principle. Beginning in the 1930s, Margaret Kennard studied the effects of motor cortex lesions in monkeys. She reported that infant monkeys appeared to have a better behavioral outcome than adult monkeys with similar injuries (Kennard, 1938, 1940). Later, Hans-Leukas Teuber concluded from Kennard's results that if you are going to have brain damage, have it early, which is what Teuber dubbed the Kennard Principle. The Kennard Principle has some intuitive appeal because it is a common observation that infants seem to recover quickly from many maladies. Because the infant brain is developing, it seems reasonable that it would compensate better than the adult brain. In fact, it is rare for children to experience lasting aphasia, which is a major problem for adults with left-hemisphere injuries. Various authors have used this observation as evidence for plasticity in the infant brain (e.g., Lenneberg, 1967).

There are two fundamental problems with the Kennard Principle. First, it assumes that all developing brains are equivalent. The brain goes through many stages of development, however, and it is a very different brain in each stage. After neurons are born, they must migrate to their appropriate location, differentiate into a particular neuron type with specific dendritic morphology, and establish area-specific connections. During these different stages, the brain is exposed to various factors, including hormones and other growth factors, each of which has specific effects on neuronal development. In addition, the brain must develop supporting structures such as glia and capillaries. Thus, injury at different stages of brain development, which is probably not complete in humans until well into adolescence, has different morphological, and thus behavioral, consequences.

Second, the Kennard principle ignores that brain development is much like building a house. You must begin with a foundation, then progress to framing, and so on. If the foundation is inadequate, there is nothing in the framing that will help. The idea that there is an important, and necessary, sequence in both brain and cognitive development was first clearly stated by Hebb, and thus I take the liberty of calling his idea the "Hebb Principle." Hebb (1949) studied children with damage to the frontal lobes in infancy, and concluded that brain damage early in life may be worse than later damage because some aspects of cognitive development are critically dependent on the integrity of particular cerebral structures at certain times in development. In other words, if certain structures do not work properly during critical periods in development, it may be that cognitive development is adversely affected and the child is never able to adequately compensate. One could imagine, for example, that if the auditory cortex is injured early in life, then language development could be compromised. Indeed, abnormal auditory processing has been proposed as an important cause of learning disabilities (e.g., Tallal, Stark, & Mellits, 1985a, 1985b).

Thus, although it seems that early brain injury can sometimes allow for better recovery than later injury, there is substantial evidence that suggest the opposite is also true. This apparent contradiction in the sequelae of early brain damage provides a conundrum for both the clinician and the scientist. There must be some basic principles that determine what the outcome of early brain damage will be. In the course of studying the effects of early brain injury in laboratory animals, my colleagues and I have identified several such principles.

THE BEHAVIORAL CONSEQUENCES OF FRONTAL LOBE INJURY IN INFANCY

Perhaps the most dramatic evidence of recovery from early childhood brain injury comes from the observations that children with frontal lobe damage early in life rarely have aphasia later in life, even when the injury is centered in the region of Broca's area. At the same time, it is a common observation that children with left-hemisphere injuries in the speech zones show unexpected deficits in right-hemisphere functions, as well as an overall drop in IQ (e.g., Woods, 1980; Woods & Teuber, 1973). Therefore, the frontal lobe appears to provide a particularly interesting region to search for principles underlying brain plasticity and behavior. Initial studies of the effects of early frontal lobe lesions in rhesus monkeys supported the general idea that there was better recovery after infant injuries than adult injuries (Harlow, Akert, & Schiltz, 1964). Subsequent studies by Goldman-Rakic and her colleagues (Goldman-Rakic, Isseroff, Schwartz, & Bugbee, 1983) suggested that the extent of recovery had been overestimated because the animals were tested when they were still young. Thus, she found that as animals with dorsolateral prefrontal lesions in early infancy developed, they became progressively more impaired at cognitive tasks known to be dependent on the integrity of the frontal lobe, such as the delayed alternation task. This result suggests that the infant brain is able to solve certain cognitive tasks using cerebral structures, such as the striatum, which develop relatively early in life. But as the cerebral cortex develops, it assumes these functions and subsequently allows more efficient performance. If the cortex is abnormal, the functions cannot be assumed by the cortex, and a deficit appears.

Similar results have been observed in children. For example, Banich, Cohen-Levine, Kim, and Huttenlocher (1990) studied the development of performance on two subtests of the Wechsler Intelligence Scale for Children (WISC; viz. vocabulary and block design) in children with congenital cerebral injuries. The authors found that at 6 years of age, there were no significant differences in performance. As the children aged, significant deficits emerged in the brain-damaged children relative to matched normal controls. Thus, it appears that as the children's brains grew, they "grew into deficits." This observation appears to confirm the Hebb Principle, and is especially problematic in making predictions regarding the prognosis for children with cerebral injuries. We are still confronted, however, with the obvious absence of aphasia in children, which means, at least under some conditions, there is good recovery after injury in infancy.

A study by Goldman and Galkin (1978) may provide some insight into this paradox. Goldman and Galkin surgically induced frontal lobe injuries in prenatal monkeys. They subsequently found that these animals showed significant sparing of performance on tests like delayed alternation, and that this sparing persisted into adulthood. Thus, it does appear that frontal injury early in development might allow significant recovery of function. However, monkeys are born embryologically more mature than humans, so it is not altogether clear exactly when this "optimal" time might be.

Another difficulty with using monkeys as subjects in studies of recovery from early cortical injury is that they are slow developing, and there is typically only one infant born at a time. Therefore, my colleagues and

I decided to investigate the effects of frontal cortical injuries in rats. Rats have large litters of pups, who develop quickly and are embryologically very young when they are born. Therefore, it is possible to surgically perturb the rat brain over a significant portion of its cortical development.

I have prepared a working timetable of cortical development in rats and humans (see Fig. 14.1), and have identified several important times as tentative markers. These include: the completion of neurogenesis, the completion of cell migration, the time of maximum dendritic growth in the superficial and intrinsic neurons, and the point of maximum synaptic density. For the human, I have taken values for visual cortex because this is probably the most studied region, and there is a substantial range in different cortical regions (Marin-Padilla, 1970a, 1970b). One conclusion to draw from Fig. 14.1 is that the cortex of the rat changes very rapidly during development. During the first week of life, cell division is largely complete, but neurons are still migrating from the ventricular zone to their appropriate region. In the second week of life, the neurons are rapidly differentiating and beginning to develop connections. This increase in connectivity reaches a peak sometime around 1 month of age. These three stages of cortical growth are substantially different in the extent to which they permit cortical plasticity after injury.

Our first task was to develop behavioral measures of frontal cortical function in the rat. With this in mind, my colleagues and I developed a neuropsychological test battery that assesses a wide variety of species-typical and learned behaviors of the rat (e.g., Whishaw, Kolb, & Suther

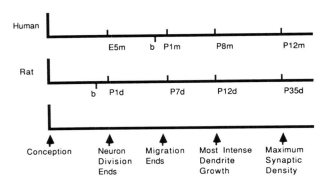

FIG. 14.1.   Tentative timetable for the comparison of brain development in the rat and human. Notice that birth is at different times in brain development. The "optimal" time for cortical injury appears to be after migration is complete, during the period of intense dendritic growth. Injury during the period of mitosis or migration leads to a miserable behavioral outcome.

land, 1983). Many of these tasks have proved especially vulnerable to the effects of damage to different regions of the frontal cortex (for reviews, see Kolb, 1984, 1990). For present purposes, I focus on two tasks that are performed poorly by adult animals with medial prefrontal cortex removals in adulthood.

The first task, which I call the *Whishaw reaching task*, measures the ability of rats to reach using their forepaws (e.g., Whishaw, O'Connor, & Dunnett, 1986). The essential features of this task are that (a) rats learn to reach through bars to retrieve small pieces of food, and (b) the animals can be forced to use just one paw by placing a bracelet around the wrist of the other arm so that it does not fit through the bars. Reaching ability can be assessed by measuring endpoint success, such as accuracy of reaching (i.e., percent of reaches in which the animal successfully retrieves food), or by videotaping the animal's behavior and doing more refine kinematic analyses on different aspects of the actual movements. Rats with medial prefrontal lesions that include the cingulate corticospinal projection are severely impaired at reaching in this task.

The second task was devised by Morris (1980). In this task, rats are trained to swim to a platform that is located just under the surface of the water in a large tank. The water is tinted with a bit of powdered milk, and thus the platform becomes invisible to the animal in the tank and can be located only by learning its location relative to a constellation of cues in the extramaze environment. Rats are aquatic animals, and thus learn to find the platform with only a few trials of practice. Performance on this task can be measured by (a) recording the time taken to swim to the platform, (b) measuring the distance swum, or (c) measuring the accuracy in heading directly to the platform (e.g., Sutherland, Whishaw, & Kolb, 1983). Rats with medial prefrontal lesions that include the prelimbic cortex are slow to learn the location of the hidden platform; if the lesions are extensive, they never learn to swim directly to it (e.g., Fantie & Kolb, 1990). Thus, by using these two measures, it is possible to identify conditions under which there is lesser or greater functional recovery after injury to the frontal cortex of rats.

Our second task was to consider what the sequelae of early frontal cortical injury in the rat might be at different times in cortical development. Over the past two decades, we have injured the frontal regions on virtually every postnatal day between birth and weaning at 3 weeks. These studies have led to three basic findings. First, cortical injury from birth to about 5 or 6 days of age is associated with a dismal functional outcome (e.g., Kolb, 1987). For example, when rats with lesions on the day of life are tested in adulthood on either the Morris water task or the Whishaw reaching task, they are more impaired than animals with similar injuries in adulthood (Fig. 14.2). Second, rats with similar injuries in

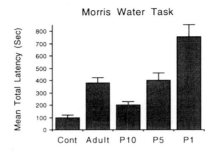

Morris Water Task

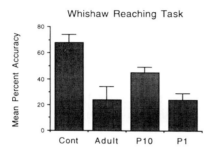

Whishaw Reaching Task

FIG. 14.2. (a) Summary of rats' performance in the Morris water task. The ordinate indicates the total time taken to find the hidden platform over 80 trials of testing. Rats with lesions on postnatal Day 10 (P10) perform significantly better than rats with lesions at other ages. Those with lesions on postnatal Day 1 (PN1) perform miserably relative to all other groups. (b) Summary of accuracy in reaching in the Whishaw reaching task. Normal rats are accurate in about 70% of their attempts, whereas rats with frontal lesions in adulthood seldom perform better than about 20%. Rats with lesions on postnatal Day 10 (P10) show some recovery on this task, whereas those with lesions on Day 1 (P1) do not.

the second week of life show almost complete recovery on some behavioral tasks, and substantial recovery on most (e.g., Kolb & Nonneman, 1978; Kolb & Whishaw, 1981). Thus, such animals perform well in the Morris task and far better than adult operates in the Whishaw task (Fig. 14.2). Third, injury to the older infant (after about Day 15) or adolescent brain allows only a small improvement in outcome relative to adult operates (e.g., Kolb, Gibb, & Muirhead, 1995; Kolb & Whishaw, 1981). Thus, it appears that cerebral injury during cell migration is particularly damaging, whereas injury only a few days later, during the time of dendritic growth, allows good recovery. This observation provides a simple explanation for Goldman's results from monkeys. Injury to the prenatal monkey brain, which was approximately equivalent embryologically to the 7- to 10-day-old rat, allowed recovery, whereas injury to the infant monkey, which is equivalent to later infancy in the rat, allowed only marginal recovery.

One lesson here is that we should not focus on the day of birth because it bears little relationship to the embryological state of the brain, which is the key consideration. I note, parenthetically, that the striking difference between cortical injury in the first and second weeks of life is not confined to the prefrontal cortex, but appears to be a general characteristic of cortical injury. We found similar results following damage to the motor, parietal, and visual cortex as well (for a review, see Kolb, 1995).

Two behavioral questions arise from our studies. First, when does the behavioral recovery occur after injury in the second week? That is, does the recovery occur quickly after the injury, does it appear in adolescence, or is it even later to develop? Second, to what extent does the lesion size influence the extent of recovery? To answer the first question, we took advantage of the fact that young rats can first solve the Morris task on postnatal Day 19. We therefore gave rats frontal lesions on Day 1 or Day 10 of life, and then began testing them in the Morris task on Day 19. To my surprise, rats with lesions at either age were impaired at the task and had failed to learn it even by Day 25 (Kolb & Gibb, 1993). We decided to give the animals more recovery time and to retest them in adolescence. We then retested the animals at Day 56 and found that, whereas the Day 1 rats were still severely impaired at the task, the Day 10 rats performed as well as normal control animals. In other words, the animals had "grown out of their deficits." Stated differently, it seems likely that what- ever plastic process supports recovery seen in adult rats, who had sus- tained injuries on Day 10, continues well after the injury. To investigate the second question, we began by making small unilateral frontal lesions at different postnatal ages and found almost complete recovery at vir- tually any age. This led us to vary the lesion size from small restricted frontal lesions to complete hemidecortication.

THE BEHAVIORAL CONSEQUENCES OF HEMIDECORTICATION IN INFANCY

I restrict my comments here to the effects of hemidecortication. Because we found that bilateral injuries to frontal, motor, or parietal cortex were all associated with the best behavioral outcome around 10 days of age, we anticipated finding the same result with hemidecortication. How- ever, this was not the case. Hemidecortication allowed the best outcome the earlier it was performed. Thus, when we removed the hemisphere on the day of birth, we found a far better outcome than when the hemisphere was removed later, such as on Day 10 (Kolb & Tomie, 1988). This result has a straightforward implication. Recovery must be medi- ated by the intact hemisphere in the hemidecorticate, and the earlier the hemisphere is recruited to support recovery, the more plastic it is.

This contrasts to the effects of bilateral lesions, and thus leads to another conclusion. In the case of bilateral injury, the recovery is being mediated by an injured hemisphere. It is likely that the poor behavioral outcome after frontal lesions on the day of birth is because development of the remaining hemisphere is severely compromised. In the case of the hemidecorticate, there is no parallel because there is no remaining hemisphere. Rather, it appears that the absence of the hemisphere may have some beneficial effect on the growth and development of the remaining normal hemisphere. This leads to a clear prediction: It is likely that any perturbation of the remaining hemisphere could be very disruptive.

To examine this possibility, we hemidecorticated animals at birth and then made either stab wounds or small sensorimotor cortex lesions in the remaining hemisphere (Kolb, Gibb, & Muirhead, 1995). The results were clear: The second lesion compromised the recovery because the animals were as behaviorally impaired as animals with hemidecortications in adulthood. Animals with only a stab wound in an otherwise normal brain were indistinguishable from normal controls. This finding is consistent with the clinical literature. For example, Vargha-Khadem, Watters, and O'Gorman (1985) showed that children with perinatal lesions of the language zones in the left hemisphere do not show a shift in language to the right hemisphere if there is a small right-hemisphere injury. Evidently recovery is dependent on the complete integrity of the hemisphere contralateral to a large lesion.

In summary, the mammalian neocortex develops through a series of stages: from the generation and migration of neurons to the appropriate location, axonal and dendritic growth, and synapse formation and pruning. The functional consequences of cortical injury vary with the developmental stage at the time of injury. Cortical injury during the end of the mitotic phase or during neuronal migration leads to a poor behavioral outcome. In rats, this period ranges from birth to about 6 days of age. In humans, it likely begins midway through the third trimester and continues through part of the first year. Cortical injury during the period of maximal dendritic differentiation and synapse formation is associated with the most complete recovery of function observed at any time in life. (I note as well that this period is also associated with maximal astrocyte development, which may turn out to be critical.) In rats, this begins at 7–10 days and probably continues into early adolescence, although this has not been determined. In humans, this period probably includes the second year of life, but the endpoint probably varies considerably with the area injured. Finally, the extent of an injury influences the likelihood of recovery. Thus, lesions that remove an entire functional area are less likely to allow recovery than lesions that leave part of a functional region intact. In addition, unilateral lesions allow better recovery than bilateral lesions, which may reflect the fact that a unilateral lesion removes only one half of a functional system.

GROSS ANATOMICAL SEQUELAE OF FRONTAL CORTEX INJURY DURING DEVELOPMENT

When we began our studies of neonatal neocortical lesions in rats, Whishaw and I were struck by three unexpected phenomena. First, adult brains of all animals with cortical lesions in the first 2 weeks of life were visibly smaller than the brains of animals with similar injury in adulthood (e.g., Kolb, Sutherland, & Whishaw, 1983; Kolb & Whishaw, 1981). When we quantified brain weight and brain dimensions, we found that both were reduced after damage to the prefrontal, motor, parietal, visual, or temporal cortex (e.g., Kolb et al., 1983). The loss in brain size is not equivalent at different ages, however, because those animals with the earliest lesions have the smallest brains. For example, rats with large frontal lesions on the day of birth have adult brains that weigh about 80% of the brains of animals with similar lesions in adulthood. Rats with lesions at 10 days of age have brains that weigh about 90% of adult operates. Thus, even the 10-day operates that show marked recovery of function had a much smaller brain than adults with similar lesions but that had a poorer behavioral outcome.

This appears to be a case of doing more with less, which is quite remarkable. Furthermore, the reduction in brain size in the youngest animals is so profound that these animals sometimes have brains that weigh less than animals with complete decortications in adulthood. We do not know the reasons for the small brains, but we have found that the decrease in brain size is immediate and can be measured 24 hours after the lesion (Kolb, 1987). In addition, the remaining cortex is visibly, and quantifiably, thinner than normal, and this too can be seen 24 hours after the lesion. This thinning of the cortex is worse the earlier the injury, and it is worse after frontal lesions than after posterior lesions. One reason for the decrease in cortical thickness is that there are fewer neurons across the thickness of the cortex. However, we do not know when the neurons disappear, nor do we know why they disappear (Kolb & Gibb, 1990).

The second unexpected finding was that when we investigated the brains of rats hemidecorticated in infancy, we found that in adulthood the cortex of the intact hemisphere was thicker than normal (e.g., Kolb et al., 1983). This is remarkable, especially because this cortex has lost its callosal connections, which would presumably tend to decrease cortical thickness. This is, in fact, the effect of hemidecortication in adulthood. In view of our finding that "earlier is best" in the hemidecorticate, we might predict that the earlier the hemidecortication, the thicker the cortex. This is indeed the case (e.g., Kolb & Tomie, 1988). The rats with the

earliest lesions—on the day of birth—had the thickest cortex. It is unlikely that the increased thickness is due to an increase in the number of
neurons in the normal hemisphere, and preliminary cell counts confirm
this hypothesis. Thus, we must look to other components of the cortex,
such as the extent of neuropil, glia, and capillaries, for an explanation of
the increased thickness.

The third unexpected finding was that when we made restricted medial frontal lesions at 7–12 days old, the lesion cavity filled in with neural
tissue (Kolb, 1995; Kolb, Petrie & Cioe, in press). That is, it appears that
the brain has regrown the lost tissue. Our studies of this phenomenon
are still ongoing but we have been able to demonstrate that new neurons
are formed after the lesions and these neurons have connections similar
to those in normal brains (Kolb, Gibb, Gorny, de Brabander & Whishaw,
1995). Furthermore, we have been able to show that if we block this
regrowth there is a reduction in functional recovery, which implies that
the new neurons contribute to the observed recovery. We have also
shown that if lesions are large, there is no regrowth. Thus, for the
studies of dendritic changes (see later) we have restricted our analyses to
rats with larger lesions.

DENDRITIC CHANGES AFTER CORTICAL
INJURIES DURING DEVELOPMENT

We have seen that injury to the cortex of newborn and 10-day-old rats
has different consequences on function as well as brain and cavity size.
In view of the puzzling finding that rats with lesions on Day 10 were
capable of showing recovery with a smaller brain, we directed our attention to changes in connectivity. Our initial studies failed to find obvious
changes in cortical inputs or outputs, therefore we focused on intrinsic
connectivity, which we inferred from changes in dendritic organization.

We began our dendritic studies by making frontal lesions in one hemisphere of newborn rats and subsequently making similar lesions in the
other hemisphere 9 days later. The animals were allowed to grow into
adulthood before being sacrificed, and their brains were prepared for
Golgi-Cox staining. If the neurons of the two hemispheres responded
differently to the lesions, there should be a clear difference in the dendritic organization of the neurons in the two hemispheres. The difference was dramatic (Fig. 14.3). Thus, when we looked at the brains of the
Day 1 and Day 10 animals, a qualitative difference was immediately
apparent. The pyramidal neurons throughout the cortex of the hemispheres with Day 10 lesions had far greater dendritic arborizations than
those in the Day 1 hemispheres. Quantification and comparison to the

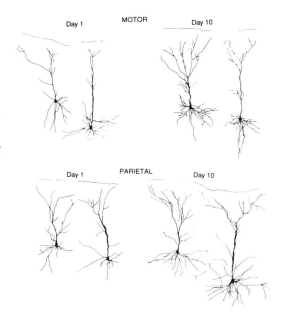

FIG. 14.3. Camera lucida drawings of Layer II/III pyramidal cells from the motor (top) and parietal (bottom) cortex of a rat with a frontal lesion in the left hemisphere on postnatal Day 1 and on the right hemisphere on postnatal Day 10. Notice that the neurons in both motor and parietal cortices are more complex in the left hemisphere, which had the lesion on Day 10. Cells from the brains of control rats are intermediate in complexity.

brains of normal littermates revealed that the rats with Day 10 lesions had more branches than normal control animals, whereas the Day 1 animals had fewer branches than normal (Kolb & Gibb, 1991, 1993; Kolb, Gibb, & van der Kooy, 1994). Furthermore, the animals with Day 10 lesions showed an increase throughout neocortex of the hemisphere. The dramatic contrast between the anatomical changes in animals with Day 1 and Day 10 frontal lesions complements the similar contrast in the functional outcomes in animals with lesions at these ages. This anatomy–behavior correlation led to the conclusion that the relationship may be causal. That is, it is possible that increased dendritic growth reflects increased synapse formation, and that this is necessary for recovery after early cortical injury (Kolb & Gibb, 1990).

The first challenge to this conclusion came from our own experiments, in which we made frontal lesions on postnatal Day 7 and then examined behavior and anatomy in adulthood (Kolb & Sutherland, 1992). Once again, we found that Day 7 lesions allowed significant recovery of function. Unexpectedly, relative to normal littermate controls, there was no increase in dendritic branching in the Day 7 operates. This result obviously compromised our hypothesis, and led us to examine spine density on the terminal branches of cortical pyramidal cells. The results showed a 15% higher density in the Day 7 frontal operates relative to their normal littermates (Kolb & Stewart, 1995). Hence, we subsequently reanalyzed the spine density in the Day 1 and Day 10 operates, and found a decrease in spine density in the Day 1 animals and a 15% increase in the Day 10 animals. Thus, it appears that both spine density and dendritic length are correlated with recovery. Because increasing both dendritic length and spine density would produce more synaptic space than just increasing spine density, it is not surprising that rats with Day 10 lesions show how better recovery than those with Day 7 lesions.

The second challenge to our dendrite–behavior correlation came from the experiment in which we examined the time course of recovery after Day 10 lesions. As described earlier, when the animals were tested in the Morris task on Days 19–22, they showed absolutely no evidence of recovery, whereas on Day 56 they showed virtually complete recovery when they were tested. If our dendrite–behavior correlation is meaningful, we had to predict that the dendritic changes were slow to develop and were not present on the first behavioral test, but were present on the second. Indeed, when we analyzed the dendritic arborization of the pyramidal cells, we found that our prediction was confirmed: The dendrites of the Day 10 animals showed no increase in either branching or spine density relative to normal brains or the brains of Day 1 operates at Day 22, but there was a dramatic difference on Day 60 (Fig. 14.4). This

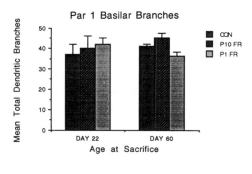

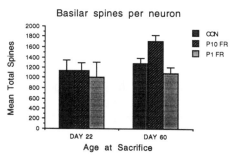

FIG. 14.4. Summary of dendritic branching and estimated spine numbers in Layer III pyramidal cells in parietal cortex of control rats (CON), and rats with frontal lesions on postnatal Day 1 (P1 FR) or Day 10 (P10 FR). Animals were sacrificed either on postnatal Day 22 or on postnatal Day 60. There is no significant dendritic remodeling on Day 22, but by Day 60 the neurons of rats with Day 10 lesions are more complex. These results suggest that the anatomical processes underlying recovery from cortical injury occur late in brain development.

result is therefore consistent with the general hypothesis that synaptic organization underlies the presence (or absence) of recovery from neocortical injury.

Our developmental result has two implications. First, the dendritic compensation to frontal lesions occurs slowly, even in developing animals. Second, in the absence of dendritic changes, there is no functional restitution. This suggests that treatments that might enhance dendritic growth, such as pharmacological or behavioral interventions, should facilitate recovery.

The correlation between dendritic growth and behavioral recovery after frontal lesions has led us to examine dendritic growth after other types of cortical lesions. In view of the marked recovery after neonatal hemidecortication, we wondered if the intact hemisphere would also show changes in dendritic growth. This question was especially interesting because we found an increase in cortical thickness after neonatal hemidecortication, and this did not appear to be due to an increase in the number of neurons. Our dendritic analysis confirmed our suspicions. Animals with hemidecortications on the day of birth showed a dramatic increase in dendritic arborization (Kolb, Gibb &, van der Kooy, 1992), but, to our surprise, this increase was restricted to motor and somatosensory cortices. We found no changes in visual or temporal cortices. This result might have been predicted because we had previously seen that the best functional recovery was in sensorimotor functions, rather than in visual or auditory functions, which showed rather poor recovery (e.g., Kolb & Tomie, 1988). That is, there was better restitution of behaviors, such as walking and reaching, than there was of visually guided behaviors, such as maze learning.

The dendritic results from the neonatal hemidecorticates led us to a prediction. I noted earlier that when we made small stab wounds in the normal hemisphere of neonatal hemidecorticates, we severely compromised recovery. It therefore follows that the stab wound must have interfered with the compensatory dendritic growth in the hemisphere. Our preliminary results support this conclusion as the stab wound blocked the cortical thickening and reduced the dendritic growth (Kolb, Gibb, & Muirhead, 1995). Thus, once again we see a correlation between increased dendritic growth and functional recovery.

We recently considered the possibility that the increased dendritic growth in the pyramidal cells of the motor cortex of neonatally hemidecorticated rats might reflect a change in the output of these neurons. It has been known for some time that neonatal hemidecortication is associated with development of an abnormal ipsilateral corticospinal pathway. We replicated this result and, in addition, were able to show an abnormal cortico-striatal pathway to the contralateral hemisphere (Kolb, Gibb, & van der Kooy, 1992). This pathway originated in the pyramidal cells of the prefrontal cortex, and may play a significant role in the recovery of behaviors such as forelimb reaching after hemidecortication (Whishaw & Kolb, 1988).

ASTROCYTES AND RECOVERY

Glia are exquisitely sensitive to cerebral injury. Thus, when rats are given even small cortical lesions, there are two distinctive types of glia (e.g., microglia and reactive astrocytes) visible throughout the cortical mantle of the ipsilateral hemisphere. The astrocyte response is among the most plastic changes seen in the brain. Astrocytes show a marked hypertrophy and a large increase in the extent of filaments made up of glial acidic fibrillary protein (GFAP). Astrocytes have been proposed to have multiple trophic functions in both the developing brain and in response to injury. In particular, astrocytes produce various soluble factors that support neuronal growth, at least in vitro (e.g, Giulian, 1993). One important feature of astrocytes in the current context is that, although some astrocytes are formed early in development, most are formed after neural mitosis is complete and reach their peak of gliogenesis somewhere around 7–10 days. The correlation between glial development and the age at which there is maximal recovery of function is intriguing. This correlation is especially interesting because the worst functional outcome from cortical injury comes after injury just after birth in rats, which is a time at which there are few astrocytes in the cortex. To examine the glial response more carefully, Gibb and I made frontal or motor cortex lesions on the day of birth, 10 days of age, or in adulthood. Animals are sacrificed at different postinjury ages, and immunohistochemical techniques are used to identify either vimentin- or GFAP-positive astrocytes. (During development, astrocytes express vimentin until about 5–10 days of age and begin to express GFAP as the vimentin decreases.) Rats with lesions at 10 days of age showed a large increase in GFAP positive cells a few days after the injury, whereas rats with Day 1 lesions showed no glial response at all. Rats with adult lesions fall in between. Because the astrocytes may produce trophic factors that support neuronal growth, our results suggest that the dramatic differences in dendritic responsivity to cortical injury at different ages may reflect the difference in astrocyte response during development. If this is so, one might expect that treatments that influence astrocyte activity will also increase functional recovery after cortical injury in development.

EXPERIENCE, RECOVERY, AND BRAIN PLASTICITY
AFTER EARLY INJURY

The idea that various types of experience or training might influence recovery from cortical injury is not new. Indeed, the use of postoperative rehabilitation for both motor and cognitive dysfunctions is based on the assumption that such treatments might be beneficial. The most extensively used paradigm has been the "enriched environment." Animals are housed in complex environments that contain "toys" and other rats, and the recovery is compared with animals living alone in standard laboratory cages. Although beneficial effects of such treatments have been shown, there have also been many reports that such experience is of little benefit (see reviews by Walsh & Greenough, 1976; Will & Kelche, 1992).

The complexity of the issue, and perhaps some insight on how to approach it, can be illustrated in an experiment by Whishaw, Sutherland, Kolb, and Becker (1986). Rats were hemidecorticated either in infancy or adulthood, and were then either placed in large tubs filled with objects, plastic pipes, branches, and so on, or were housed in standard laboratory cages. After 90 days, the animals were trained in Morris water task. Rats with neonatal hemidecortications showed no benefit of the enrichment, whereas rats with adult hemidecortications benefited significantly from the experience. Thus, we see in the same experiment that hemidecorticate rats both did and did not benefit from the treatment. The critical predictor was whether the hemidecorticate animal already showed evidence of recovery. Neonatal hemidecorticates already showed recovery relative to the adult operates, and enrichment did not enhance this recovery. This result suggests that there might be limits to the plasticity of the brain, and that enrichment is most beneficial under conditions in which there is normally little recovery of function. A practical implication of this conclusion is that it appears that people who show the worst outcome from cerebral injury might show the greatest gains from rehabilitation. If this is true, they should also show the most change in synaptic organization. The nature of these changes, and the issue of what constrains changes in animals with relatively good "spontaneous" recovery, have formed the basis of a series of studies over the past decade.

The results of the Whishaw experiment suggest that rats with frontal lesions on the day of birth might show the greatest benefit from enrichment, and this was indeed the case. Rats with lesions on Day 1 or Day 5 showed dramatic functional improvement after 3 months of enriched rearing, whereas rats with Day 10 lesions showed no beneficial effect (e.g., Kolb & Elliott, 1987). In fact, the enriched rats with lesions on postnatal Day 5 were functionally equivalent to rats with lesions on postnatal Day 10. This functional recovery was correlated with a remarkable 16% increase in cortical thickness in the early operates, which was nearly threefold greater than the 6% increase in unoperated rats. Evidently the brain of the perinatally brain-injured rat is capable of significant plasticity, but it apparently does not occur without environmental stimulation. This result implies that behavioral therapies may indeed play an important role in treating cortical injuries that are normally associated with a poor behavioral outcome. This conclusion is further supported by an experiment in which we tried a different form of enrichment.

Field reported that premature babies grow more quickly and are released from the hospital sooner if they are stimulated by stoking with a brush for 15 minutes three times a day (Field et al., 1986; Schanberg & Field, 1987). We reasoned that if tactile stimulation in premature babies could affect brain growth, a similar treatment in infant brain-damaged rats might facilitate recovery and increase plastic changes in the cortex. After all, newborn rats are embryologically equivalent to premature humans. Rats were given frontal lesions on Days 3–5 after birth, and were stroked for 15 minutes three times daily until weaning at 21 days. The results were dramatic. The stimulated frontal rats grew faster than unstimulated frontal rats, and they were significantly better at the Morris water task and the Whishaw reaching task when tested in adulthood. Furthermore, the brains of the stroked rats were heavier, and there was an increase in dendritic arborization in cortical pyramidal cells relative to the unstroked rats. These results imply that human infants with perinatal injury may benefit from extensive tactile experience during infancy. In addition, the fact that we obtained similar results with both stroking in infants and rearing in enriched environments in older rats suggests that there is more than one way to stimulate cortical plasticity after early injury. We are not yet in a position to determine which type of treatment may prove to be more beneficial.

CONCLUSIONS

Our studies of brain plasticity following cortical injury during development led to several general conclusions:

1. Damage to the developing brain has different functional consequences at different developmental stages. Injury during the period of neuronal migration, and prior to astrocyte development, appears to lead to poor functional outcome. In contrast, injury during the period of

maximal dendritic growth, which in the rat correlates with the period of maximal astrocyte growth, leads to good functional outcome.

2. Functional recovery following complete removal of one hemisphere during development follows different rules of recovery. In this case, the earlier the injury, the better the recovery. The better functional restitution after hemidecortication in the young brain probably reflects that the recovery is being mediated, at least in part, by an intact hemisphere. In contrast, bilateral injury to the developing brain necessarily requires that recovery is mediated by an injured hemisphere.

3. Rats with lesions on postnatal Day 10 have smaller brains than normal, but they are capable of doing more functionally than animals with larger brains who have had similar lesions in adulthood. This appears to be accomplished by having more synapses per cortical neuron. Thus, it is likely that it is the intrinsic organization of the cortex that is responsible for the functional recovery, rather than the growth of novel cortical afferents or efferents.

4. We have seen a consistent correlation between dendritic growth, spine density, and recovery of function. For example, rats with either Day 10 frontal lesions or Day 1 hemidecortications show significant sparing of functions, and this is associated with increased dendritic growth. Rats with Day 1 frontal lesions have a poor functional outcome and a decrease in dendritic arborization.

5. The development of abnormal cortico-subcortical connections is correlated with recovery when there is an increase in dendritic growth in the pyramidal cells and with an absence of recovery when there is no increase in dendrites or spines. In other words, changing the long afferent or efferent connections of the cortex is not enough in itself to ensure recovery.

6. Unilateral lesions allow more dendritic growth and better functional outcome than bilateral lesions. Even small perturbations of the hemisphere contralateral to hemidecortication appear to interfere with both recovery and dendritic growth.

7. Behavior does not recover after early lesions until the dendritic changes take place. This does not occur quickly, and appears to take at least 1 month, although the precise time course has not been determined.

8. There is a correlation between the intensity of the astrocytic response to injury and the extent of functional recovery. Rats with frontal lesions on Day 10 have an exaggerated astrocyte response, whereas those with Day 1 lesions have no astrocyte response. It is proposed that astrocytes may produce some type of trophic factor(s) that may contribute to both synaptic growth and functional recovery.

9. Experience can have profound effects on both functional recovery

and synaptic plasticity after cerebral injury in developing animals. The effects of experience appear to be most dramatic in those cases in which outcome is worst, which is the animals with injury at the earliest ages. 10. Under optimal circumstances it is possible to regrow lost brain tissue. Rats with restricted medial frontal lesions on Day 10 regrow the lost brain and this is associated with dramatic functional recovery.

REFERENCES

Banich, M. T., Cohen-Levine, S., Kim, H., & Huttenlocher, P. (1990). The effects of developmental factors on IQ in hemiplegic children. *Neuropsychologia, 28,* 35–47.

Broca, P. (1965). Siege de la faculte de langage articule dans l'hemisphere gauche du cerveau, *Bullutin de Societe Anthropologie, 6,* 377–393.

Fantie, B., & Kolb, B. (1990). An examination of prefrontal lesion size and the effects of cortical grafts on performance of the Morris water task by rats. *Psychobiology, 18,* 74–80.

Field, T., Schanberg, S. M., Scafidi, F., Bauer, C. R., Vega-Lahr, N., Garcia, R., Nystrom, J., & Kuhn, C. M. (1986). Tactile/kinesthetic stimulation effects on preterm neonates. *Pediatrics, 77,* 654–658.

Giulian, D. (1993). Reactive glia as rivals in regulating neuronal survival. *Glia, 7,* 102–110.

Goldman, P. S., & Galkin, T. W. (1978). Prenatal removal of frontal association cortex in the fetal rhesus monkey: Anatomical and functional consequences in postnatal life. *Brain Research, 152,* 451–485.

Goldman-Rakic, P. S., Isseroff, A., Schwartz, M. L., & Bugbee, N. M. (1983). The neurobiology of cognitive development. In P. H. Mussen (Ed.), *Handbook of child psychology: Biology and infancy development* (pp. 311–344). New York: Wiley.

Harlow, H. F., Akert, K., & Schiltz, K. A. (1964). The effects of bilateral prefrontal lesions on learned behavior of neonatal, infant and preadolescent monkeys. In J. M. Warren & K. Akert (Eds.), *The frontal granular cortex and behavior* (pp. 126–148). New York: McGraw-Hill.

Hebb, D. O. (1949). *The organization of behavior.* New York: McGraw-Hill.

Kennard, M. (1938). Reorganization of motor function in the cerebral cortex of monkeys deprived of motor and premotor areas in infancy. *Journal of Neurophysiology, 1,* 477–496.

Kennard, M. (1940). Relation of age to motor impairment in man and in subhuman primates. *Archives of Neurology and Psychiatry, 44,* 377–397.

Kolb, B. (1984). The functions of the frontal cortex of the rat: A comparative perspective. *Brain Research Reviews, 8,* 65–98.

Kolb, B. (1987). Recovery from early cortical damage in rats: I. Differential behavioral and anatomical effects of frontal lesions at different ages of neural maturation. *Behavioural Brain Research, 25,* 205–220.

Kolb, B. (1990). The prefrontal cortex. In B. Kolb & R. Tees (Eds.), *The cerebral cortex of the rat* (pp. 537–562). Cambridge, MA: MIT Press.

Kolb, B. (1995). *Brain plasticity and behavior.* Hillsdale, NJ: Lawrence Erlbaum Associates.

Kolb, B., & Elliott, W. (1987). Recovery from early cortical damage in rats: II. Effects of experience on anatomy and behavior following frontal lesions at 1 or 5 days of age. *Behavioural Brain Research, 26,* 47–56.

Kolb, B., & Gibb, R. (1990). Anatomical correlates of behavioural change after neonatal prefrontal lesions in rats. *Progress in Brain Research, 85,* 241–256.

Kolb, B., & Gibb, R. (1991). Sparing of function after neonatal frontal lesions correlates with increased cortical dendritic branching: A possible mechanism for the Kennard effect. *Behavioural Brain Research, 43,* 51–56.

Kolb, B., & Gibb, R. (1993). Possible anatomical basis of recovery of spatial learning after neonatal prefrontal lesions in rats. *Behavioral Neuroscience, 107,* 799–811.

Kolb, B., Gibb, R., Gorny, G., de Brahander, J., & Whishaw, I. Q. (1995). Cerebral regrowth after cortical lesions in rats. *Society for Neuroscience Abstracts, 21,* 311.

Kolb, B., Gibb, R., & Muirhead, D. (1996). *Recovery from neonatal hemidecortication is blocked by perturbation of the intact hemisphere.* Manuscript submitted for publication.

Kolb, B., Gibb, R., & van der Kooy (1992). Cortical and striatal structure and connectivity are altered by neonatal hemidecorticaition in rats. Journal of Comparative Neurology, 322, 311–324.

Kolb, B., Gibb, R., & van der Kooy, (1994). Neonatal frontal cortical lesions in rats alter cortical structure and connectivity. *Brain Research, 645,* 85–97.

Kolb, B.,& Nonneman, A. J. (1978). Sparing of function in rats with early prefrontal cortex lesions. *Brain Research, 151,* 135–148.

Kolb, B., Petrie, B., & Cioe, J. (1995). *Recovery from early cortical damage in rats: VII. Comparison of the behavioural and anatomical effects of medial prefrontal lesions at different ages of neural maturation.* Behavioral Brain Research, in press.

Kolb, B., & Stewart, J. (1995). Changes in neonatal gonadal hormonal environment prevent behavioral sparing and alter cortical morphogenesis after early frontal cortex lesions in male and female rats. *Behavioral Neuroscience, 109,* 285–294.

Kolb, B., & Sutherland, R. J. (1992). Noradrenaline depletion blocks behavioral sparing and alters cortical morphogenesis after neonatal frontal cortex damage in rats. *Journal of Neuroscience, 12,* 2221–2330.

Kolb, B., Sutherland, R. J., & Whishaw, I. Q. (1983). Neonatal hemidecortication or frontal cortex ablation produce similar behavioral spring but opposite effects upon morphogenesis of remaining cortex. *Behavioral Neuroscience, 97,* 154–158.

Kolb, B., & Tomie, J. (1988). Recovery from early cortical damage in rats: IV. Effects of hemidecortication at 1, 5, or 10 days of age. *Behavioural Brain Research, 28,* 259–274.

Kolb, B., & Whishaw, I. Q. (1981). Neonatal frontal lesions in the rat: Sparing of learned but not species-typical behavior in the presence of reduced brain weight and cortical thickness. *Journal of Comparative and Physiological Psychology, 95,* 863–879.

Lenneberg, E. (1967). *Biological foundations of language.* New York: Wiley.

Marin-Padilla, M. (1970a). Prenatal and early postnatal ontogenesis of the human motor cortex: A Golgi study: I. The sequential development of the cortical layers. *Brain Research, 23,* 167–183.

Marin-Padilla, M. (1970b). Prenatal and early postnatal ontogenesis of the human motor cortex: A Golgi study: II. The basket-pyramidal cell system. *Brain Research, 23,* 185–191.

Morris, R. G. M. (1980). Spatial localization does not require the presence of local cues. *Learning and Motivation, 12,* 239–261.

Schanberg, S. M., & Field, T. M. (1987). Sensory deprivation stress and supplemental stimulation in the rat pup and preterm human neonate. *Child Development, 58,* 1431–1447.

Sutherland, R. J., Whishaw, I. Q., & Kolb, B. (1983). A behavioral analysis of spatial localization following electrolytic, kainate-, or colchicine-induced damage to the hippocampal formation of the rat. *Behavioural Brain Research, 7,* 133–153.

Tallal, P., Stark, R. E., & Mellits, E. D. (1985a). The relationship between auditory temporal analysis and receptive language development: Evidence from studies of developmental language disorder. *Neuropsychologia, 23,* 527–534.

Tallal, P., Stark, R. E., & Mellits, E. D. (1985b). Identification of language-impaired children on the basis of rapid perception and production skills. *Brain and Language, 25,* 314–322.

Teuber, H. -L. (1975). Recovery of function after brain injury in man. In Ciba foundation Symposium 34, *Outcome of severe damage to the central nervous system* (pp. 159–196). Amsterdam: Elsevier.

Vargha-Khadem, F., Watters, G., & O'Gorman, A. M. (1985). Development of speech and language following bilateral frontal lesions. *Brain and Language, 37*, 167–183.

Walsh, R., & Greenough, W. T. (1976). *Environments as therapy for brain damage.* New York: Plenum.

Whishaw, I. Q., & Kolb, B. (1988). Sparing of skilled forelimb reaching and corticospinal projections after neonatal motor cortex removal or hemidecortication in the rat: Support for the Kennard doctrine. *Brain Research, 451*, 97–114.

Whishaw, I. Q., Kolb, B., & Sutherland, R. J. (1983). The behavior of the laboratory rat. In T. E. Robinson (Ed.), *Behavioral approaches to brain research* (pp. 141–211). New York: Oxford University Press.

Whishaw, I. Q., O'Connor, W. T., & Dunnett, S. B. (1986). The contributions of motor cortex, nigrostriatal dopamine and caudate putamen to skilled forelimb use in the rat. *Brain, 109*, 805–843.

Whishaw, I. Q., Sutherland, R. J., Kolb, B., & Becker, J. (1986). Effects of neonatal forebrain noradrenaline depletion on recovery from brain damage: Performance on a spatial navigation task as a function of age of surgery and postsurgical housing. *Behavioral and Neural Biology, 6*, 285–307.

Will, B., & Kelche, C. (1992). Environmental approaches to recovery of function from brain damage: A review of animal studies (1981 to 1991). In F. D. Rose & D. A. Johnson (Eds.), *Recovery from brain damage: Reflections and directions* (pp. 79–104). New York: Plenum.

Woods, B. T. (1980). The restricted effects of right-hemisphere lesions after age one; Wechsler test data. *Neuropsychologia, 18*, 65–70.

Woods, B. T., & Teuber, H. -L. (1973). Early onset of complementary specialization of cerebral hemispheres in man. *Transactions of the American Neurological Association, 98*, 113–117.

15

Outcome Following Traumatic Brain Injury: An Australian Study

Jennie L. Ponsford
John H. Olver
Carolyn Curran

From the results of numerous follow-up studies, there is now a growing recognition of the significant and lasting impact of traumatic brain injury (TBI). The most comprehensive longitudinal studies conducted to date include those of Brooks, Campsie, Symington, Beattie, and McKinlay (1986); Brown and Nell (1992); Oddy, Coughlan, Tyerman, and Jenkins (1985); and Thomsen (1984). Follow-up interviews were conducted with the relatives of TBI patients and, in some cases, the injured individuals themselves. Although the degree of ongoing disability varied somewhat, according to the severity of the injuries, there were many similarities in the findings. Physical disabilities persisted in the most severe cases, but most recovered to an independent level of mobility. However, there was a far higher frequency of lasting changes in cognitive, behavioral, and emotional functioning. These psychosocial sequelae presented the most serious ongoing difficulties, leading to a decline in personal and social relationships, leisure pursuits, and employment status. Although functional independence continued to improve in the most severe cases, there was not a great deal of change in psychosocial functioning over time. Social isolation was a significant and lasting problem.

There have been no prospective longitudinal studies of outcome following TBI conducted in Australia to date, particularly examining factors that predict outcome, how the problems and needs of those who sustain TBI and their families change over time, and whether they deteriorate after discharge from rehabilitation. Moreover, the subjects in the Brooks et al. (1986), Oddy et al. (1985), and Thomsen (1984) studies had either no access to rehabilitation facilities or were treated within a general neurological rehabilitation service. Over the past decade, there have been significant improvements in the comprehensiveness and specialization of rehabilitation services available to TBI individuals, with a greater emphasis on psychosocial issues. There have been significant developments in Australia in this respect. The long-term impact of the provision of such services on outcome is, as yet, unknown.

BETHESDA HOSPITAL HEAD INJURY
REHABILITATION PROGRAM

Since 1983, Bethesda Hospital in Melbourne, Australia, has had a specialized head-injury rehabilitation program that annually admits an average of 120 TBI patients, usually age 13 years or over. All those admitted to Bethesda's Head Injury Unit have sustained TBI as a result of either motor vehicle or work-related accidents. The State of Victoria has a no-fault accident compensation system, which provides funding for the rehabilitation of those injured in motor vehicle and work-related accidents. TBI patients are admitted to Bethesda from acute hospitals, subject to bed availability, when they are medically stable and emerging from coma, but usually still in posttraumatic amnesia (PTA).

Bethesda offers a comprehensive, interdisciplinary rehabilitation program at both inpatient and outpatient levels. The program's aim is to overcome disabilities and handicaps caused by physical, cognitive, behavioral, and emotional impairments. It provides psychosocial support for patient and family, as well as assistance in obtaining an optimal level of community reintegration (e.g., in terms of living situation, vocational productivity, and social and recreational activities). A significant amount of support is available for return to work or study, including funding for supported work trials. For those returning to study, there are integration aides, tutoring, and ongoing individual support. The average length of time spent in the rehabilitation program is 10 months. However, length of stay is obviously influenced by many factors, including severity, so there is a broad range in this respect.

Follow-Up

Following discharge from the program, patients are followed up at 6-month intervals in the first 2 years, and again at 3 and 5 years. The aim of these interviews is to document change over time and the nature of ongoing difficulties, and to identify areas in need of further intervention. Such assistance is provided by the Bethesda rehabilitation team, or referral is made to relevant community-based resources.

Questionnaire

A structured questionnaire is administered at each follow-up interview. The patients are invited to bring someone with them to the follow-up interview. However, this is not always possible. Therefore, responses reported in the studies discussed in this chapter are based on self-report by the injured patients. The questionnaire covers the following:

• Neurological complaints—including epilepsy, headaches, dizziness, and visual disturbances.
• Mobility—level of mobility, exercise tolerance.
• Communication difficulties—as reported by the injured person, including comprehension, word finding, and motor speech problems (dysarthria/dyspraxia).
• Cognitive, behavioral, and emotional changes—also as reported by the TBI individual. Cognitive changes include the areas of planning, memory, concentration, speed of thinking, and mental fatigue. Behavioral problems include irritability, impulsiveness, socially inappropriate behavior, reduced initiative, and self-centeredness. Emotional problems include the presence of anxiety, depression, and thoughts of suicide.
• Relationship issues—including marital status, support from close others, social isolation, and sexual changes.
• Activities of daily living (ADL)—performance of personal ADL (e.g., feeding, dressing, hygiene), light domestic ADL (e.g., meal preparation, washing up, dusting) heavy domestic ADL (e.g., heavy cleaning, gardening, laundry), community ADL (e.g., shopping, banking), and use of transport.
• Leisure pursuits.
• Employment or study.

OUTCOME AT 2 YEARS POSTINJURY

Ponsford, Olver, and Curran (1995) presented a comprehensive profile of outcome for the first 175 TBI individuals who attended the follow-up interview 2 years (+/−4 weeks) after injury, the details of which are set out later. This group consisted of 109 males and 66 females, with a mean age of 27.4 years ($SD = 11.9$ years, range = 11–69 years). The group had an average of 10.3 years of education ($SD = 2.3$ years). Only 61% of the sample were employed (101 full time, 5 part time). A further 15% were students. Twenty-four percent of the group were unemployed at the time of injury.

This sample represented 48% of consecutive admissions to the head-injury rehabilitation program at Bethesda Hospital between March 1985 and January 1989. There were no significant differences between the group of subjects who attended the follow-up interview and those who failed to attend in terms of age, gender, Glasgow Coma Scale (GCS) score on acute hospital admission, duration of posttraumatic amnesia (PTA), or location of dwelling (Melbourne metropolitan area or country). There was a small, but significant, group difference in terms of years of education (see Tables 15.1 & 15.2).

Seventy-four percent of the group were injured in motor car or motorcycle accidents. Eighteen percent were pedestrians, and 5% were cyclists. Others were injured by a fall or a blow to the head in the workplace. The majority of patients (89%) sustained severe injuries, as classified by GCS scores of 3–8 on acute hospital admission. However, it must be noted that GCS scores were missing for 39 cases. PTA duration was documented in all but one case. All patients had a PTA duration exceeding 24 hours, and in 51% of cases PTA exceeded 4 weeks. Patients were admitted for rehabilitation an average of 47 days postinjury (SD = 27, range = 7–159). The mean time spent in the rehabilitation program was 253 days (SD = 160, range = 10–1088).

Neurological Complaints

A significant proportion of the group experienced neurological problems, including headaches (36%) and dizziness (26%). Six percent developed epilepsy. Almost half of the sample (48%) reported visual difficulties. The most common problems included blurred vision, double vision, and acuity impairment.

TABLE 15.1
T Tests Comparing Patients Who Did and Did Not Attend
for Follow-Up Review

Variable	Subjects Mean (SD)[a]	Comparison Mean (SD)[b]	t value	df	p
Age	27.4 (11.9)	27.0 (11.4)	0.35	364	.724
Glasgow Coma Scale score	5.3 (2.9)	6.0 (4.3)	−1.69	244	.092
PTA duration	45.9 (44.4)	39.0 (42.7)	1.51	355	.132
Years of education	10.3 (2.3)	10.8 (2.2)	−2.09	336	.037

Note. From "A Profile of Outcome: 2 Years after Traumatic Brain Injury" by J. Ponsford, J. Olver, and C. Curran, 1995, *Brain Injury.* Copyright 1995 by Taylor & Francis. Reprinted by permission.
[a]n = 175.
[b]n = 191.

TABLE 15.2
**Patients Who Did and Did Not Attend for Follow-Up: Breakdown
by Gender and Location of Dwelling**

Variable	Subjects[a]	Comparison group[b]	χ^2
Gender			
Male	109	133	1.88 (1), $p = .170$
Female	66	58	
Location			
Melbourne metro	127	124	2.14 (1), $p = .144$
Country/rural	38	67	

Note. From "A Profile of Outcome: 2 Years After Traumatic Brain Injury" by J. Ponsford,
J. Olver, and C. Curran, 1995, *Brain Injury.* Copyright 1995 by Taylor & Francis. Reprinted
by permission.
[a]$n = 175.$
[b]$n = 191.$

Mobility and Exercise Tolerance

Only 3% of the sample were confined to a wheelchair or bed at 2 years.
Many were at their previous level of mobility, or were at least able to
walk, run, and jump (60%; see Table 15.3). However, 59% still fatigued
more easily when exercising than before the injury.

Activities of Daily Living (ADL)

As can be seen from Table 15.4, most TBI patients were independent in
personal and domestic ADL at 2 years. However, a significant number
(34%) still required supervision or assistance with community activities

TABLE 15.3
**Level of Mobility and Tolerance of Exercise
2 Years Postinjury**

Mobility and exercise tolerance[a]	%
Nonambulant or wheelchair	3
Walks independently, unable to run or jump	37
Able to walk, run, and jump	60
Tires more easily than preinjury	59

Note. From "A Profile of Outcome: 2 Years After Traumatic Brain
Injury" by J. Ponsford, J. Olver, and C. Curran, 1995, *Brain Injury.*
Copyright 1995 by Taylor & Francis. Reprinted by permission.
[a]$n = 175.$

TABLE 15.4
Independence in Activities of Daily Living Including
Use of Transport at 2 Years Postinjury

Activities[a] (Independence with or without aids)	%
Daily living	
Feeding	93
Dressing	87
Personal hygiene	88
Light domestic chores (e.g., cooking, dusting)	79
Heavy domestic chores (e.g., laundry, gardening)	68
Community skills (e.g., shopping, banking)	66
Transport	
Transport—fully dependent	21
Limited use of public transport	14
Independent use of public transport	27
Able to drive a car	38

Note. From "A Profile of Outcome: 2 Years After Traumatic Brain Injury" by J. Ponsford, J. Olver, and C. Curran, 1995, *Brain Injury*. Copyright 1995 by Taylor & Francis. Reprinted by permission.
[a]$n = 175$.

of daily living, such as shopping and banking. Thirty-eight percent of the TBI patients were able to drive. A further 25% were unable to drive, but were independent in the use of public transport. This group also included 12 patients who were too young to obtain a driver's license.

Communication

More than two thirds of the group (68%) reported experiencing word-finding difficulties at 2 years. Thirty-four percent said they had problems following conversation. Twenty-six percent reported motor speech difficulties.

Cognitive, Behavioral, and Emotional Changes

As can be seen in Table 15.5, more than two thirds of the sample reported negative changes in memory, concentration, speed of thinking, and tendency to fatigue mentally. Almost half of the group was aware of changes in planning ability. Behavior changes were also commonly reported, with irritability being the most frequent complaint (67%). Increased impulsivity and reduced initiative were acknowledged by almost half of the subjects. Self-centeredness and inappropriate social behavior were reported by 28% and 26% of the sample, respectively.

TABLE 15.5
Percentage of Patients Who Reported
Cognitive, Behavioral, and Emotional
Problems at 2 Years Postinjury

Problems[a]	%
Cognitive	
Memory	74
Planning	48
Speed of thinking	64
Concentration	62
Fatigue	72
Word-finding difficulties	68
Behavioral	
Initiative	44
Self-centered	28
Irritable/short-tempered/aggressive	67
Impulsive	43
Inappropriate social behavior	26
Social isolation	50
Emotional	
Anxious	58
Depressed	59

Note. From "A Profile of Outcome: 2 Years After Traumatic Brain Injury" by J. Ponsford, J. Olver, and C. Curran, 1995, *Brain Injury.* Copyright 1995 by Taylor & Francis. Reprinted by permission.
[a]$n = 175$.

Emotional changes were present in a majority of cases. Fifty-eight percent said they felt more anxious than prior to injury, and 59% said they
felt more depressed than prior to injury.

Relationship Issues

When asked who was the most significant person in their life, 48% of the
sample nominated parents and 28% indicated a spouse. Sixty-four percent of the subjects reported requiring more support from close friends
or family than prior to injury. There had been no changes in marital
status at 2 years relative to preinjury status. Sixty-one percent of the
group had never married, 30% were married, and 9% were separated,
divorced, or widowed. About 40% reported sexual changes. Most of
those reporting a change in interest in sex indicated that there was a
decrease in interest rather than an increase (75%). Half of the group
reported that they had lost friends or had become more socially isolated
since the injury.

Leisure Interests

Many of the patients pursued alternative leisure interests with or without assistance. At 2 years, 73% were reporting changes in this respect.

Employment/Study

It is most appropriate to examine employment figures for those subjects who were employed at the time of injury. Of the 106 patients who were employed on a full- or part-time basis at the time of injury, 44 (42%) were employed at 2 years (35 full time, 9 part time). Of the 27 subjects who were students prior to injury, 48% were still studying, 8% were working, and 44% were unemployed.

To summarize these findings, in this group of severe TBI individuals, headaches and visual disturbances appeared to be an ongoing problem for a significant proportion of cases at 2 years postinjury. Most had recovered to an independent level in terms of mobility and ability to perform personal and domestic activities of daily living. However, about a third of the sample continued to require some assistance with activities in the community, such as shopping, banking, and use of transport. More than half the group still received more support from others than before the injury.

In contrast to the relatively good physical recovery, a majority of the sample was reporting cognitive, behavioral, and emotional changes at 2 years. Figures regarding the frequency of cognitive, behavioral, and emotional changes following TBI are remarkably similar to those reported by the relatives of severe TBI subjects 2 years postinjury in a number of other studies, (e.g., Brown & Nell, 1992; Dikmen, Machamer, & Temkin, 1993; Jacobs, 1988; Lezak, 1987; Weddell, Oddy, & Jenkins, 1980). In most of these studies, responses were based on reports from relatives. Although the reliability of self-report in TBI individuals has been questioned on the grounds that they lack self-awareness (Prigatano & Fordyce, 1986), the high proportion of patients reporting cognitive, behavioral, and emotional changes at 2 years in this study suggests a growing awareness of changes by this stage. What was not clear from the subjects' responses was the precise nature and severity of the difficulties experienced, and the extent to which specific problems were interfering with these individuals' ability to get on with their lives.

The high proportion of psychological changes reported at 2 years was somewhat disappointing, considering the intensity of the rehabilitation received by the patients in the Bethesda sample relative to that received by TBI individuals in earlier studies. This suggests that such intensive rehabilitation is successful in maximizing physical recovery and independence in activities of daily living, but that many TBI individuals may require ongoing support and assistance with cognitive, behavioral, and emotional problems.

More than half of the sample was unable to return to employment by 2 years postinjury. A significant proportion of those studying at the time of injury was also unemployed. Most patients pursued alternative leisure interests. There is an obvious need for provision of ongoing assistance in establishing a vocation and/or developing alternative social and recreational interests after TBI individuals return to the community.

FACTORS PREDICTING EMPLOYMENT OUTCOME

In the next phase of the study, we attempted to identify factors that predicted or influenced outcome at 2 years. The results of this research, outlined here, have been published by Ponsford, Olver, Curran, and Ng (1995). In recent years, the outcome measure most commonly studied has been return to employment. This is so because employment status is relatively easy to define and measure. Although return to employment is clearly only one of a number of significant aspects of outcome, vocational productivity has been found to be strongly associated with physical and emotional well-being (Melamed, Groswasser, & Stern, 1992).

In previous studies, a number of individual variables have shown significant correlations with outcome. These include GCS scores, PTA duration, age, presence of multiple trauma, and neuropsychological measures of psychomotor speed (Bishara, Partridge, Godfrey, & Knight, 1992; Klonoff, Costa, & Snow, 1986; Moore, Stambrook, Peters, Cardoses, & Kassum, 1990; Vollmer et al., 1991). These findings suggest that a multivariate approach may result in more accurate predictions.

Therefore, a multivariate approach was used to examine which of a number of variables—relating to demographic factors, injury severity, and degree of disability on admission to rehabilitation—were, in combination, the best predictors of employment status 2 years after TBI. Although several previous studies have taken a multivariate approach to the prediction of future employment and productivity status (e.g., Ruff et al., 1993; Vogenthaler, Smith, & Goldfader, 1989), there has been no cross-validation of findings, which is essential to verify the predictive value of a given set of variables. Some previous studies have also included subjects who were not employed prior to injury. This can confound the influence of other factors on employment outcome.

The subjects studied for the purpose of determining predictors were drawn from 254 TBI patients who had attended the follow-up review clinic. This group consisted of the initial sample of 175 patients, whose outcome was described in the previous section. To allow for cross-validation, a second sample of the next 79 TBI individuals attending the follow-up clinic was also studied.

To study predictors of employment outcome at 2 years, we examined only those patients who had been employed at the time of injury. For the initial study, 106 of the 175 patients who attended the follow-up interview were selected because they were employed either full time or part time at the time of injury. Valid information for all of the variables being studied was available for 74 of these 106 subjects. The group of 74 subjects consisted of 48 males (65%) and 26 females (35%). The mean age of the sample at the time of injury was 29.5 years (SD = 10.6, range = 16–59 years). The group had an average of 10.7 years of education (SD = 2.5, range = 5–18 years). The mean GCS score on acute hospital admission was 5.5 (SD = 3.1, range = 3–15). The mean PTA duration was 42.7 days (SD = 42.2, range = 2–183 days). Sixty-nine of these subjects were employed on a full-time basis at the time of injury, and 5 were employed part time.

The cross-validation sample comprised the next group of 79 patients who were seen in the follow-up clinic. Of this group, 62 had been employed on a full-time basis and none on a part-time basis at the time of injury. Valid information on all of the variables under study was available for 50 of these 62 subjects. Thus, the cross-validation sample consisted of 43 (86%) males and 7 (14%) females, with a mean age of 29.3 years (SD = 11.5, range = 18–54) and an average of 10.8 years of education (SD = 2.2, range = 6–18). The mean GCS score on acute hospital admission was 6.9 (SD = 3.7, range = 3–14), and the mean PTA duration was 41.8 days (SD = 38.5, range = 3–183 days).

Employment Rates at 2 Years

Of the first sample of 74 TBI patients who had been working at the time of injury, 30 (40%) were employed in either full- or part-time work at 2 years. Only one of the five who were employed part time prior to injury returned to part-time employment. The others were not employed at 2 years. Of those employed full time at the time of injury, 24 (35%) returned to full-time work, 5 (7%) returned to part-time work, and 40 (58%) were not employed.

Of the 50 subjects in the cross-validation sample, all of whom were working full time at the time of injury, 32 (64%) were employed on either a full- or part-time basis at 2 years. Twenty-five (50%) were employed full time, 7 (14%) were employed part time, and 18 (36%) were not employed. More comprehensive data regarding the nature of employment were available for this group. Sixteen of the 25 full-time employees had returned to their previous position with the same duties, 4 had alternative duties with the previous employer, and 5 returned to full-time work with a new employer. Only one part-time worker had returned to the previous position. The other six in part-time employment had been working full-time previously, and were working part-time in alternative employment.

There were 263 subjects who failed to attend the follow-up interview during this time period. We were interested to see how employment rates in this group compared with those in the samples who did participate. One hundred and eighty of these 263 patients were able to be contacted by telephone to check their employment status. Of this group of 180, 138 had been working at the time of injury. Sixty of these 138 subjects (43.5%) were employed on a full- or part-time basis at 2 years. The rates of return to employment in the groups that did and did not attend the interviews were thus quite comparable [$\chi^2(1) = .07, p > .05$].

Establishing Predictors

Eight predictor variables were chosen on the basis of results from previous studies. The demographic variables studied were age, gender, years of education, and employment. Earlier studies found a substantially lower rate of return to work in TBI individuals over the age of 40 years (Bruckner & Randle, 1972; Humphrey & Oddy, 1981). Therefore, we coded subjects dichotomously on the variable of age, according to whether they were under or over 40. Injury-related variables included the GCS score on acute admission to hospital, PTA duration, and presence of limb fractures. Functional disability on admission to the rehabilitation program was represented by the total score on the Disability Rating Scale (DRS; Rappaport, Hall, Hopkins, Belleza, & Cope, 1982).

Point-biserial correlation coefficients were calculated between each of the predictor variables and employment status for the entire group of 254 subjects from the initial and cross-validation samples. The results are set out in Table 15.6. The four variables that showed statistically significant correlations with employment status at 2 years were age, GCS score on acute admission, PTA duration, and total score on the DRS.

A stepwise discriminant function analysis was conducted using the first sample of 74 subjects employed at the time of injury, with these four variables as the input variables. The aim was to determine the best linear combination of variables that discriminated between the group of subjects employed at 2 years and the group that was not employed.

This analysis gave a discriminant function consisting of three variables: total score on the DRS, initial GCS score, and age. Pooled within-groups correlations of each variable with the canonical discriminant

TABLE 15.6
Point-Biserial Correlation Coefficients
Between Predictor Variables
and Employment Status at 2 Years

Variable	r	p
Gender	.0824	.144
Age	.2140	.003
Years of education	−.1127	.086
Employment category	.0028	.487
GCS score	−.2540	.002
PTA	.3186	.000
Fractured limbs	−.0869	.188
Total DRS score	.3438	.000

Note. From "Prediction of Employment Status 2 Years After Traumatic Brain Injury" by J. Ponsford, J. Olver, C. Curran, and K. Ng, 1995, *Brain Injury.* Copyright 1995 by Taylor & Francis. Reprinted by permission.

function are set out in Table 15.7. The function discriminated significantly [$\chi^2(3) = 15.4$, Wilks' $\lambda = .768$, $p = .0015$]. Table 15.8 shows the classification results indicating how well the final set of discriminating variables discriminated between groups. These three variables correctly classified 74% of grouped cases.

For the purpose of cross-validation, the original discriminant function was used to classify the second group of subjects. It correctly classified 68% of the second sample. Classification results for the cross-validation sample are set out in Table 15.9. Results of a chi-square analysis comparing the correct and incorrect classifications for the two samples indicated

TABLE 15.7
Pooled Within-Groups Correlations Between
Discriminating Variables and Canonical
Discriminant Function

Variable	Correlations
Total DRS score	.85366
PTA	.71364
GCS score	−.46225
Age	.30837

Note. From "Prediction of Employment Status 2 Years After Traumatic Brain Injury" by J. Ponsford, J. Olver, C. Curran, and K. Ng, 1995, *Brain Injury.* Copyright 1995 by Taylor & Francis. Reprinted by permission.

TABLE 15.8
Classification Results: Original Sample

Actual group	Number of cases	Predicted group membership (Employed)	Predicted group membership (Not employed)
Employed	30	23 (77%)	7 (23%)
Not employed	44	12 (27%)	32 (73%)

Note. From "Prediction of Employment Status 2 Years After Traumatic Brain Injury" by J. Ponsford, J. Olver, C. Curran, and K. Ng, 1995, *Brain Injury*. Copyright 1995 by Taylor & Francis. Reprinted by permission.

no statistically significant difference [$\chi^2(1) = 0.59, p > .05$]. The three variables (viz. score on the DRS on admission to rehabilitation, GCS score on acute hospital admission, and age) were thus confirmed as predictors of employment outcome in the second group of TBI subjects. No previous study has confirmed the reliability of a set of predictors of employment outcome through cross-validation across different samples.

The score on the DRS was by far the greatest contributor to the discriminant function, with a correlation of .86. This scale appears to be a clinically useful tool, which may assist in the prediction of outcome. PTA duration was not included in the canonical discrminant function by virtue of its high correlation (.76) with total score on the DRS, but it showed a high correlation (.71) with the discriminant function. It is important, therefore, not to interpret the inclusion of GCS score in the discriminant function as indicative of its being necessarily a "better" predictor of future employment status than PTA duration.

Examination of misclassified subjects suggests a variety of contributing factors. Negative influences included: preexisting personality or social problems, presence of multiple trauma, behavior problems, lack of employer support, availability of financial support from a spouse, or other intervening social circumstances. Positive factors included: employer

TABLE 15.9
Classification Results: Cross-Validation Sample

Actual group	Number of cases	Predicted group membership (Employed)	Predicted group membership (Not employed)
Employed	32	21 (66%)	11 (34%)
Not employed	18	5 (28%)	13 (72%)

Note. From "Prediction of Employment Status 2 Years After Traumatic Brain Injury" by J. Ponsford, J. Olver, C. Curran, and K. Ng, 1995, *Brain Injury*. Copyright 1995 by Taylor & Francis. Reprinted by permission.

support with availability of alternative duties, and determination and adaptability on the part of the injured individual. It was apparent that a broad range of factors, other than those included in the analysis, potentially affect employment outcome following TBI. These should be taken into account when considering individual cases. Although a multivariate approach appears to aid prediction of outcome, the clinical usefulness of such prediction equations remains uncertain.

Further study needs to be made of qualitative aspects of employment status in TBI survivors who return to work, including worker satisfaction, nature of duties being performed, opportunities for promotion, job stability, and retention in the workforce over time. Findings from a study on 103 of the 254 TBI subjects, who have now been interviewed 5 years after injury, have indicated a significant decline in employment rates between 2 and 5 years. This decline is disappointing in view of the intensity of vocational assistance initially provided to these individuals.

The limitations of the use of employment as a sole outcome variable also need to be acknowledged. Other less tangible aspects of a person's lifestyle, such as the capacity to form and sustain personal and social relationships, and the ability to pursue recreational interests, are also very important. From the 2-year outcome profile, these appear to be even more vulnerable to the impact of TBI than employment. However, there are current limitations in the measurement of these variables that may potentially complicate and obscure the outcome picture further— most notably limitations in the use of self-report (McKinlay & Brooks, 1984; Prigatano & Fordyce, 1986). These need to be resolved before being tested against possible predictors.

From these findings, it seems clear that ongoing assistance and support should be available to TBI individuals for many years after injury. Rehabilitation systems and funding support need to be adapted to provide for this. Although acute rehabilitation is important, some aspects of it might be made more efficient and cost-effective by providing therapy less intensively in certain areas, but making it available over an extended period of time. This is particularly true in the domains of cognitive, behavioral, and emotional problems. Without ongoing support services, intensive rehabilitative efforts directed at those who have sustained severe TBI may have a limited impact on long-term outcome.

ACKNOWLEDGMENTS

The authors acknowledge the support of the Australian Rotary Health Research Fund and gratefully acknowledge the assistance of Professor Kim Ng for his advice on the statistical analyses.

REFERENCES

Bishara, S. N., Partridge, F. M., Godfrey, H., & Knight, R. G. (1992). Post-traumatic amnesia and Glasgow Coma Scale related to outcome in survivors in a consecutive series of patients with severe closed head injury. *Brain Injury, 6,* 373–380.

Brooks, N., Campsie, L., Symington, C., Beattie, A., & McKinlay, W. (1986). The five year outcome of severe blunt head injury: A relative's view. *Journal of Neurology, Neurosurgery and Psychiatry, 49,* 764–770.

Brown, D. S. O., & Nell, V. (1992). Recovery from diffuse traumatic brain injury in Johannesburg: A concurrent prospective study. *Archives of Physical Medicine & Rehabilitation, 73,* 758–770.

Bruckner, F. E., & Randle, A. P. H. (1972). Return to work after severe head injuries. *Rheumatology and Physical Medicine, 51,* 344–348.

Dikmen, S., Machamer, J., & Temkin, N. (1993). Psychosocial outcome in patients with moderate to severe head injury: 2-year follow-up. *Brain Injury, 7,* 113–124.

Humphrey, M., & Oddy, M. (1981). Return to work: A review of post war studies. *Injury, 12,* 107–114.

Jacobs, H. (1988). The Los Angeles head injury survey: Procedures and initial findings. *Archives of Physical Medicine & Rehabilitation, 69,* 425–431.

Klonoff, P., Costa, L., & Snow, W. (1986). Predictors and indicators of quality of life in patients with closed head injury. *Journal of Clinical and Experimental Neuropsychology, 8,* 469–485.

Lezak, M. (1987). The relationship between personality disorders, social disturbances and physical disabilities following traumatic brain injury. *Journal of Head Trauma Rehabilitation, 2,* 57–69.

McKinlay, W. W., & Brooks, D. N. (1984). Methodological problems in assessing psychosocial recovery following severe head injury. *Journal of Clinical Neuropsychology, 6,* 87–99.

Melamed, S., Groswasser, Z., & Stern, M. J. (1992). Acceptance of disabilities, work involvement and subjective rehabilitation status of traumatically brain injured (TBI) patients. *Brain Injury, 6,* 233–244.

Moore, A. D., Stambrook, M., Peters, L. C., Cardoses, E. R., & Kassum, P. A. (1990). Long-term multidimensional outcome following isolated traumatic brain injuries and traumatic brain injuries associated with multiple trauma. *Brain Injury, 4,* 379–389.

Oddy, M., Coughlan, T., Tyerman, A., & Jenkins, D. (1985). Social adjustment after closed head injury: A further follow-up seven years after injury. *Journal of Neurology, Neurosurgery, and Psychiatry, 48,* 564–568.

Ponsford, J. L., Olver, J. H., & Curran, C. (1995). A profile of outcome: 2 years after traumatic brain injury. *Brain Injury, 9,* 1–10.

Ponsford, J. L., Olver, J. H., Curran, C., & Ng, K. (1995). Prediction of employment status 2 years after traumatic brain injury. *Brain Injury, 9,* 11–20.

Prigatano, G. P., & Fordyce, D. J. (1986). Cognitive dysfunction and psychosocial adjustment after brain injury. In G. P. Prigatano, D. J. Fordyce, J. R. Roueche, H. K. Zeiner, M. Pepping, & B. Case Wood (Eds.), *Neuropsychological rehabilitation after brain injury* (pp. 1–7). Baltimore: John Hopkins University Press.

Rappaport, M., Hall, K. M., Hopkins, K., Belleza, T., & Cope, D. N. (1982). Disability rating scale for severe head trauma. Coma to community. *Archives of Physical Medicine and Rehabilitation, 63,* 118–123.

Ruff, R. M., Marshall, L. F., Crouch, J., Klauber, M. R., Levin, H. S., Barth, J., Kreutzer, J., Blunt, B. A., Foulkes, M. A., Eisenberg, H. M., Jane, J. A., & Marmarou, A. (1993). Predictors of outcome following severe head trauma: Follow-up data from the Traumatic Coma Data Bank. *Brain Injury, 7,* 101–111.

Thomsen, I. V. (1984). Late outcome of very severe blunt head trauma: A 10–15 year second follow-up. *Journal of Neurology, Neurosurgery and Psychiatry, 47,* 260–268.

Vogenthaler, D. R., Smith, K. R., & Goldfader, P. (1989). Head injury, a multivariate study: Predicting long-term productivity and independent living outcome. *Brain Injury, 3,* 369–385.

Vollmer, D. G., Torner, J. C., Jane, J. A., Sadovnic, B., Charlebois, D., Eisenberg, H. M., Foulkes, M. A., Marmarou, A., & Marshall, L. F. (1991). Age and outcome following traumatic coma: Why do older patients fare worse? *Journal of Neurosurgery, 75* (Suppl.), 537–549.

Weddell, R., Oddy, M., & Jenkins, D. (1980). Social adjustment after rehabilitation: A two year follow-up of patients with severe head injury. *Psychological Medicine, 10,* 257–263.

16

Psychosocial Outcome After an Intensive, Neuropsychologically Oriented Day Program: Contributing Program Variables

Anne-Lise Christensen
Carla Caetano
Gitte Rasmussen

Neuropsychology has had a major influence on rehabilitation in the postacute phase of brain injury. Various rehabilitation centers have published results indicating efficacy of treatment. It may be argued that a general acceptance has been reached regarding the value of such treatment. However, many questions remain unanswered, particularly those pertaining to variables that affect outcome.

The psychosocial outcome of a specific intensive day program, (viz. that of the Center for Rehabilitation of Brain Injury [CRBI] at the University of Copenhagen, Denmark) is briefly reviewed, and three program variables that influence outcome are considered: (a) program philosophy that influences the planning of the rehabilitation course, (b) specific content of the treatment program, and (c) length of contact with patients.

PSYCHOSOCIAL DATA FROM CRBI

Data from our program of a 3-year follow-up study of 69 patients have been presented and described in detail (Teasdale & Christensen, 1994). Briefly restated, results were derived from patients from the following categories: 53% suffered cranial trauma and had a coma duration, as measured by the Glasgow Coma Scale (GCS), of 8 days (i.e., moderate to severe level of head injury); 30% suffered stroke; and the remaining 17%

sustained injuries due to encephalitis, meningitis, or tumor. There was a predominance of males (61%), and median age at injury was 24 years. The median time interval between injury and entry into the program was over 2 years.

The data were obtained from (a) interviews with patients, (b) reference to medical records, and (c) discussions with relatives and social workers at five time intervals (viz. preinjury, preprogram, postprogram, 1-year follow-up, and 3-year follow-up). Psychosocial outcome was categorized as type of domestic situation, occupational or educational involvement, and leisure activities. Results, particularly at 1-year follow-up, indicated substantial improvement in independent living, employment/education, and leisure activities. These improvements were generally sustained at 3-year follow-up.

Specifically, domestic situation was combined into three categories: (a) dependent (i.e., living with significant others), particularly characteristic for the younger patients; (b) living alone; (c) living with a spouse or other partner in a stable cohabiting relationship. Prior to injury, 40% of patients were living in situations involving dependence. From preinjury to preprogram—a period of a little over 2 years—the proportion of patients living in dependent situations remained almost the same, but the proportion living alone more than doubled (in part due to dissolution of marital relationships). However, up to 1 year after the program, the number of patients living in dependent situations declined to half of what it was at entrance to the program, and the numbers living in marital relationships increased to more than 50%. This increase was sustained between 1 year and 3 years after completion of the program, with only a small decline in the proportion of marital relationships.

Occupational distribution included competitive employment (i.e., either part time or full time), state-subsidized work, and education. All but one of the patients were either employed or in educational programs prior to injury. Following injury, however, and at entry into the program, almost none (15%) was in employment or educational programs. Those who were working were under threat of losing their jobs if not rehabilitated. Following completion of the program, the numbers in employment and the proportion entering education programs increased: At 1-year follow-up, 65% of the patients were either in employment or educational programs; at 3-year follow-up, the numbers were practically identical.

Leisure activities consisted of three broad categories: patients who reported no pastimes or hobbies, those whose leisure activities were either solitary and/or engaged at home, and finally those whose leisure activities took individuals out of the home and into the company of others. At preinjury, about 85% of the patients had some leisure activities, and over 70% included social activities outside the home. Following injury, however, and at entry into the program, over 50% of patients reported engaging in no real leisure activities. At the 1- and 3-year follow-ups, the proportion engaged in leisure activities almost reached the preinjury level, although social activities outside the home remained lower.

Currently, we are conducting a survey of all the students who have completed our program since 1990. Although our data are not yet complete, 22% of former patients are in competitive employment (i.e., unsubsidized employment), and a further 19% are in some form of subsidized work. In addition, 33% are in educational programs. This combined figure of 74% is in contrast to Thomsen's (1984) 10- to 15-year follow-up study of 40 young, severely head-injured Danish patients (posttraumatic amnesia more than 3 months for over half the sample) who did not receive intensive treatment, but did receive some treatment (e.g., for communication disorders). Results indicate only 15% of patients at the 2- to 5-year follow-up, and 14% of patients at the 10- to 15-year follow-up to be in competitive employment or attending courses. Thus, is little doubt that the rate of return to work or education in the present program represents a considerable improvement on what could have been expected in the absence of postacute rehabilitation, even if it were argued that Thomsen's sample had predominantly more severely head-injured patients than those admitted to the CRBI.

The outcome results from the CRBI are promising. The data show a success rate that is increasingly consistent with the literature, particularly as regards vocational functioning (e.g., Ben-Yishay, Silver, Piasetsky, & Rattock, 1987; Prigatano, Fordyce, Zeiner, Roueche, Pepping, & Wood, 1986). The key question seems to be this: Can we specify the content of the program, and can we identify the core elements of the program philosophy that influence effective planning of the rehabilitation course? To do so adequately, it is necessary to identify the theoretical underpinnings that influence the planning of a program's general character and its individual aspects regarding intervention.

PROGRAM PHILOSOPHY

From the program's start in 1985, its theoretical basis has been the Luria approach to assessment (Christensen, 1984) and the training of cognitive functions (Luria, 1948/1963; Luria, Naydin, Tsvetkova, & Vinarskaya, 1969). However, psychotherapeutic treatment has become an increasingly important part of the program due to the influence of Goldstein's (1952) writings and his successors in the United States (e.g., Yehuda

Ben-Yishay; see Ben-Yishay & Larkin, 1989), for a discussion of group treatment in rehabilitation). In particular, Prigatano has been instrumental in further developing and elaborating on the importance of therapeutic treatment (Prigatano et al., 1986). The core elements of the program philosophy may be summarized by illucidating the key characteristics of Luria's approach to rehabilitation, and by defining the specific elements of the rehabilitative process.

Key Characteristics of Luria's Rehabilitation Approach

The following characteristics provide the main guidelines for the daily work and atmosphere at the CRBI:

1. Recognizing the individuals' uniqueness in diagnosis and treatment, which, from a neuropsychological perspective, incorporates the understanding of functional systems. Thus, flexible and individualized adaption of treatment strategies is encouraged, and, where possible, Lurian theory of brain functioning is adhered to in terms of a theoretical base. Obviously, advances in research theory of brain functioning are incorporated to supplement Luria's model.

2. Allowing for a therapeutic relationship that is trusting, collaborative, and problem solving. It may be argued that this characteristic is intrinsic to most psychotherapeutic approaches. However, in regard to rehabilitation, the emphasis is on encouraging the brain-injured person to become a coworker in the rehabilitation process, rather than a passive recipient of "treatment."

3. Encouraging continual development in rehabilitation planning and treatment based on the previous ideas. At the CRBI, this typically occurs in a multifaceted manner (e.g., initially through the use of test data, behavioral observations, and information from the family; later through the use of feedback from the primary therapist, staff, and other patients in the group).

Thus, the process by which these characteristics occurs is cyclical, resting on a therapeutic relationship that has been nurtured and developed so as to facilitate change. Essentially, the aim of the relationship is to reformulate the patient's identity in correspondence with abilities and deficits that the initial assessment has revealed. This goal is achieved by the feedback being timed in accordance with the level of insight that the patient has gained, such that an inner balance may be developed. Ultimately, the aim is for the person to adequately deal with the successes and failures of normal life.

Specific Elements of the Lurian-Based Rehabilitation Process

Luria's rehabilitation process promoted a realistic attitude by providing feedback on behaviors, (i.e., strengths and weaknesses), as well as comparing the final behavior to the original plan. Furthermore, although Luria did not specifically address the following elements in his primary rehabilitation writings, they were nonetheless implied by his approach to rehabilitation (Christensen & Caetano, in press): (a) facilitating acceptance of changes in previous identity, and (b) assisting in the reformation of identity subsequent to injury.

Currently, one aspect of brain-injury rehabilitation that has received increasing interest is that of the influence of previous personality on functioning subsequent to brain injury (see, e.g., Prigatano, 1994). It has been our experience that the rehabilitation process can be promoted if knowledge about the features identifying the person before the injury is available. Thus, the individual's culture, class (i.e., economic, social, and educational aspects) and occupation should be considered. Of equal importance is the individual's experience of role or self-definition within the family of origin and current family, within peer groups past and present, in sexual relationships, at work, and at play.

Thus, the treatment program's content must correspond to these demands for ongoing dynamic development. The program also has to be especially sensitive to the identification of appropriate timing for change. Furthermore, it seems advantageous for treatment if the program mirrors reality (i.e., it must be meaningful and stimulating, challenging interest and motivation).

SPECIFIC CONTENT OF THE CRBI PROGRAM

The exact nature of the CRBI program has been described elsewhere (Christensen, 1993; Christensen & Teasdale, 1993). The program's development has been influenced by Luria's theory, as well as a number of other variables. First, it should be emphasized that a psychosocial, rather than a medical, model predominates at the CRBI. The staff consists of psychologists, physical therapists, a speech and language therapist, a special education teacher, and a voice therapist. Psychologists act as primary therapists/case managers for one or, at most, two patients at a time. Medical and psychiatric resources are provided on a consultant basis.

Second, the CRBI is located at a university in one of the wings of the humanities faculty. Thus, patients have access to all the facilities the university has to offer, such as the cafeterias, libraries, sitting areas, and university bookstore. Furthermore, a number of the CRBI staff teach at the university, and practicum students regularly participate in the program. This provides an invigorating environment with an emphasis on learning. The patients are called *students* in the program, in accordance with the environment and model of the program.

Third, the program may be described as multifaceted and holistic in orientation, with highly intensive relationships developing between staff and students. Essentially, the program is composed of a number of elements where cognitive functions, emotional reactions, and psychosocial adaptation are handled at various levels—either in isolation (i.e., individual therapy) or in an integrated manner (i.e., program group activities or family meetings). The primary therapist has the overall information and general responsibility for one or two of the students each semester. The students work alone with their primary therapist, and in groups that vary in content and size according to each student's specific demands and needs.

The following trends exist in the program: (a) blending of participatory group activities that require individual responsibility; (b) opportunity for highly individualized individual therapy; (c) meeting of specific needs through special education, language therapy, or voice training; (d) provision of a diverse and specialized form of physical training; (e) incorporation of significant others; and (f) opportunity for integrating postprogram education, occupational, or leisure needs while participating in the program or at follow-up. Each of these aspects is briefly discussed here, providing examples from the program.

Group Activities: Individual Responsibility

The first program element—which provides perhaps the best example of this aspect of the program, which has been given much consideration, and which has been elaborated on through the years—is the morning meeting. The morning meeting is 1 hour every day, all students are present, and it is highly appreciated by them. The therapeutic purpose is centered around activation, orientation, cognition, and development of social skills and rules. Tasks for 5 of the 15 students are delegated in turn, on a weekly basis, creating an active and productive atmosphere. This provides the opportunity for individual responsibility to be taken within a group context. The meeting is chaired by a student who is responsible for the agenda, including choosing a song from a song book found in most Danish homes.

The second element is morning gymnastics, led by another student. The program is short, but comprehensive, including all parts of the body from top to bottom in a logical pattern, calling for planning and remembering. The minutes from the day before are read by the chair of the meeting, and the review of the day's program follows before a third student presents the news of the day (i.e., world and/or local news). This presentation has a personal stand and ends with a question leading to a general discussion.

The third element is presenting a definition or explanation of a topic that may have caused disagreement during the previous day's discussions. The meeting ends with a call for feedback to everybody who has been in charge of a task. Minutes are taken by a fifth student.

A spirited and intimate level of interaction is most often characteristic following the meeting. A psychologist and physiotherapist are responsible for the course of the meeting. However, primary therapists of students with specific tasks are often present to coach their student, and to be informed about all aspects of the psychological interaction in the group.

Further examples of individual responsibility within a group context occur in weekly cognitive and project groups. In both, students are expected to take turns on a day-by-day basis, take minutes of the group activities, and actively participate in providing feedback and offering suggestions during "evaluation" periods. The students in cognitive groups may also be expected to complete assignments at home. The project groups require students as a group, with individual responsibilities, to deliver one presentation a semester on a topic of interest, which is attended by the staff and the rest of the students. At a weekly "joint meeting," students and staff meet for a general evaluation of the week's program, where an open feedback forum is provided.

Besides the training of specific cognitive functions (i.e., concentration, attention, tempo, learning capacity, problem solving, and memory), individualized cognitive training is also provided. Thus, tasks of specific relevance to the individual are provided in individual and group treatment. An example is a former guitarist who was working at a music conservatory before her injury. During her training, music lessons were prepared with her primary therapist, where upon she acted as a teacher for one of the CRBI's psychologists. She was asked to evaluate her own performance, which was later compared with her pupil's evaluation. In another case, a Danish/Spanish translator was taught a new generation of a computer word processor that had succeeded the one he had learned and used before his injury.

Psychotherapy

Psychotherapy plays an important role in the CRBI's work. The 15 students are divided into two groups that meet twice a week. Individual psychotherapy is undertaken by each student's primary psychologist. The theory and adaptation are much in congruence with the American tradition of psychotherapy with brain-injured patients (see Ellis, 1989, for an example of developments in this regard).

Special Needs

Special education is provided as needed. Aphasia training with a speech and language therapist is also available. Voice training is offered where dysarthria is the problem (i.e., specifically where difficulties such as modulation of speech, pitch, tempo, and volume occur). This typically occurs on a weekly basis.

Physical Training

An area in which much development has taken place is physical training. An evolution from a more traditional neurological treatment approach (i.e., based on acute rehabilitation in a hospital setting) to one that encompasses education and the role of cognition has occurred at the CRBI (Rasmussen, 1995). This change in orientation (i.e., from "treatment" to "training") is a result of a number of factors: (a) the relationship of cognitive dysfunction to physical activity, (b) the time of onset of injury—students at the CRBI are typically 2 years postinjury, (c) the decrease in level of fitness since injury such that cardiovascular functioning and endurance are reduced, and (d) the fact that the CRBI is housed at Copenhagen University, which does not have good facilities for physical training. Thus, the fitness club of a nearby large hotel is used, where students mingle freely with hotel guests and former students. This provides a "natural," rather than a "medical," setting.

The physical training at the CRBI is in accordance with other activities inspired by Luria's methodology. Specifically, the functional reorganization principles of inter- and intrasystemic reorganization are considered (Luria, 1948/1963). Thus, for motor deficits following injuries at lower cortical levels of integration (e.g., pareses and disorders of tone and coordination), early implementation of compensatory strategies is provided. Lesions at higher cortical levels, which cause disorders such as apraxia, permit reorganization strategies through intersystemic reorganization.

Therefore, treatment is individualized for each student within the guidelines of the structured program. Each student working at the fitness club is provided with a schedule of activities to follow, as well as being required to make the necessary calculations to determine their "physical output." This provides information on their physical functioning, as well as a broad range of cognitive functions (e.g., planning, structuring abilities, ability to sequence information, memory skills, basic arithmetic skills, etc.), which may be incorporated into the overall treatment plan.

Furthermore, other activities, such as aerobics, volleyball, dance, and jogging, are provided to assist in psychosocial functioning while simultaneously strengthening abilities in coordination, balance, and so on. Emphasis is also placed on cognitive dysfunction, which might contribute to difficulties in this regard. Such activities (e.g., squash, bowling, etc.), which the individual student might have been interested in, are also included. The aim is to develop leisure activities that may be continued subsequent to the program.

In summary, the goal of physical training is to provide the individual with an integrated understanding of the relationship between cognitive dysfunction and difficulties with physical activities, as well as to improve the individual's general fitness level. The role of physical activities as a means to improve psychosocial interaction is also emphasized, particularly in relation to leisure activities subsequent to program completion.

Significant Others

Our student's relatives are considered partners in the rehabilitative process, as well as family members who are in need of therapeutic support. They are included in the treatment as part of the individual psychotherapy process and/or support groups.

Weekly Presentations

Being part of the university environment also means that weekly presentations are part of the program. A lecture is given by either a university teacher or other visiting guests known for their special areas of expertise (e.g., a journalist from a TV station, a chef who has special ideas regarding food, a painter or an art specialist, etc.). Topics must be relevant to the general interests characterizing the program milieu. Previous students of the program may also be presenters. Further, students may attend general university presentation given by other facilities or departments, open to the public, when of interest.

Preparation for Program Completion

In the last month of the program, planning for the student's future is focused on, both in regard to living situation (e.g., where the person is to live, interpersonal relationships, etc.) and in the planning for work or educational activities subsequent to treatment. Interpersonal contacts within the groups have often spontaneously developed into socialized activities outside the group. Participation in sports or other leisure activities has also been encouraged both during and subsequent to the program.

LENGTH OF CONTACT WITH STUDENTS

The length of contact with students has been an issue for thought and discussion since the CRBI started. A planned 6-month follow-up period has been issued from the beginning, where the students are followed individually by their primary therapist according to their need. They also meet as a group once a month, and an open-door policy has been practiced by the staff—where students can call or show up as they feel inclined.

We were concerned that this approach might not work, but experience has shown that students' true need is to manage their own lives. Hence, they only ask for support when the situation is particularly serious. In this event, the problems can most often be solved more easily than would be the case if a new therapist were to be involved.

The reactions of several former students when our latest survey was made suggest the importance of length of contact as a variable influencing change. The telephone contact consisted of questions being asked regarding work or education, and ended with a broader statement regarding well-being. The reactions in many cases were that people felt good about the renewed contact and the possibility of expressing their feelings and talking about their current situation. One commented: "It is challenging to be asked . . . maybe the "push" this provides could mean another step forward." Thus, it could be argued that contact subsequent to the program provides an impetus for change: It motivates students to account for their current context and planning of future needs as a result of the previous relationship developed with the rehabilitation staff and program.

CONCLUSIONS

In summary, psychosocial outcome data have been presented, and three program variables that may affect outcome have been proposed: the theoretical basis of a program, specific content of a program, and length of contact maintained with students. These program variables, among others, may be intrinsic to outcome results in other rehabilitation programs. However, the difficulty remains in defining the manner in which these variables may be adequately evaluated.

We believe that the first variable discussed, namely that of program philosophy, is perhaps the most important. It provides the framework on which the specific elements of a program are built. Rehabilitation literature frequently comments on the lack of a model from which to develop and evaluate assessment and treatment strategies, although authors have attempted to define premises on which intervention is based (see, e.g., Ben-Yishay & Prigatano, 1990; Diller, 1994).

Thus, a clear description of premises that guide treatment, rather than the specific elements of the treatment program itself, may provide a more realistic appraisal of program outcome variables. As can be seen from the CRBI program, where there is individualization of treatment, flexibility, and consistently occurring change, the specific elements of the program may be secondary to effective treatment. The definition of the process elements of a rehabilitation program may be more important than defining only the specific contributory elements.

REFERENCES

Ben-Yishay, Y., & Larkin, P. (1989). Structured group treatment for brain injury survivors. In D. W. Ellis & A.-L. Christensen (Eds.), *Neuropsychological treatment after brain injury* (pp. 271–296). Norwell, MA: Kluver Academic Publishers.

Ben-Yishay, Y., & Prigatano, G. P. (1990). Cognitive remediation. In M. Rosenthall, E. R. Griffith, M. R. Bond, & J. D. Miller (Eds.), *Rehabilitation of the adult and child with traumatic brain injury* (pp. 393–409). Philadelphia: F. A. Davis.

Ben-Yishay, Y., Silver, S. M., Piasetsky, E. B., & Rattok, J. (1987). Relationship between employability and vocational outcome after intensive holistic cognitive rehabilitation. *Journal of Head Trauma Rehabilitation. 1*, 35–49.

Christensen, A.-L. (1984). *Luria's neuropsychological investigation* (2nd ed.). Copenhagen: Munskgaard.

Christensen, A.-L. (1993). Outpatient management and outcome in relation to work in traumatic brain injury patients. *Acta Neurologica Scandinavica, 85*, 32–38.

Christensen, A.-L., & Caetano, C. (in press). Alexander Romanovitsch Luria (1902–1977): Contributions to neuropsychological rehabilitation. *Neuropsychological Rehabilitation.*

Christensen, A.-L., & Teasdale, T. W. (1993). A comprehensive and intensive program for cognitive and psychosocial rehabilitation. In F. J. Stachowiak, R. D Bleser, G. Deloche, R. Lasejae, H. Kremin, P. North, L. Pizzamiglia, I. Robertson, & B. Wilson (Eds.), *Developments in the assessment and rehabilitation of brain-damaged patients.* (pp. 465–467). Tubingem: Gunter Narr Verlag.

Diller, L. (1994). Finding the right treatment combinations: Changes in rehabilitation over the past five years. In A.-L. Christensen & B. P. Uzzell (Eds.), *Brain injury and neuropsychological rehabilitation: International perspectives* (pp. 1–16). Hillsdale, NJ: Lawrence Erlbaum Associates.

Ellis, D. W. (1989). Neuropsychotherapy. In D. W. Ellis & A.-L. Christensen (Eds.), *Neuropsychological treatment after brain injury* (pp. 241–270). Norwell, MA: Kluwer Academic Publishers.

Goldstein, K. (1952). Effects of brain damage on personality. *Psychiatry, 15,* 245–260.

Luria, A. R. (1963). *Restoration of function after brain injury* (B. Haigh, Trans.). London: Pergamon. (Original work published 1948).

Luria, A. R., Naydin, V. I., Tsvetkova, L. S., & Vinarskaya, E. N. (1969). Restoration of higher cortical function following local brain damage. In P. J. Vinken & G. W. Bruyn (Eds.), *Handbook of clinical neurology* (pp. 368–433). Amsterdam: North-Holland.

Prigatano, G. P. (1994). Individuality, lesion location and psychotherapy after brain injury. In A.-L. Christensen & B. P. Uzzell (Eds.), *Brain Injury and neuropsychological rehabilitation: International perspectives* (pp. 173–186). Hillsdale, NJ: Lawrence Erlbaum Associates.

Prigatano, G. P., Fordyce, D. J., Zeiner, H. K., Roueche, J. R., Pepping, M., & Wood, B. (1986). *Neuropsychological rehabilitation after brain injury.* Baltimore: Johns Hopkins University Press.

Rasmussen, G. (1995). Aerobics with hemiplegic patients: Results of physical aerobic fitness training in stroke rehabilitation. In M. Harrison & R. Rustad. (Eds.), *Physiotherapy in stroke management.* Edinburgh: Churchill Livingston.

Teasdale, T. W., & Christensen, A.-L. (1994). Psychosocial outcome in Denmark. In A.-L. Christensen & B. P. Uzzell (Eds.), *Brain injury and neuropsychological rehabilitation: International perspectives* (pp. 235–244). Hillsdale, NJ: Lawrence Erlbaum Associates.

Thomsen, I. V. (1984). Late outcome of very severe blunt head trauma: A 10–15 year second follow up. *Journal of Neurology, Neurosurgery and Psychiatry, 47,* 260–268.

17

Medical Rehabilitation Outcomes for Persons with Traumatic Brain Injury: Some Recommended Directions for Research

Marcus J. Fuhrer
J. Scott Richards

To summarize at the onset, this chapter is devoted to: (a) describing a recent conference on outcomes research in medical rehabilitation organized by the National Center for Medical Rehabilitation Research (NCMRR), (b) communicating some of the recommendations eminating from that conference that are especially relevant to the rehabilitation of persons with traumatic brain injury (TBI), and (c) presenting a background sketch of NCMRR to provide a setting for the conference description and recommendations.

The past two decades have been marked by a dramatic expansion of clinical services and other resources devoted to the rehabilitation of persons who have sustained TBI. Characteristic of an area undergoing rapid development, alternative treatment techniques and models of organizing services have proliferated. Many of the most commonly practiced interventions rest on an extremely fragile scientific foundation. This reflects, in part, that the genesis and subsequent development of these interventions took place almost exclusively in the service arena, rather than as part of a formal research endeavor. The need to assess the effectiveness of these practices takes on heightened importance because of their frequently daunting costs and unsure benefits, and the need for dependable means of reducing the burden of TBI, both to individuals and society at large.

THE NATIONAL CENTER FOR MEDICAL
REHABILITATION RESEARCH

In view of the situation outlined previously, it is hardly surprising that the rehabilitation of persons with TBI is one of the emphasis areas of NCMRR. Indeed, the center's expressed mission is to develop the scientific knowledge required to improve the effectiveness of medical rehabilitation practices, and promote and maintain the health of persons with disabilities throughout their lives. Recently, NCMRR devoted effort to fleshing out a sense of the outcomes research that is called for in many areas of medical rehabilitation, including rehabilitation of persons with TBI. The remainder of this chapter describes that effort.

The legislation that created NCMRR at the National Institutes of Health (NIH) was passed by the Congress in the fall of 1990. Establishment of the center corrected the long-standing anomaly that, although rehabilitation-related research was being sponsored by many of the institutes and centers comprising NIH, no organizational focus existed for the support and planning of such research. Lacking the program activities and budget to warrant being an independent center within NIH, NCMRR was placed within the National Institute of Child Health and Human Development.

The legislation that founded NCMRR also established the National Advisory Board on Medical Rehabilitation Research. The Advisory Board is composed of 12 individuals involved in medical rehabilitation representing scientists or service providers, and 6 individuals representing persons with disabilities. That same legislation called for development of a research plan for the new center—a task that was undertaken by the Advisory Board. The result of that effort, the *Research Plan for the National Center for Medical Rehabilitation Research* (National Institutes of Health, 1993), emphasizes a distinctly inclusive view of medical rehabilitation research (Fig. 17.1). The interaction between the person and the rehabilitation process is conceived as being influenced by biological, psychosocial, and environmental factors, and as being reflected in life domains that encompass survival, productivity, as well as social and work relationships. Further, that interaction is understood to take place across the individual's life span.

Research aimed at assessing the efficacy and effectiveness of medical rehabilitation practices is one of seven emphasis areas described in the research plan. The other emphasis areas are: improving functional mobility; promoting behavioral adaptation to functional losses; developing improved assistive technology; understanding whole-body system responses to physical impairments and functional changes; developing more precise methods of measuring impairments, disabilities, as well as

The Rehabilitation Process:
A Systems Approach

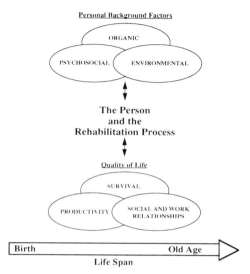

FIG. 17.1. The interaction of the individual with the medical rehabilitation process.

societal and functional limitations; and training research scientists in the field of medical rehabilitation.

CONFERENCE BACKGROUND

Because the NCMRR research plan was intended to provide a sense of direction and not a detailed road map, each area was broadly formulated. Subsequently, effort has been devoted to explicating these areas more concretely, using means that are characteristic of NIH. A conference or workshop is conducted in which internationally acknowledged experts develop recommendations for needed research initiatives. Those recommendations are disseminated widely by reports, journal articles, and edited volumes in an effort to stimulate investigators to undertake the relevant research. The recommendations also may be drawn on by organizational components of NIH in formulating solicitations for grant applications.

During August 29–31, 1994, a conference was conducted to develop recommendations regarding needed initiatives in medical rehabilitation outcomes research. Organized by NCMRR and cosponsored by the Agency for Health Care Policy and Research (AHCPR), the conference was entitled "An Agenda for Medical Rehabilitation Outcomes Research." The invited presenters were individuals who have contributed to medical rehabilitation outcomes research, and who represented the spectrum of disciplines that collaborate in the conduct of medical rehabilitation services and research. Other participants represented federal agencies interested in medical rehabilitation services or research, professional organizations whose memberships provide rehabilitation services, voluntary health organizations that are advocates for the recipients of medical rehabilitation services, and the National Advisory Board on Medical Rehabilitation Research.

To facilitate communication, presenters were asked to use the language of the *International Classification of Impairments, Disabilities, and Handicaps* (ICIDH; World Health Organization, 1980). A number of presentations were grouped under four rubrics concerning issues applicable to many disabling conditions: (a) "Philosophic Issues in Medical Rehabilitation Outcomes Research," (b) "Strategy and Design Issues in Medical Rehabilitation Outcome Studies," (c) "Measurement of Disability and Handicap in Medical Rehabilitation Outcome Studies," and (d) "Measurement of Quality of Life and of Health Status in Medical Rehabilitation Outcome Studies." These categories were the basis of four work groups that were charged with developing recommendations for future research in each area. Five additional work groups generated recommendations relevant to various groupings of specific disabling conditions, including: conditions related to the central nervous system (CNS), cardiovascular conditions, musculoskeletal conditions, conditions related to early development, and aging-related conditions. The recommendations from the work groups were presented in a plenary session for comment by the attendees.[1]

The balance of this chapter describes the recommendations pertinent to CNS-related conditions, in general, and TBI, in particular. The chairperson of this work group was J. Scott Richards, Ph.D. (University of Alabama Spain Rehabilitation Center), whose report provided the basis of the recommendations outlined next.

RECOMMENDATIONS

The group's recommendations were guided by the objective of improving the scientific basis for rehabilitation interventions by identifying which practices work, for which patients, with what specific problems, at which times. Importance was attached to: (a) developing and evaluat-

---

[1]Information about the conference agenda, presenters, and other participants are available from the first author on request.

ing interventions according to sound theoretical formulations (e.g., from neuroscience, learning theory, and cognitive theory), and (b) assessing those interventions in terms of their place in and implications for the continuum of domains in which CNS insult is embedded (e.g., from pathophysiology through impairment, disability, handicap, and quality of life). It was suggested that researchers seeking funding from sources such as NCMRR, for the development of interventions at the levels of pathophysiology and impairment, should accept the burden of convincing reviewers of the likelihood that those interventions will have positive impacts at the levels of disability or handicap. It was also suggested that researchers working with interventions at the level of disability or handicap need to be aware of how potential outcomes are likely to be influenced by determinants at the levels of pathophysiology or impairment. Last, attention was directed to the importance of encompassing cost considerations in evaluating the efficacy or effectiveness of rehabilitation practices and, therefore, of assigning priority to the conduct of cost-effectiveness, cost-benefit, and cost-utility analyses.

The recommendations were in three areas: (a) acute rehabilitation effectiveness; (b) postacute rehabilitation effectiveness, community living, and secondary prevention; and (c) development of an infrastructure for CNS outcomes research.

Acute Rehabilitation Effectiveness

Acute rehabilitation services for persons with TBI, as distinguished from postacute services, are typically provided by a multidisciplinary team in an inpatient setting located in a free-standing medical rehabilitation hospital or a unit of a general hospital. The individualized treatment goals include: stabilizing the patient medically, treating associated conditions such as fractures, preventing development of secondary conditions such as pressure ulcers or contractures, teaching adjustive skills necessary to compensate for individuals' impairments and disabilities, and equipping family members to facilitate patients' resumption of life at home and in the community. Apropos of this stage of the comprehensive rehabilitation process, the following recommendations were made:

- Evaluate interventional procedures and technology with the potential for alleviating disability or handicap by reducing tissue damage, facilitating functional reorganization of the nervous system, or stimulating compensatory neural mechanisms.
- Determine the degree to which treatments directed at improving functioning at the level of impairment, disability, or handicap depend on the nature, location, and extent of CNS damage.

- Compare imaging techniques such as functional magnetic resonance imaging (MRI), single photon emission computerized tomography (SPECT), or positron emission tomography (PET) against less expensive, conventional techniques, such as the clinical examination or multidimensional predictive models based on functional measures for predicting outcomes of rehabilitative interventions.
- Continue development and validation of procedures aimed at encouraging patients' active, sustained participation in the rehabilitation regimen.
- Evaluate the effectiveness of cognitive remediation.
- Evaluate techniques to prevent or reverse the secondary complications of CNS injury that are encountered during acute rehabilitation (e.g., spasticity, contractures, and the neurogenic bowel and bladder).
- Assess the effectiveness and efficiency of rehabilitation therapies intended to facilitate the learning process by which patients become more independent in important life activities.
- Develop and evaluate theoretically grounded techniques to enhance transfer of training among hospital services and between hospital and home settings.

Postacute Rehabilitation Effectiveness

These recommendations were prefaced by the observation that medical rehabilitation services for persons with severe injury of the brain or spinal cord are increasingly being shifted from hospital or residential facilities to outpatient settings or the home. This shift in the context of services, driven largely by demands for cost containment, may adversely affect the effectiveness of those services, although not always. For example, it is likely that activities of daily living and coping skills taught in the home, rather than the hospital, will transfer better to the variety of situations encountered in daily life in the community. Effectiveness research is required to determine whether these kinds of positive outcomes prevail, as opposed to the less desirable ones, which can be readily imagined. The specific recommendations were as follows:

- Evaluate the comparative effectiveness of postacute TBI services and settings, including various treatment-oriented programs versus custodial or nursing home programs.
- Determine the relationship between the adequacy of postdischarge primary care and outcomes, including maintenance of rehabilitation gains and reduction of secondary conditions.

- Assess the effectiveness of interventions designed to reduce or eliminate secondary conditions, such as sexual dysfunction, depression, and pressure sores.
- Evaluate the effectiveness of interventions aimed at enhancing treatment adherence relevant to the rehabilitation process.
- Assess the effectiveness of hospital- or community-based treatment methods for alcohol or drug abuse by persons with CNS trauma.
- Determine how outcomes such as social reintegration following rehabilitation are affected by stigma such as that associated with dysarthria or aphasia.
- Evaluate methods for providing consumers of rehabilitation services with easily understood, objective data about outcomes achieved by service providers in their community.

Development of a CNS Outcomes Research Infrastructure

These recommendations reflect the fact that medical rehabilitation outcomes research is a sufficiently new endeavor that some of the research infrastructure for the efficient execution of studies is not in place. Some of that needed capability requires collaboration among research centers. Such cooperation can be effective in dealing with the problems of: (a) limitations in the number and kinds of patients in particular service settings to constitute study samples of adequate size, (b) difficulties in accessing subjects for control groups, and (c) expenses in monitoring patients in long-term follow-up studies who reside in remote locations. The group's specific recommendations included the following:

- Develop cooperative arrangements among a sufficient number of centers so that well-delineated patient groups can be rapidly assembled for clinical trials.
- Evaluate methods empirically for maximizing the success of follow-up evaluations.
- Validate self-report instruments widely used in rehabilitation against objective, observationally based data.
- Develop better methods of modeling and measuring the pathophysiological severity of CNS disease, disease stage, and impairment.
- Develop more adequate routine outcome-monitoring systems specific to CNS diseases or conditions.
- Adapt commonly used self-report scales that assess disability, handicap, or quality of life for use by persons with cognitive or communication deficits.

POSSIBLE USES OF THE RECOMMENDATIONS

Recommendations like the ones outlined here may serve a number of purposes. One is to reinforce the nascent interests of investigators who may move on to formulate concrete research plans and to seek funding for those plans. This is not to suggest that capable investigators passively await direction and stimulation from funding agencies. Rather, most investigators envision a variety of directions that their previous or ongoing research might take. Discovering that their peers assign special importance to specific issues may be exactly what is needed to elect a particular direction and to initiate concrete research planning.

Research funding organizations such as NCMRR, AHCPR, the National Institute on Disability and Rehabilitation Research within the Department of Education, as well as some voluntary health organizations have long established provisions for funding investigator-initiated applications with such a history. Funding agencies also may draw on conference recommendations to stimulate research necessary to address the knowledge needs that are highlighted. For NCMRR, this may take the form of a request for applications (RFA) or a program announcement (PA). Both involve the solicitation of research grant applications that address designated research questions, and both are widely disseminated by being published in the *NIH Guide* that announces scientific initiatives of NIH. A principal difference between the PA and RFA is that a specific amount of funds is set aside to fund meritorious applications in response to an RFA. Funds for applications stimulated by a PA come from the overall portion of the budget reserved for investigator-initiated applications. That does not eliminate the possibility that these applications will enjoy a competitive advantage. Given a set of applications of similar scientific soundness, according to peer review evaluations, final funding decisions may well favor applications that address issues identified in a PA as opposed to applications that address other issues.

In conclusion, the recommendations presented in this chapter represent the collective judgments of a select group of investigators and service providers, as well as representatives of rehabilitation-related professional organizations and voluntary health agencies. The recommendations relate to the kinds of research that merit priority to establish the outcomes of medical rehabilitation services for persons with CNS dysfunction, in general, and TBI, in particular. The encouragement provided is only one impetus among many that are required to establish a credible knowledge base for future rehabilitation practices for persons with TBI.

REFERENCES

National Institutes of Health. (1993). *Research plan for the national center for medical rehabilitation research*. Bethesda, MD: Author.

National Institutes of Health. NIH guide for grants and contracts. Bethesda, MD: Author.

World Health Organization. (1980). *International classification of impairments, disabilities, and handicaps: A manual of classification relating to the consequences of disease*. Geneva: Author.

18

Traumatic Brain Injury: Work Outcome and Supported Employment

Paul Wehman

Traumatic brain injury (TBI) is rapidly becoming recognized as a national problem of epidemic proportions. Annually, approximately 400,000–500,000 individuals sustain a brain injury of sufficient degree to require treatment (Frankowski, 1986), with anywhere from 44,000 to 90,000 sustaining injury that results in severe, chronic, debilitating impairments (Jennett; Snoek, Bond, & Brooks, 1981; Traphajan, 1988). Survivors of severe brain injury typically exhibit cognitive, physical, or psychosocial impairments that inhibit a return to employment and other activities of daily living, and adversely affect these individuals' quality of life (Klonoff, Costa, & Snow, 1986; Vogenthaler, 1987a, 1987b).

Medical technology has decreased mortality rates for severe head injury and increased life expectancies of survivors, albeit at great cost (Levin, Benton, & Grossman, 1982). Because a significant proportion of brain-injury survivors are young adults who are either entering or about to enter their peak earning years (Frankowski, 1986), and because of decreased mortality rates due to complications from trauma, brain injury frequently results in long-term economic hardship on victims, their families, and society (McMordie & Barker, 1988). The costs of traumatic brain injury—including acute care, rehabilitation efforts, lost earnings and productivity, reduced savings, and extended medical and income maintenance—are staggering (Kalsbeek, McLaurin, Harris, & Miller, 1980; McMordie & Barker, 1988).

A significant portion of these costs to victims, their families, and society can be directly linked to poor rates of postinjury employment for survivors of severe TBI. A number of follow-up surveys have found that these individuals are unlikely to enter or reenter the workforce following injury (Brooks, Campsie, Symington, Beattie, & McKinlay, 1987; Stapleton, 1986; Weddell, Oddy, & Jenkins, 1980). Many who do return to the workforce do so in less demanding work, with fewer hours, at less pay, or in sheltered workshops or volunteer positions (McMordie, Barker, & Paolo, 1990; Peck, Fulton, Cohen, Warren, & Antonello, 1984).

One strategy used recently to overcome this unemployment problem is supported employment. *Supported employment* is defined as paid employment for persons with developmental disabilities, for whom competitive employment at or above the minimum wage is unlikely and who, because of their disabilities, need ongoing support to perform their work. Support is provided through activities such as training, supervision, and transportation. Supported employment is conducted in a variety of settings, particularly work sites in which persons without disabilities are employed. This approach is targeted toward severely disabled populations, who traditionally have been difficult to place into competitive employment (e.g., Wehman, Sale, & Parent, 1992).

Supported employment is a combination of employment and ongoing services. It is a type of employment, rather than a method of employment preparation or a type of service activity. It is a powerful and flexible way to (a) ensure normal employment benefits, (b) provide ongoing and appropriate support, (c) create opportunities, and (d) achieve full participation, integration, and flexibility. New employment initiatives in the United States have created a climate of opportunity to develop new work options for all people with severe disabilities. Furthermore, in October 1992, representatives of European countries met in Norfolk, Virginia, with the author to discuss the establishment of a European consortium on supported employment. There is a growing interest internationally, as well as in the United States, on how supported employment can be utilized.

FEATURES OF SUPPORTED EMPLOYMENT

Six features of supported employment programs explain how they differ from a traditional service approach.

1. Employment. The purpose of these programs is employment with the regular outcomes of having a job. Wages, working conditions, and job security are key considerations.

2. Ongoing support. The focus is on providing the ongoing support required to get and keep a job, rather than on getting a person ready for a job sometime in the future.

3. Jobs, not services. Emphasis is on creating opportunities to work, rather than just providing services to develop skills.

4. Full participation. People who are severely disabled are not excluded. The assumption is that all persons, regardless of the degree of their disability, have the capacity to undertake supported employment if appropriate ongoing support services can be provided.

5. Social integration. Contact and relationships with people without disabilities who are not paid caregivers are emphasized. Social integration with coworkers, supervisors, and others occur at work, near work, during lunchtimes or breaks, or during nonwork hours as a result of wages earned.

6. Variety and flexibility. Supported employment does not lock programs into one or two work options. It is flexible because of the wide range of jobs in the community and the many ways of providing support to individuals in those jobs.

To best illustrate how supported employment can be applied to the work reentry of persons with TBI, data compiled over the past 6 years from the Virginia Commonwealth University program are presented next, along with a descriptive case study.

METHODOLOGY

Setting and Participating Clients

The supported employment program for traumatically brain-injured persons is based at a university in the southeastern United States. The program has been fully operational since January 1987, although one client was seen for services before that time. Funding for 10 employment specialists is derived from the state rehabilitation agency, insurance companies, and, periodically, federal or state grants.

All clients are under medical supervision of a physiatrist on referral to the supported employment program. One hundred and fifteen clients have been referred for supported employment services. Virtually all have been initially accepted for potential placement, provided they are between 18 and 64 years of age and have a history of severe TBI. *Severe TBI* is defined as an insult to the brain caused by a direct or indirect force and resulting in a Glasgow Coma Scale (GCS) score of ≤ 8 for ≥ 6 hours. To be considered a candidate for the program, there must also be a strong indication that the person cannot work successfully without ongoing job support. This indication is determined by (a) documented previous employment failures postinjury, or (b) reports from the family, physician, referring rehabilitation counselor, or client indicating concern about independent work ability. It has been a policy of the program to not exclude patients from the referral pool based on cognitive, physical, or psychosocial impairments.

An initial neuropsychological examination is completed on every referral. Measures of intellectual, cognitive, and psychomotor ability include the Galveston Orientation Amnesia Test, as well as portions of the Wechsler Adult Intelligence Scale–Revised (WAIS–R), the Wide Range Achievement Test–Revised (WRAT–R), and the Halstead–Reitan. Every effort was made to incorporate neuropsychological tests that measure skill areas relevant to vocational functioning. Once results are summarized, they are reviewed with program placement staff. The client's relative strengths and weaknesses are noted, particularly in regard to his or her expressed vocational interests.

In January 1987, three "job coaches," also known as employment specialists, provided job development, job placement, job site training, and ongoing job retention services to clients with TBI. By 1989, this number doubled to seven. These staff did travel training, made initial and ongoing home visits, worked with local Social Security personnel, and arranged for payment for services from rehabilitation and insurance carriers. Each employment specialist was assigned approximately 8–10 cases for placement and training, which were usually accumulated over a period of several months. All cognitive training, adaptations, and other interventions occurred during employment at the job site. Tables 18.1 and 18.2 provide demographic, neuropsychological, and occupational profiles of the individuals who were referred to the program.

As can be observed in Table 18.1, the mean age at injury was 25 years, with the mean age of referral being 31 years. Time unconscious averaged 48 days, with a range of 0–182 days. Approximately one fifth of the referrals had not finished high school. One third were high school graduates. Approximately one fourth of all individuals (27%) had some college, and 13% were college students. Approximately 9% of persons in the initial group of referrals were on medication for seizure control, and 27.5% reported physical weakness.

Descriptive data from neuropsychological test were in the impaired range (less than 6th percentile) for the following skill areas: attention, motor speed, verbal learning, verbal memory, visual memory, and visuoconstruction. With regard to academic skills, performance ranged from the 9th percentile (Arithmetic WRAT–R) to the 25th percentile (arithmetic Reasoning WAIS–R and Gray Oral Reading Test–R). Spelling was at the 16th percentile. In the area of problem-solving skills (Category Test), the mean number of errors obtained indicated performance at approximately the 20th percentile. Performance was at the 16th percentile in the skill area of fund of information. Performance was in the average range (greater than 25th percentile) on only one of

TABLE 18.1
Demographic Information

Demographic Characteristic		%
Sex		
Male		82.5
Female		17.5
Race		
Black		21.2
White		75.0
Other		3.8
Chronological age		
Mean at injury	(range = 5–64)	24.8 years
Mean at referral	(range = 17–65)	30.9 years
Mean at placement	(range = 18–65)	31.5 years
Educational level		
Less than high school		22.5
High school graduate		36.6
Some college classes		26.8
College graduates		12.7
Postgraduate		1.4
Etiology of brain injury		
Automobile accident		49.3
Motorcycle/bicycle accident		10.7
Pedestrian accident		10.7
Fall		9.3
Sprots injury		1.3
Assault		5.3
Gunshot		4
Abuse		2.7
Other		6.7
Residential at time of referral		
Parent's/other relative's home		58.3
Own home		25.4
Domiciliary care/supervised living		10.5
Other		5.8
Concomitant significant disabilities (medical)		
Physical impairments		11.3
Seizures		8.8
Visual impairments		13.8
Physical weaknesses		27.5
Hearing impairments		2.5
Duration of unconsciousness		Mean = 48 days
		Range = 0–182
Mean length of time since injury		6.1 years
Recipients of Supplemental Security Income and /or Social Security Disability Income		61

Note. Number of placed TBI clients is 80.

261

TABLE 18.2
Occupational Information

	%
Company type	
Commercial (e.g., retailers)	44.1
Food service	16.9
Industrial	12.7
Health care	8.5
Service provider	5.9
Lodging	5.1
Education	3.4
Other	2.5
Janitorial/custodial	0.8
Company affiliation	
Profit for profit	87.3
State government	5.9
Private nonprofit	3.4
Local government	2.5
Federal government	0.8
Type of work	
Stock clerk/warehouse	23.7
Clerical/office work	19.5
Food service	16.9
Janitorial/custodial	11.0
Bench work/assembly	9.3
Groundskeeping	7.6
Laundry	4.2
Human services	2.5
Transportation	2.5
Unskilled labor	2.5
Level of integration in the workplace	
Frequent work-related interaction	55.9
Moderate level of work-related interaction	27.1
No work-related interaction	11.0
General physical separation	5.1
Complete segregation	0.8

the tests administered: Controlled Oral Word Association Test was at the 29th percentile.

DISCUSSION

Based on the results of this investigation and other related studies (Wehman et al., 1989, 1990), the supported employment approach to promoting vocational outcomes for persons with TBI should be viewed with cautious optimism. It appears that supported employment is as effective, if not more so, than other approaches currently being used to assist people in returning to work. We now know that many people with severe TBI can return to some form of competitive employment. Although this may require several hundred hours of direct, one-to-one intervention provided by a trained employment specialist, there is every reason to be encouraged that persons with significant functional limitations can obtain and maintain part- or full-time employment within the community and earn at least minimum wage.

In this descriptive study, 80 individuals returned to competitive employment through participation in a supported employment program. The demographic data reveal that these individuals had significant physical and cognitive disabilities as a result of severe TBI. Neuropsychological evaluation revealed a diverse pattern of cognitive impairment. Results indicate that individuals in the supported employment program showed significant neuropsychological deficits in a number of important areas. Individuals displayed the largest deficits in the areas of attention and concentration, learning and memory, motor speed/dexterity, and visuoconstruction. These abilities were severely impaired by injury. Notably, performance was in the average range on only 1 of the 13 tests administered (a measure of verbal fluency). Impaired abilities in attention, memory, and motor skills greatly affect work performance. Thus, compensating for deficits in these areas, as well as addressing neurobehavioral dysfunction, are important challenges in working with individuals with TBI.

Current job site data support that, when individuals are willing to use compensatory strategies, each of the deficit areas cited previously can be effectively addressed. In the area of defective motor speed, implementation of assistive technology and job restructuring can help increase an individual's production level. In addition, information obtained through a job analysis, prior to placement, can be compared with client assessment data to ensure that an individual's vocational strengths are utilized.

Prior to participation in supported employment, all referrals had been unable to either obtain or maintain employment, working only 13% of the total months during which they could have worked. Participation in supported employment revised this figure to 67% of total months worked postinjury. It should be noted, however, that the monthly employment ratio of 67% represents a slight decrease from the rate of 75% reported in our 1990 study (Wehman et al., 1990).

The number of individuals served through the program increased from 43 in 1990 to 80 in the present investigation. We continue to obtain more information about this approach's effectiveness. Results consistently indicate that supported employment participation has a positive effect on an individual's ability to enter and remain in the workforce, even if not at the same job. Monthly employment ratios during the period between injury and entry into supported employment are consistently low, but rise close to 70% levels after involvement in supported employment. This is particularly noteworthy because, for this specific sample, referral to supported employment occurred about 6 years after injury. The data also reflect an increase over the preinjury monthly employment rate, where individuals of working age were employed only 40% of the total months they could have been working. It may be that persons referred to the program had not developed stable, ongoing work histories prior to injury. The monthly employment ratio should not be seen as the only outcome measure of program effectiveness, but it does provide additional information about how clients are doing vocationally.

What follows next is a case study of one person who has benefited from the use of a supported employment approach.

Case Study—Lee

Lee is a 37-year-old man who experienced a Grade III TBI as a result of falling asleep while driving. His automobile struck a tree, and he remained undiscovered for nearly 12 hours. Lee was in a coma for 21 days, and remained hospitalized for 5 months.

Before his injury, Lee graduated from college with a degree in journalism and worked as a sportswriter for two major newspapers. At 9 months postinjury, Lee attempted to return to work as a sportswriter, but was unsuccessful due to his inability to meet story deadlines. As a client of the Department of Rehabilitative Services (DRS), Lee then attended a state residential rehabilitation center and received certification as an office aide. He was placed into a mail processing position by the DRS, but left the job 1 month later because he could not meet the production standards. Lee was unable to locate employment on his own, and thus had been working as a volunteer at outpatient rehabilitation center as a physical therapy aide when he was referred for supported employment services by his state rehabilitation counselor.

Job Placement

At the time of Lee's referral to the supported employment program, neuropsychological evaluation results revealed strengths in his verbal skills, such as written and spoken communication. Lee's areas of weakness included visual perception, visual–motor integration, and memory functioning. Assessment activities revealed that Lee would do best in an employment setting that required communication skills and had minimal demands on visual and motor skills, and new learning. Lee displayed good social skills, thus it was able to get along well with coworkers and the public. Also, due to Lee's distractibility, it was thought that he would likely function best in environments with little extraneous noise or background stimuli. Lee informed the employment specialist that he would be dissatisfied with repetitive work and wanted to work "helping people." Additionally, he desired a part-time position so his Social Security benefits would not be jeopardized. Eight months after being referred to the supported employment program, Lee was placed in a position as an activities aide at a convalescent center. The job duties involved one-to-one visitations with room-bound residents, documentation of visits on a patient interaction report, and assisting the activities director in planning and implementing other activities as needed.

Lee had good communication skills. His preference for nonrepetitive work in the human services field, plus his desire for part-time employment, made him a good candidate for the position. In addition, the position would also place minimal demands on visual–motor skills, and the working environment was fairly quiet, increasing Lee's ability to concentrate and perform his job duties.

After the interview and 3 days prior to Lee's first day at work, the assistant activities director telephoned the employment specialist with concerns about placing an individual with TBI in the position. She stated that they needed someone who had common sense, was capable of thinking for him or herself, and was a quick thinker. The assistant activities director also stated that she was reluctant to allow Lee to have one-to-one contact with residents. The week before, a resident with Alzheimer's disease had wheeled himself down the second-story stairs; she questioned how Lee would have responded if faced with such a situation. The employment specialist reassured the employer that she would be there 100% of time to train Lee, and that if Lee failed to meet the job requirements independently the program would seek a more suitable job for him. The employment specialist also reemphasized Lee's strengths and reiterated why he was the "man for the job." Next, the director of activities called the employment specialist and stated that she too had concerns. Over the next 3 days, the director vacillated about whether to hire Lee for the job. Finally, the activities director agreed to give Lee a shot. He was hired to work 20 hours per week at $3.55 per hour.

One of Lee's difficulty areas with memory functioning. The employment specialist structured and organized the visitation and documentation procedures. Also, books with daily readings were purchased so Lee would not have to keep track of the previous day's readings. Lee's distractibility and poor concentration were areas of concern during training too. The employment specialist trained Lee to create a "quiet environment" during a visit by always asking the resident whether he could lower the volume of the TV or radio, and by shutting the door. Modeling was a major teaching strategy used during initial training activities. The employment specialist modeled appropriate ways to interact with residents during room visits, and provided Lee with feedback on his performance.

Work Outcome

To date, the employment specialist continues to contact Lee and/or the employer at least twice a month to enhance job retention and proactively identify potential areas that may require further intervention. Situations that have arisen during the follow-along phase have included: turnover in supervisors, Lee's occasional desire to terminate employment and seek a new job, changes in his physical ability, and reports of a decrease in job performance.

There has been high turnover in the activities directors: In the past 2 years, there have been six changes in supervision. The employment specialist has returned to educate the new director on the supports available to Lee through the program, and to address any initial concerns. On occasion, Lee has expressed a desire to terminate his employment, reportedly due to feeling depressed because the individuals he visits may be close to death and die. The employment specialist has lended an open ear and talked with Lee about death and dying. In addition, the employment specialist advocated for Lee to become more actively involved with healthier residents during daily activities. Lee now conducts Bible study groups, calls the weekly Bingo game, and transports residents to activities.

Once during a follow-along visit, it was noticed that Lee was losing his balance and having spastic movements. The employment specialist brought this to the attention of Lee and his family members, and recom-·mended they seek medical assistance. Based on the employment specialist's request, the family arranged for Lee to see his neurologist and have his medications reevaluated. His medications were changed and improvement was evident.

Last, situations have arisen when the supervisor was not pleased with the quality or the number of visits Lee's was performing. The employment specialist, who regularly collects data on Lee's performance, was able to determine whether the concern was warranted, and gave an accurate appraisal of his performance. Once the employment specialist discovered that Lee was taking additional unauthorized smoking breaks. The onsite intervention included discussions with Lee on why this should not occur and the natural consequences of the behavior if it was not modified. Lee agreed to reduce the number of breaks.

On another occasion, the supervisor reported that Lee had been slacking off on his documentation—he was recording the same case note for each resident's visit. The employment specialist met with Lee and together they designed and implemented a checklist, which Lee used to become more creative during a visit.

Whenever production was reported as a concern, the employment specialist investigated the situation by calculating the number of minutes required to provide the number of visits requested. This calculation has been presented to the supervisor; on each occasion, the supervisor has had to decide about the quality versus quantity of visits.

To date, Lee has been working as a part-time activities aide for 5 years and 7 months. Total staff intervention time to date has been approximately 580 hours, and Lee has earned approximately $19,500. Lee and the most recent supervisor have been working together since September 1991. The employer is reportedly satisfied with Lee's performance at this time, and Lee is content with his job.

DISCUSSION

The value of specialized intervention and ongoing assistance has been demonstrated in this chapter. As medical technology advances, there will be increasing bioethical dilemmas over how much service can be provided to postacute patients. This chapter shows that supported employment is a vocational intervention that yields real work outcomes. At the same time, the issue of long-term funding and support underwriting specialized vocational interventions such as these is raised. Substantial amounts of money are spent to help patients return to relatively low-paying jobs. Increasingly more rehabilitationists and health care providers are asking for ways to pay for these services.

Long-Term Support Services

Although it is clear that supported employment has not yet been established as the definitive vocational rehabilitation approach for clients with severe neurological injuries, there are now sufficient data to encourage study of long-term funding for the community service needs of this group. For example, we now know that a number of individuals can be reemployed, but need protracted services to maintain their employment status. When looking at long-term funding issues, it is helpful to recognize that the federal and state vocational rehabilitation service systems are the primary means by which persons with TBI can access rehabilitative services, including supported employment, regardless of the state, province, or country. Therefore, what are the major issues in crafting a funding strategy?

Long-Term Funding: Key Issues

Perception of Rehabilitation Potential. Rehabilitation counselors may be reluctant to offer services to individuals with severe neurological injuries because of a historical pessimism regarding these patients' rehabilitation potential. Indeed, some researchers found an inverse relationship between severity of injury and likelihood of receiving significant levels of rehabilitative services. Other investigators have found that few persons with severe brain injury are enrolled in work retraining, sheltered, or volunteer activities.

Perceptions of Vocational Rehabilitation Services. The enduring concept of vocational rehabilitation services is that they are time limited and purely vocational. This continues to be the focus of state programs. Many professionals agree that the vocational rehabilitation service system can be beneficial to individuals who have sustained mild injuries and who can make a successful transition from medical rehabilitation to their home communities without specialized services. Persons with severe TBI generally have more complex, varied, and multifaced deficits and needs that require long-term service obligations. Moreover, the service process (i.e., vocational evaluation, work hardening, work adjustment, etc.) presupposes that clients can remember and build on their experiences during service phases and generalize their training to actual work environments—abilities frequently impaired by severe head injury. Finally, the time-limited nature of vocational rehabilitation services does not address the episodic occurrences of emotional/behavioral impairments, which frequently accompany severe TBI.

Funding Sources for Extended Services. The coordination of funding from time-limited to extended services has been problematic for agencies serving persons with TBI who did not fall under the traditional mental health/mental retardation umbrella. For example, a group of researchers found that, of the 27 states that awarded system change grants in 1986–1987 to develop supported employment as a service option, only 5 identified funding sources for extended services for this population. Further, they only did so for those individuals who also met the additional criteria of the state mental health, mental retardation, or developmental disability agency.

Types of Availability of Services.   Although recent years there has been progress in developing services for persons with severe neurological injury, the majority of programs continue to focus on acute medical care and acute rehabilitation, according to the U.S. Head Injury Foundation. Specialized postacute vocational, neurobehavioral, and independent-living services are limited in number, and demand for services far exceeds availability. These services also tend to be expensive, and therefore are beyond the means of most survivors and their families, as well as beyond the willingness of most public and private funding sources.

Implications and Research Needs

The issues described in this chapter underscore both the paucity of knowledge regarding employment for persons with severe neurological injuries, and the limited commitments of public expenditures (time, effort, and money) to resolve the problems that persons with TBI experience in attempting to enter or reenter the workforce. These issues also suggest directions in the research and public policy areas for improving the vocational outlook for these individuals. The literature notes that it is difficult to predict which survivors of severe injuries will become employed and which will not. Available research is contradictory and typically has not included individuals involved in intensive interventions. Research is needed to address the following areas:

1. There is a need for a better understanding of the reasons why some members of this population fail to achieve long-term employment success, even within a program of supported employment. For example, Sale, West, Sherron, and Wehman (1991) analyzed data that show that, once clients with TBI stay employed at least 6–9 months, their long-term vocational stability improves. The high-risk time period is in the first several months of employment.

2. There is also a need to examine the types of interventions that are most effective in addressing specific vocational and social deficits, including job-placement strategies, employer–coworker preparation, compensatory strategies, crisis intervention, and effective use of counseling, medical, neuropsychological, behavioral, respite, and other support services. More specifically, what is the most efficient and cost-effective way to arrange these services?

3. Research on the impact of rehabilitation efforts is confounded by

the difficulty in determining, retrospectively, the types of rehabilitation services that individuals have received and the effects of specific services. Program outcome research must attempt to identify and address the effects of prior services, as well as the effects of spontaneous recovery over time through the brain's natural recovery and compensation processes.

4. Research and demonstration efforts are also needed on the efficacy of using group models or modifications of individual-supported employment, such as industrial-based enclaves or clustered placements. Are these viable alternatives for individuals who need relatively permanent monitoring and intervention, and who repeatedly fail to achieve stabilization in individual placement? If so, how can group models be designed and implemented so as to achieve maximum integration and earnings while minimizing stigma?

5. There is virtually no information on the costs and benefits of providing necessary interventions that allow individuals with severe neurological injuries to become employed and stay employed, or cost-effectiveness comparisons across various return-to-work methods. Likewise, there is limited information on the costs of not providing vocational services, including alternative day-support services, permanent income maintenance, and loss of contributions to the tax base from both the brain-injured person and family members who must forego or limit their own employment to provide daily care for their injured loved one. West et al. (1991) reported that 291 hours of staff intervention time were necessary for each person placed, with costs to stabilization averaging $6896 and annual costs of extended services being $2476. However, this report tells us nothing about the benefits accrued for clients with TBI.

Addressing these research needs should improve services to the client group, as well as encourage expenditures of vocational rehabilitation case service dollars and access to vocational services as well.

In summary, integrated, community-based services are still in their infancy for people with severe TBI. There are a number of steps that state and federal agencies can take to spur development of services. First and foremost, state and federal funding agencies should begin the arduous process of developing a comprehensive, coordinated system of services for persons with severe brain injury—from the acute medical stage, through acute rehabilitation, to long-term services. Funding dollars should be earmarked specifically for programs to meet the unique needs of this population, and should include supported and independent living, respite care management, and social/recreational development, as well as extended supported employment services.

REFERENCES

Brooks, D. N., Campsie, L., Symington, C., Beattie, A., & McKinlay, W. (1987). The effects of severe head injury on patient and relative within seven years of injury. *Journal of Head Trauma Rehabilitation, 2*(3), 1–13.

Frankowski, R. (1986). Descriptive epidemiologic studies of head injury in the United States: 1974–1984. In L. Karger & T. Basel, *Trauma treatment in practice: The head injured patient* (pp. 152–172).

Jennett, B., Snoek, J., Bond, M., & Brooks, N. (1981). Disability after severe head injury: Observations on the use of the Glasgow Coma Scale. *Journal of Neurology, Neurosurgery, and Psychiatry, 44*, 285–293.

Kalsbeek, W. D., McLaurin, R. L., Harris, B. S. H., & Miller, J. D. (1980). The national head and spinal cord injury survey: Major findings. *Journal of Neurosurgery, 53*(Suppl.), S19–S43.

Klonoff, P. S., Costa, L. D., & Snow, W. G. (1986). Predictors and indicators of quality of life in patients with closed-head injury. *Journal of Clinical and Experimental Neuropsychology, 8*, 469–485.

Levin, H. S., Benton, A., & Grossman, R. G. (1982). *Neurobehavioral consequences of closed head injuries.* New York: Oxford University Press.

McMordie, W. R., & Barker, S. L. (1988). The financial trauma of head injury. *Brain Injury, 2*, 357–364.

McMordie, W. R., Barker, S. L., & Paolo, T. M. (1990). Return to work (RTW) after head injury. *Brain Injury, 4*, 57–69.

Peck, G., Fulton, C., Cohen, C., Warren, J. R., & Antonello, J. (1984, October). *Neuropsychological, physical, and psychological factors affecting long-term vocational outcomes following severe head injury.* Paper presented at the annual meeting of the International Neuropsychological Society, Houston, TX.

Sale, P., West, M., Sherron, P., & Wehman P. (1991). Exploratory analysis of job separations from supported employment for persons with traumatic brain injury. *Journal of Head Trauma Rehabilitation, 6*(3), 1–11.

Stapleton, M. B. (1986). Maryland Rehabilitation Center closed head injury study: A retrospective survey. *Cognitive Rehabilitation, 4*, 34–42.

Traphajan, J. (1988). *Community re-entry.* Southborough, MA: National Head Injury Foundation.

Vogenthaler, D. R. (1987a). An overview of head injury: Its consequences and rehabilitation. *Brain Injury, 1*, 113–127.

Vogenthaler, D. R. (1987b). Rehabilitation after closed head injury: A primer. *Journal of Rehabilitation, 53*(4), 15–21.

Weddell, R., Oddy, M., & Jenkins, D. (1980). Social adjustment after rehabilitation: A two year follow-up of patients with severe head injury. *Psychological Medicine, 10*, 257–263.

Wehman, P., Kreutzer, J., West, M., Sherron, P., Diambra, J., Fry, R., Groah, C., Sale, P., & Killam S. (1989). Employment outcomes of persons following traumatic brain injury: Pre-injury, post-injury, and supported employment. *Brain Injury, 3*(12), 397–412.

Wehman, P., Kreutzer, J., West, M., Sherron, P., Zasler, N., Groah, C., Stonnington, H., Burns, C., & Sale, P. (1990). Return to work for persons with traumatic brain injury: A supported employment approach. *Archives of Physical Medicine and Rehabilitation, 71*, 1047–1052.

Wehman, P., Sale, P., & Parent, W. (1992). *Supported employment: Strategies for integration of workers with disabilities. From research to practice.* Andover, MA: Andover Medical Publishers.

West, M., Wehman, P., Kregel, J., Kreutzer, J., Sherron, P., & Zasler, N. (1991). An analysis of costs associated with operating a return to work program for traumatically brain injured individuals. *Archives of Physical Medicine and Rehabilitation, 72*, 127–131.

IV

Family and Community

19

Family Transactions and Traumatic Brain Injury

Janet E. Farmer
Renée Stucky-Ropp

The occurrence of a significant traumatic brain injury (TBI) typically precipitates a life crisis for families. Family members are generally unprepared for changes observed in the person with TBI and must grapple with an uncertain course of recovery. TBI often demands new ways of coping, alterations in patient and family self-definitions, and lengthy or lifelong adaptation. The individual with TBI may experience multiple losses, including impaired physical health and cognitive functioning, change in roles or responsibilities, decreased autonomy, and loss of future expectations. Family members also experience losses, sometimes acquiring the perception that they are unlike "normal, healthy families" (McDaniel, Hepworth, & Doherty, 1992).

The dramatic and sometimes devastating effects of a TBI on individual family members, and on the family as a whole, have become increasingly evident (Kreutzer, Gervasio, & Camplair, 1994a; Waaland, 1990). Although the influence on the family is not always entirely negative (Mauss-Clum & Ryan, 1981; Sachs, 1985), families almost inevitably experience a period of turmoil and chaos (Maitz, 1991). Changes in the individual's functional abilities and personality, and subsequent changes in the family's financial resources and lifestyle, may occur, producing significant emotional strain and practical daily burdens for family members (Kreutzer et al., 1994a; Lezak, 1988; Livingston & Brooks, 1988).

A less studied, but equally important, aspect of family functioning is the impact of family characteristics on the outcome of the person with TBI. Not only does the occurrence of TBI shape families, but the family's structure, interaction style, and coping resources also have a reciprocal influence on the course of the individual's recovery (Leach, Frank, Bouman, & Farmer, 1994; Rivara et al., 1993, 1994). If preinjury family functioning was unhealthy, or if the family system begins to break down under the strain associated with the injury, its ability to meet individual family members' needs is jeopardized (Maitz, 1991).

This chapter briefly reviews the relationship between TBI and family functioning. First, the challenges and burdens experienced by family members are reviewed, and the sequelae of TBI most likely to create family problems are discussed. Because the effect of TBI varies depending on the relationship of the family member to the survivor, the perspectives of the spouse, parent, child, sibling, and extended family are explored. Second, the family system's influence on the individual's adaptation is discussed. Finally, directions for future research are suggested. This chapter is not intended to be a comprehensive review of TBI's effect on family systems, but rather a highlight of the most pertinent issues involving families. More comprehensive reviews of this area exist for the interested reader (Camplair, Kreutzer, & Doherty, 1990; Kay & Cavallo, 1994; Kreutzer, Marwitz, & Kepler, 1992; Lezak, 1988; Maitz, 1991; Urbach & Culbert, 1991).

THE EFFECT OF TBI ON THE FAMILY

Families are social systems with relationships and roles that develop to maintain effective daily functioning and to meet a series of developmental tasks, such as childrearing or caring for aging relatives (Kay & Cavallo, 1994; Leaf, 1993; Minuchin, 1974). Each family has a unique pattern of relating that optimally balances the needs of all its interconnected members. This homeostasis is upset when one person in the family system sustains a brain injury. The family's efforts to restore itself and institute a new balance following TBI may be viewed as parallel to the process of rehabilitation and adaptation in the injured person. To the extent that recovery is incomplete for the individual following brain injury, the family system can never return to its former "self" (Kay & Cavallo, 1994).

Any catastrophic injury/illness is accompanied by profound demands on the family system. However, TBI differs from other traumatic injuries in terms of effect on family functioning by the following elements: (a) the constellation of cognitive, emotional, and behavioral sequelae of TBI; (b) the often permanent nature of the deficits, which requires ongoing alterations in family functioning to accommodate the needs of the member with TBI; and (c) the demographics of TBI, which primarily occurs in young adult males, and affects either relatively mature families in the process of launching a youth into greater independence or young families in the early stages of their development (Kay & Cavallo, 1994).

These characteristics of TBI produce elevated levels of psychological distress among relatives and caregivers. Researchers have found a high need for tranquilizers or sleep medications among family members (Panting & Merry, 1972), marital dysfunction and a high divorce rate among spouses (Thomsen, 1974, 1984), breakdown in family cohesion (Bond, 1975), persistent depression and perceptions of stress 1 year postinjury (McKinlay, Brooks, Bond, Martinage, & Marshall, 1981; Oddy, Humphrey, & Uttley, 1978), and feelings of being trapped and isolated (Lezak, 1988). Livingston, Brooks, and Bond (1985) established that families of more severely injured persons show more adjustment problems than those with mildly injured members. These reports may have actually underestimated coping problems. Family members have sometimes displayed what has been described as "command performance syndrome," where they mask their emotional distress in the presence of the individual with TBI and health care professionals (Sbordone, Kral, Gerard, & Katz, 1984). This often creates the erroneous impression that they are effectively coping with the increased burdens and do not require psychological intervention.

More recently, Kreutzer and colleagues (1994a) found that nearly half (47%) of the caregivers of adult outpatients with TBI reported clinically significant levels of emotional distress on a standardized assessment of personal adjustment, or approximately twice the rate of distress reported by the normative sample. Almost one third of the respondents reported high levels of anxiety, and 25% of the sample indicated significant concerns in the areas of depression, hostility/irritability, and somatic complaints. Consistent with previous research, caregivers also endorsed items reflecting chronic stress, feelings of isolation and social alienation, and a sense of being overwhelmed and unappreciated. On global measures of family functioning, 74% identified problems with communication and approximately 50% reported a decrease in expressions of positive affection of caring among family members. Thus, although persons with TBI have described their families as more cohesive following injury (Frank, Haut, Smick, Haut, & Chaney, 1990), caregivers have often experienced less emotional closeness and greater frustration in their communication efforts.

Sequelae Most Likely to Create Family Problems

Although at times quite severe and requiring definite alterations in family routines, physical problems following TBI generally are not strongly associated with subjective family burden (Brooks & McKinlay, 1983; Brooks, Campsie, Symington, Beattie, & McKinlay, 1987; Kay & Cavallo, 1994). Physical injuries are usually dealt with effectively by the family over time. Such obvious impairments are manageable because they are relatively stable, allow accommodations to be planned, are usually within the awareness of the person with the brain injury, and are visible to and acknowledged by others. Cognitive problems, including impaired attention, memory, speed of processing, and problem solving, frequently create greater challenges because they are less predictable, can influence all aspects of interaction, and may be outside the awareness of the person with TBI. Despite these complications, families often can effectively compensate for such deficits in daily life.

However, it is the emotional, behavioral, and personality alterations, such as angry outbursts, self-centeredness, impulsivity, disinhibition, and social insensitivity, that are extremely taxing for families (Kay & Cavallo, 1994; Lezak, 1988; Urbach & Culbert, 1991). Such problems can erupt unexpectedly, have an explicit emotional consequence on the recipient, are often embarrassing to others, and may create a crisis in management. These behavioral difficulties elevate stress in family life, and also induce family isolation. As social contacts and outings decrease, the immediate family bears increasing responsibility for the social network of the person with a brain injury (Kay & Cavallo, 1994). As time passes, subjective family burden actually increases (Brooks et al., 1987), becoming more strongly associated with these personality alterations and less strongly associated with neurological deficits (Brooks & McKinlay, 1983).

Lezak (1988) described the most burdensome problems encountered by families living with a person with TBI. These emotional, social, and behavioral changes are briefly reviewed.

Impaired Social Perception and Social Awareness.   Individuals with TBI commonly exhibit a childlike egocentricity, similar to the social perspective of a 4- or 5-year-old child. They may exhibit a decreased capacity to empathize with others or to recognize others' emotional reactions and needs. They may consistently place demands on the caregiver due to the inability to be socially sensitive and considerate of others. Additionally, the family may experience social and emotional abandonment because the individual with TBI can no longer provide emotional support or encouragement. The caregiver is often worn out, and others who could provide needed social support no longer come around due to the individual's inappropriate behaviors.

Impaired Self-Regulation.   Self-regulation difficulties can be exhibited in various ways, each particularly burdensome to the family. Impulsivity is the prominent feature of such impaired control, and poor anger management is the most commonly reported form of impulsivity.

Almost any activity can be affected by impulsivity, such as eating behavior, sexuality, spending money, and substance abuse. Control problems can also emerge as general restlessness and agitation.

Dependency. The family member with TBI may be physically, financially, and/or emotionally dependent on relatives. Physical and financial aspects of the individual's dependency may exceed the family's capacity to provide for care, creating feelings of guilt, shame, or failure. In addition, individuals with TBI may become increasingly emotionally and socially dependent on family members if former social support networks dissolve.

Inability to Learn from Experience. The individual's inability to profit from mistakes may create a cycle of failure. Although inappropriate behavior may repeatedly result in difficulties, many individuals do not alter their actions. Therefore, the family must confront each situation as if it were new, and attempt to anticipate potential problems to prevent their reoccurrence.

Specific Emotional Alterations. Prominent changes in emotional control that families find difficult to understand or endure are apathy, silliness, heightened reactivity, and irritability. Moreover, family members frequently assume that the individual's problematic reactions could be controlled if the person were motivated to do so. If families hold the belief that the individual's inappropriate behaviors are deliberate, then members often experience a high level of distress.

Reactive Psychological Disturbances. Psychological disturbances, such as anxiety, paranoia, and depression, may occur in response to the experience of loss, whether that loss is physical, cognitive, or social. Anxiety may arise from the individual's awareness of diminished abilities and disintegrating self-confidence. These feelings may produce extreme caution, a sense of inadequacy, confusion, and fears of going crazy or being perceived as mentally retarded. The individual may appear withdrawn, fearful, agitated, and moody, and the family may experience frustration over an inability to improve matters.

Impaired social–perceptual capabilities, combined with a lack of insight, feelings of worthlessness due to incompetencies, and fears of rejection, create a productive environment for the development of paranoia. Paranoid suspiciousness frequently is exhibited in concerns over spousal fidelity and the management of the individual's money.

Most persons who have experienced loss as a result of brain injury experience at best a transient depression, and commonly are burdened with more severe, chronic depression. In addition to presenting the family with emotional behavior that is disturbing and difficult to manage, depression also tends to exacerbate the individual's other emotional and social problems. Obviously, TBI disrupts normal family interaction patterns and places the family at risk for serious adjustment problems.

Problems Associated with Specific Family Relationships

Family members vary in their response to TBI, depending on their relationship to the injured person and the roles that the individual fulfilled in the family. The following section reviews information regarding the impact of TBI on the spouse, parent, child, sibling, and extended family members.

Marital Relationships.   In many ways, the spouse bears the greatest burden when his or her partner sustains a brain injury because an equal adult partnership has been broken, thereby creating the loss of the primary companion and source of emotional support at the very time that he or she is most needed (Kay & Cavallo, 1994; Kreutzer et al., 1994a; Lezak, 1988; Peters, Stambrook, Moore, & Esses, 1990). The uninjured spouse is generally placed into the role of primary caregiver—both for the injured spouse and the family when there are children. The uninjured spouse's complex feelings about the former relationship, combined with guilt and fears of social rejection, may make it difficult for him or her to consider divorce, although psychological impairments in the person with TBI may limit the reestablishment of a satisfying marital relationship. Furthermore, there is no social support for the spouse to mourn the loss of the loved one, although the person loved by the spouse is not the same (Lezak, 1988).

When marriages do survive, sexuality and intimacy are generally greatly impaired (Kay & Cavallo, 1994; Kreutzer, Zasler, Camplair, & Leininger, 1990; Lezak, 1988). The person with the brain injury may have diminished capacity for intimacy, altered sexual drive, and impaired ability to perform sexually (for physiological or psychological reasons). The noninjured partner frequently experiences social and emotional isolation. He or she may find it difficult to participate in social activities with married couples, yet cannot resort to singles activities for social contact. Finally, as the primary caregiver, the noninjured partner must take on most, if not all, of the household and family responsibilities, and may experience verbal and even physical abuse from the injured partner (Kay & Cavallo, 1994; Lezak, 1988). For these reasons, depression is pervasive in partners of persons with TBI (Kreutzer et al., 1994a; Lezak 1988).

Parental Relationships. Parental stressors differ somewhat depending on whether the injured child was a minor or an independent adult. Regardless of the injured child's age, parents may experience dashed hopes, along with the realization that their responsibility for the care and well-being of that child may be long term—that they will neither acquire the freedom associated with retirement years, nor experience uninterrupted privacy and independence (Lezak, 1988). When a young child is injured, the mother generally acquires the primary responsibility of nurturer and caregiver, possibly creating competition between the remaining children and the other parent for the mother's limited attention and resources (Kay & Cavallo, 1994; Lezak, 1988). Marital conflicts are commonplace and may result from disagreements over care of the child (Lezak, 1988), neglect of the marital relationship, or isolation from adult social activities (Kay & Cavallo, 1994). It is common for marriages to dissolve within 1–2 years following onset of TBI in a child (Lezak, 1988).

Significant brain injury in a minor child tends to arrest the normal evolution of the family, hindering successful completion of normal developmental family stages. Parents may be so involved in caring for a perpetually dependent family member that they are unable to participate fully in their other children's gradual progression to independence (Lezak, 1988). When the injury occurs to a grown child, parents frequently are thrust back to an earlier developmental phase of caring for a dependent child. Parents may find themselves trapped physically and financially by the needs of their dependent adult child, who may frequently resent and resist the dependency (Kay & Cavallo, 1994).

Child Relationships. Children of parents with TBI are confronted with special problems over which they have minimal control. Younger children may suddenly discover that the nurturance and guidance of a previously loving and competent parent is lost (Kay & Cavallo, 1994). The injured parent may be irritable, unpredictable, and even in competition for the uninjured parent's attention. Children may experience a sharp increase in responsibility, feelings of shame or inability to bring peers home, and decreased opportunities to participate in school and community activities requiring a parent because that noninjured parent is occupied with the injured parent's care (Lezak, 1988). Additionally, children encounter numerous losses, and may experience anger and frustration at having a "different" family, and at the absence of previously enjoyed family activities. Urbach and Culbert (1991) posited that children of a parent with TBI represent a true high-risk group for emotional and behavioral difficulties.

Sibling Relationships.   Similar to being the child of a parent with TBI, siblings of injured children typically experience diminished parental attention, as parents reorient their attention and energy toward the child with the brain injury (Kay & Cavallo, 1994; Waaland, 1990). Older children at home may have more household responsibilities, and may also find themselves in socially awkward situations due to the inappropriate behavior of the sibling with TBI. Premorbid relationships between siblings, as well as personality styles of siblings, likely influence postinjury relationships, perhaps creating a closer attachment to the injured sibling or an angry distant relationship.

Extended Family Relationships.   Little is known about the effect of TBI on extended family members. In today's mobile society, family ties are less certain than in previous generations, and extended family members seldom participate in the care of the individual with a TBI (Kay & Cavallo, 1994). Kay and Cavallo discussed the benefits to the nuclear family of involving the extended family whenever possible in learning about the injury and the recovery process. Immediate family members who can obtain support from extended families, even occasionally for respite care, are at great advantage. However, families frequently have difficulty obtaining the support of relatives because extended family members who do not live with the person with TBI typically have minimal understanding and may be less sympathetic to the family stresses (Kay & Cavallo, 1994).

In summary, a primary difficulty for families is the integration of a behaviorally and psychologically different person into the family. Reintegrating the different person into the family requires each family member to let go of previous expectations of the person with TBI. More realistic perceptions and interactions need to be established. "Families who continue to treat significantly changed patients as they remember them encounter frustrations, misunderstandings, and disappointments at every point of contact" (Lezak, 1988, p. 123).

THE IMPACT OF THE FAMILY ON THE PERSON
WITH TBI

Although there is a growing body of research about the effects of TBI on family functioning, only recently has there been evidence of the family's effect on outcomes of survivors of TBI (Leach et al., 1994; Rivara et al.,

1993, 1994). Previous studies have focused primarily on injury severity and residual impairments as determinants of outcome following TBI, with little attention given to the role of the family and other social/environmental factors as contributors to outcome. Farmer and Peterson (1995) stressed the need to move toward an ecological systems approach to the study of outcomes following TBI. That is, they proposed that adaptation in the person with TBI be viewed as the product of multiple transactions between the individual and his or her environment. This idea certainly is not new (Coie et al., 1993; Pless, Roghmann, & Haggerty, 1972), but has had minimal influence on the study of outcomes following TBI, perhaps because the direct effect of TBI on the individual can be so dramatic and concerning.

The majority of investigations examining the family's influence on recovery following TBI have been conducted with injured children and their families. An early study by Brown, Chadwick, Shaffer, Rutter, and Traub (1981) found that children with severe injuries and preinjury family adjustment problems were twice as likely to show psychiatric disorders 1 year after TBI, compared with severely injured children whose families did not have these problems.

Rivara and colleagues (1993, 1994) recently extended these findings using more sophisticated measures of child and family functioning. They first assessed 94 children with TBI to determine academic, cognitive, and behavioral outcomes 1 year postinjury. They then examined injury severity and preinjury family functioning as predictors of these outcomes. Children whose families had better global ratings of preinjury family functioning, more positive family relationships, and a less rigid family structure showed better academic performance and fewer behavior problems 1 year postinjury. Severity of TBI and preinjury ratings contributed in different ways to the prediction of child outcomes. Injury severity had the greatest impact on academic and cognitive performance. In contrast, preinjury family functioning variables were better predictors of child behavior ratings than injury severity. When children's preinjury functioning was included in the prediction equation, the child measures replaced family functioning as stronger predictors of outcome. This was not particularly surprising because the preinjury child and family functioning measures were highly correlated. These studies underscore the important contribution of families to child adjustment, both before and after injury.

Others have also found that family factors are related to outcome following TBI. For example, Greenspan and MacKenzie (1994) reported that injured children from poor or near-poor families were more likely to need special education services, show impairments in physical health, and exhibit behavioral problems than similarly injured children from families of higher socioeconomic status (SES). Children of families living in poverty are clearly at greater risk of poor outcomes if injured.

In a separate study of adults with TBI, Leach and colleagues (1994) found that more effective family coping strategies predicted lower levels of depression in persons with TBI. Specifically, a family's ability to access social support was strongly associated with better emotional adjustment in the survivor. Thus, although TBI is a significant stressor for families, the family's structure and coping resources can either positively or negatively influence adjustment in all family members, including the person with TBI.

DIRECTIONS FOR FUTURE RESEARCH

Although studies that examined family reactions to TBI appeared during the 1970s, considerable attention to the family was not apparent until the 1980s. In the early to mid-1980s, individual family members were the primary focus of research (Kay & Cavallo, 1994). In the latter years of that decade, the focus shifted from individual family members to families as systems, and the affect of TBI on roles, relationships, and the family's status in society. Most recently, there have been increasing efforts to understand the moderating effects of pre- and postinjury family functioning on the functional outcomes of the persons with TBI.

Although researchers have begun to address the relationship between injury occurrence and family factors, numerous areas require further investigation and elaboration. First, additional research is needed to identify the characteristics of families at risk and, conversely, families that are more resilient under the strain of changes wrought by TBI (Coie et al., 1993). Increasingly severe injury has been implicated as one factor that increases risk of poor outcomes in families (e.g., Peters et al., 1990). Other factors that warrant further attention include: (a) demographic characteristics, such as family size, economic resources, and race; (b) family coping strategies and styles of interaction, both pre- and postinjury; (c) family knowledge about TBI and expectations for recovery in their member; (d) family members' ability to access intrafamiliar and community supports; and (e) developmental stage of the family (e.g., early marriage vs. retirement years). How these family factors influence outcomes in persons with TBI also remains an open question for empirical investigation.

Second, a major goal of future studies should be to characterize family outcome over time (Camplair et al., 1990). To date, the majority of research investigating family adaptation has addressed only the first year postinjury. Ideally, studies should (a) focus on reactions within the same families over time, and (b) follow families for several years to chart family coping patterns.

A third rich area for future studies is the assessment of the family unit as a whole, instead of focusing on reactions of a particular family informant (Camplair et al., 1990). Family researchers have developed assessment instruments that provide quantitative information on family functioning. For example, Epstein, Baldwin, and Bishop (1983) developed the Family Assessment Device (FAD). Kreutzer and colleagues (1994a, 1994b) successfully used this measure in recent studies examining patterns of family interactions after TBI. A second self-report instrument likely to contribute to a better understanding of family outcome is the Family Adaptability and Cohesion Evaluation Scales (FACES II; Olson, Sprenkle, & Russell, 1979; FACES III; Olson, Portner, & Lavee, 1985). There is also a need to supplement such self-report measures with standardized clinical interviews, behavioral observations of family interactions during problem-solving tasks, and ratings of family functioning by rehabilitation professionals (Camplair et al., 1990; Kreutzer et al., 1994a).

Fourth, there are only a few studies documenting the effectiveness of family interventions following TBI, despite the increasing emphasis on including family members in the rehabilitation process. For example, Muir, Rosenthal, and Diehl (1990) described a 10- to 12-session program developed to educate families about TBI during rehabilitation. They observed that persons with TBI and their families increased their involvement in rehabilitation planning. In addition, family members showed increased knowledge about TBI and ways to better manage patient care. This study provided preliminary evidence that educational interventions have a positive influence on families after TBI, and highlighted the need for continuing evaluation of family treatment efforts.

The development and evaluation of such family treatment interventions must be guided by input from family members about their perceived needs (see Kreutzer, Serio, & Bergquist, 1994), clinical experience, and the growing body of research identifying factors that promote or impede positive outcomes in persons with TBI and families. As noted by Frank (1994), such interventions need to go beyond direct treatment of patients and families to modifications in community supports and public policies that provide resources for families following TBI.

Once effective family treatments are identified, strategies for implementing them need to be developed and evaluated. For example, having a superior treatment to improve adjustment in the siblings of persons with TBI is worth little if treatment providers have few opportunities to interact with the siblings. This is particularly challenging if the family lives in a rural community, has few financial resources, or feels separated from rehabilitation specialists due to racial, ethnic, or cultural differences.

CONCLUSIONS

TBI affects both the individual who directly sustains the injury and family members. Following TBI, family systems undergo changes ranging from relatively mild adjustments to severe compromises that result in significant alterations in the system's functioning. Individual roles and interpersonal expectations may be blurred or altered (Muir et al., 1990). Yet the impact of the injury is, in part, defined by the response of the family system, making it at once the recipient of burden and the moderator of the patient's and individual family member's outcomes. To optimize the family's ability to function adaptively, clinicians and researchers must continue to study ways to reduce risk and enhance resilience in both the person with TBI and his or her caregivers.

REFERENCES

Bond, M. R. (1975). Psychosocial outcome after severe head injury. *CIBA Foundation Symposium, 34*, 145–153.

Brooks, N., Campsie, L., Symington, C., Beattie, A., & McKinlay, W. (1987). The effects of severe head injury upon patient and relative within several years of injury. *Journal of Head Trauma Rehabilitation, 2*, 1–13.

Brooks, N., & McKinlay, W. (1983). Personality and behavioral change after severe blunt head injury: A relative's view. *Journal of Neurology, Neurosurgery and Psychiatry, 46*, 336–344.

Brown, G., Chadwick, O., Shaffer, D., Rutter, M., & Traub, M. (1981). A prospective study of children with head injuries: III. Psychiatric sequelae. *Psychological Medicine, 11*, 63–78.

Camplair, P. S., Kreutzer, J. S., & Doherty, K. R. (1990). Family outcome following adult traumatic brain injury. In J. S. Kreutzer & P. Wehman (Eds.), *Community integration following traumatic brain injury* (pp. 207–223). Baltimore, MD: Paul H. Brooks.

Coie, J. D., Watt, N. F., West, S. G., Hawkins, J. D., Asarnow, J. R., Markman, H. J., Ramey, F. L., Shure, M. B., & Long, B. (1993). The science of prevention: A conceptual framework and some directions for a national research program. *American Psychologist, 48*, 1013–1022.

Epstein, N. B., Baldwin, L. M., & Bishop, D. S. (1983). The McMaster Family Assessment Device. *Journal of Marital and Family Therapy, 9*, 171–180.

Farmer, J. E., & Peterson, L. (1995). Pediatric traumatic brain injury: Promoting successful school re-entry. *School Psychology Review, 24*, 230–243.

Frank, R. G. (1994). Families and rehabilitation. *Brain Injury, 8*(3), 193–195.

Frank, R. G., Haut, A. E., Smick, M., Haut, W., & Chaney, J. M. (1990). Coping and family functions after closed head injury. *Brain Injury, 4*(3), 289–295.

Greenspan, A. I., & MacKenzie, E. J. (1994). Functional outcome after pediatric head injury. *Pediatrics, 94*(4), 425–432.

Kay, T., & Cavallo, M. M. (1994). The family system: Impact, assessment, and intervention. In J. M. Silver, S. C. Yudofsky, & R. E. Hales (Eds.), *Neuropsychiatry of traumatic brain injury* (pp. 533–567). Washington, DC: American Psychiatric Press.

Kreutzer, J. S., Gervasio, A. H., & Camplair, P. S. (1994a). Primary caregivers' psychological status and family functioning after traumatic brain injury. *Brain Injury, 8*(3), 197–210.

Kreutzer, J. S., Gervasio, A. H., & Camplair, P. S. (1994b). Patient correlates of caregivers' distress and family functioning after traumatic brain injury. *Brain Injury, 8*(3), 211–230.

Kreutzer, J. S., Marwitz, J. H., & Kepler, K. (1992). Traumatic brain injury: Family response and outcome. *Archives of Physical Medicine and Rehabilitation, 73,* 771–778.

Kreutzer, J. S., Serio, C. D., & Bergquist, S. (1994). Family needs after brain injury: A quantitative analysis. *Journal of Head Trauma Rehabilitation, 9*(3), 104–115.

Kreutzer, J. S., Zasler, N. D., Camplair, P. S., & Leininger, B. E. (1990). A practical guide to family intervention following adult traumatic brain injury. In J. S. Kreutzer & P. Wehman (Eds.), *Community integration following traumatic brain injury* (pp. 249–273). Baltimore, MD: Paul H. Brooks.

Leach, L. R., Frank, R. G., Bouman, D. E., & Farmer, J. E. (1994). Family functioning, social support and depression after traumatic brain injury. *Brain Injury, 8*(7), 599–606.

Leaf, L. E. (1993). Traumatic brain injury: Affecting family recovery. *Brain Injury, 7*(6), 543–546.

Lezak, M. D. (1988). Brain damage is a family affair. *Journal of Clinical and Experimental Neuropsychology, 10,* 111–123.

Livingston, M. G., & Brooks, D. N. (1988). The burden on families of the brain injured: A review. *Journal of Head Trauma Rehabilitation, 4,* 6–15.

Livingston, M. G., Brooks, D. N., & Bond, M. R. (1985). Three months after severe head injury: Psychiatric and social impact on relatives. *Journal of Neurology, Neurosurgery, and Psychiatry, 48,* 870–875.

Maitz, E. A. (1991). Family systems theory applied to head injury. In J. M. Williams & T. Kay (Eds.), *Head injury: A family matter* (pp. 65–79). Baltimore, MD: Paul H. Brooks.

Mauss-Clum, N., & Ryan, M. (1981). Brain injury and the family. *Journal of Neurosurgical Nursing, 13,* 165–169.

McDaniel, S. H., Hepworth, J., & Doherty, W. J. (1992). *Medical family therapy: A biopsychosocial approach to families with health problems.* New York: Basic Books.

McKinlay, W. W., Brooks, D. N., Bond, M. R., Martinage, D. P., & Marshall, M. M. (1981). The short-term outcome of severe blunt head injury as reported by relatives of injured persons. *Journal of Neurology, Neurosurgery, and Psychiatry, 44,* 527–533.

Minuchin, S. (1974). *Families and family therapy.* Cambridge, MA: Harvard University Press.

Muir, C. A., Rosenthal, M., & Diehl, L. N. (1990). Methods of family intervention. In M. Rosenthal, M. R. Bond, E. R. Griffith, & J. D. Miller (Eds.), *Rehabilitation of the adult and child with traumatic brain injury* (2nd ed., pp. 433–448). Philadelphia, PA: F. A. Davis Company.

Oddy, M., Humphrey, M., & Uttley, D. (1978). Stresses upon the relatives of head-injured patients. *British Journal of Psychiatry, 133,* 507–513.

Olson, D. H., Portner, J., & Lavee, Y. (1985). *FACES-III: Family Adaptability and Cohesion Evaluation Scales.* St. Paul: University of Minnesota, Family Social Science.

Olson, D. H., Sprenkle, D., & Russell, C. (1979). Circumplex model of marital and family systems: I. Cohesion and adaptability dimensions, family types and clinical applications. *Family Process, 18,* 3–28.

Panting, A., & Merry, P. H. (1972). The long-term rehabilitation of severe head injuries with particular reference for the need for social and medical support for the patient's family. *Rehabilitation, 38,* 33–37.

Peters, L. C., Stambrook, M., Moore, A. D., & Esses, L. (1990). Psychosocial sequelae of closed head injury: Effects on the marital relationship. *Brain Injury, 4*(1), 39–47.

Pless, I., Roghmann, K., & Haggerty, R. (1972). Chronic illness, family functioning, and psychological adjustment: A model for the allocation of prevention mental health services. *International Journal of Epidemiology, 1*, 271–277.

Rivara, J. B., Jaffe, K. M., Fay, G. C., Polissar, N. L., Martin, K. M., Shurtleff, H. A., & Liao, S. (1993). Family functioning and injury severity as predictors of child functioning one year following traumatic brain injury. *Archives of Physical Medicine and Rehabilitation, 74*, 1047–1055.

Rivara, J. B., Jaffe, K. M., Polissar, N. L., Gay, G. C., Martin, K. M., Shurtleff, H. A., & Liao, S. (1994). Family functioning and children's academic performance and behavior problems in the year following traumatic brain injury. *Archives of Physical Medicine and Rehabilitation, 75*, 369–379.

Sachs, P. (1985). Beyond support: Traumatic head injury as a growth experience for families. *Rehabilitation Nursing, January–February*, 21–23.

Sbordone, R. J., Kral, M., Gerard, M., & Katz, J. (1984). Evidence of a "command performance syndrome" in the significant others of the victims of severe traumatic head injury. *The International Journal of Clinical Neuropsychology, 6*, 183–185.

Thomsen, I. V. (1974). The patient with severe head injury and his family: A follow-up study of 50 patients. *Scandinavian Journal of Rehabilitation Medicine, 6*, 180–183.

Thomsen, I. V. (1984). Late outcome of severe blunt head trauma: A 10–15 year follow-up. *Journal of Neurology, Neurosurgery, and Psychiatry, 47*, 260–268.

Urbach, J. R., & Culbert, J. P. (1991). Head-injured parents and their children: Psychosocial consequences of a traumatic syndrome. *Psychosomatics, 32*, 24–33.

Waaland, P. K. (1990). Family response to childhood traumatic brain injury. In J. S. Kreutzer & P. Wehman (Eds.), *Community integration following traumatic brain injury* (pp. 225–247). Baltimore, MD: Paul H. Brooks.

20

The Development of Grassroots Support for Research and Services in Brain Injury

Fred J. Krause

In 1980, the year the National Head Injury Foundation (NHIF) was founded, the founders, including parents and siblings, along with a handful of professionals, were concerned about obtaining basic medical and family support services for persons with traumatic brain injury (TBI). Little did they dream that one day there would be international meetings on the study of brain injury.

Although we have come a long way since then, there is still a long way to go. NHIF, as envisioned by Marilyn Spivack and founders from across the country, was to serve as the catalyst for services, research, and support for persons with TBI and their families. In 1980, there were only a handful of programs serving persons with TBI: few training programs, little in the way of educational and community services, and, in general, a complete lack of awareness about the demographics of TBI. This lack of awareness and support by the public led to the phrase the "silent epidemic."

It is rather sad when you think about it. According to the U.S. Department of Health and Human Services, the reported number of persons sustaining TBI per year in the United States is 2 million. In the rest of the world, the numbers continue to climb, especially with increased motor vehicle use around the globe. If the number of persons sustaining a TBI every year is so large, why the "silent epidemic," and what can we do about it? This chapter discusses the development of grassroot support for research and services for persons with TBI.

Every great movement in the world has started at the grassroots level because someone was concerned enough to get involved with others with similar needs. Every movement has been identified with a cause or purpose, and therefore has had champions of this cause who provided the leadership needed to start a movement. The early leaders were usually parents who had the support of the few professionals who cared enough about family issues.

One of the earliest grassroot movements in the United States was started by parents of children with mental retardation. These parents organized at the family and community levels, meeting in their homes, churches, and synagogues. Their major goal was to support each other and to get services for their children. Now, over 40 years later, the Association of Retarded Citizen (ARC) is still active in advocacy, in community-based services for persons with mental retardation, and in empowerment of persons with mental retardation. As a result of this important grassroots movement, in 1963 the U.S. Congress enacted legislation providing for the construction of mental retardation research centers, which later led to the development of the University Affiliated Centers for Mental Retardation. Today, the congressional support for the mental retardation research centers is $10.4 million and $18 million for the university-affiliated programs. Perhaps the most significant legislation resulting from this grassroots movement was the Education for all Handicapped Children's Act in 1975, which provided for free and appropriate public education for all children 21 years old and under with disabilities. Other acts that have followed include the Developmental Disabilities Assistance Act and the Bill of Rights Act of 1975, which established legal rights for all persons with developmental disabilities and created a federally supported protection and advocacy system.

The act most identified with grassroots movement is the American with Disability Act, (ADA) which was enacted in 1990. The ADA ensures the right for all people with disabilities to have access to public buildings, forbids discrimination in employment and housing, and provides for redress of grievances arising from discrimination.

One may ask how all of this was accomplished by grassroots movements. The answer is creating public awareness, using the media to carry the message, and getting the public and politicians to support the cause.

One of the first international support organizations—the International League of Societies for people with Mental Handicaps (ILSMH)—was founded in 1969. It brings together parent-sponsored associations from all over the world. More than 100 member societies participate with ILSMH. These societies all have the desire to obtain services for persons with disabilities. All of these voluntary support associations work to get the following services: (a) educational, (b) vocational, (c) medical, (d) residential, and (e) guardianship.

To secure these services, the ILSMH learned that parents or concerned friends must (a) band together with other parents; (b) keep the pressure on public officials and legislators; and (c) enlist the aid of professionals in the field, the support of civic organizations, and the support of the corporate and business world if they are to succeed. It is this basic similarity of their needs and concerns that has provided the strong impetus for parent organizations; it has made them the most visible and potent consumer groups in the field of human services throughout the world, including the former Soviet Union states. The ILSMH is an action-oriented organization that serves as an exchange of information and a clearinghouse for model service and legislation. This service orientation distinguishes the League from "professional" organizations. The most notable of its accomplishments was the *Declaration of Rights of Mentally Retarded Persons,* adopted by the United Nations (UN) in the latter part of 1976.

I turn now to the development of the NHIF in the United States. As is well known, NHIF was founded on April 20, 1980, when 13 people (e.g., doctors, psychologists, and parents of head-injured children) gathered at the home of Marilyn Price Spivack. Spivack, the founder of NHIF, started the organization out of the same frustration and concern for the lack of services for people with head injuries, as did the parents of persons with mental retardation some 41 years earlier. However, much had changed in terms of social acceptance and public policy. NHIF was established for the same purposes as well: (a) to make the public aware of head injury, (b) to provide a clearinghouse for information, (c) to develop support groups for families, and (d) to establish rehabilitation services and programs.

Today, 14 years later, NHIF has grown to be an association of more than 25,000 members, chapters or affiliated groups in every state, and a multimillion dollar budget. The primary mission of NHIF continues to be to improve the quality of life for persons with head injury and their families, and to promote prevention. However, NHIF has become more sophisticated with time. With the move to Washington, DC, it has developed a strong public policy program, an effective lobbying effort using professionals, and a strong public awareness and public education program. This has resulted in increased federal funding, passage of safety and prevention legislation, and creation of community-based, regional brain-injury centers.

In addition, NHIF has worked to involve people with brain injury in all aspects of the association, including membership on the board of directors and all standing committees. NHIF has convened international groups, brought international experts to speak at the NHIF National Symposium, and hosted international guests. In addition, NHIF has participated in conferences throughout the world.

To strengthen the work of NHIF, the association is working in close association and collaboration with other professional organizations, such as the Neurotrauma Society, the Academy of Rehabilitation Medicine, the Congress of Rehabilitation Medicine, the American Association of Neurological Surgeons, the National Coalition for Research in Neurological Disorders, and the National Institutes of Health. NHIF has served as a model for the development of similar support associations throughout the world.

As a voluntary support organization that conducts professional seminars, symposia, and other forms of education, NHIF has learned first and foremost that it must: (a) keep the pressure on public officials and legislative bodies; (b) enlist the support of professionals and providers of service; and (c) use the media, especially television, for public awareness and acceptance of head injury as an important cause that needs public support. Most of all, NHIF has learned to support persons with TBI—to include them at all levels and to provide choices.

In 1993, an International Brain Injury Association (IBIA) was established. IBIA is an international voluntary support organization composed of voluntary brain-injury organizations, professionals, providers, and brain-injured persons and their families. The major function of IBIA is to:

- serve as a clearinghouse for information;
- serve as an international exchange of information and people;
- serve to stimulate world support through media and multinational corporations;
- serve to create an international "Be HeadSmart" prevention campaign;
- lobby for safe cars, gun control, helmet use, seatbelt use, and so on;
- promote international laws on safety through the UN;
- conduct family support and empowerment conferences;
- advocate for rights of all people with TBI;
- educate the public about TBI as the number one killer of young people through multicultural educational programs;
- publish an international family support journal;
- work with the governing bodies of member nations to develop community services and to support research;
- use the "Decade of the Brain" to move an international agenda on TBI forward;
- convene a world congress with delegate representatives to develop an international Bill of Rights for persons with TBI, and gain international support and acceptance via the UN to adopt this declaration of rights; and
- develop a forecast of how brain injury in the year 2000 might look if research and services are developed and supported.

The IBIA will work with the World Health Organization (WHO), the UN, the scientific community, national governments, and other brain-injury organizations. It will not duplicate services of other organizations; rather, it will support and enhance those opportunities.

To increase awareness and support for services, research, and prevention, we must come together to raise the level of public awareness about TBI. This can best be done by creating an international support association that provides the leadership required to get the job done. Is an international support organization needed? In response to this question, the following is offered:

First, the most important reason for international support is the increasing number of persons sustaining a brain injury around the world. For example, in the United States, a head injury occurs every 15 seconds, resulting in 2 million such injuries a year. In the Bronx, New York area, the incidence rate is 407 head injuries per 100,000, which yields annual costs exceeding $25 billion. Second, the proliferation of motor vehicle use around the world is leading to increased numbers of accidents, resulting in higher incidence rates of head injury. Third, with violence against persons on the increase, there is a concomitant increase in head injury. Fourth, there are no international public policies or support services. Fifth, there is the need for multicultural public education programs. Sixth, there is a need for multicultural prevention programs. Seventh, through collaboration and by banding together, there is strength.

To date, IBIA has been very successful. A major prevention conference is planned for November 1994 in Bangalore, India, and the First World Congress on Brain Injury will be held in Copenhagen, Denmark, from May 14 to 17, 1995. The Congress is being sponsored by IBIA, the WHO, the Danish Brain Injury Association, and the NHIF. This is a good example of how IBIA intends to work cooperatively. We invite your participation. IBIA's major goals are to sponsor grassroots organizations worldwide. At the conference in Bangalore, India, there will be the announcement of the establishment of the Indian Brain Injury Association.

In addition to this, IBIA has participated in programs in Italy, Hungary, Lithuania, and the former Soviet Union. Plans are underway to begin an exchange program. Truly, IBIA is just at the beginning stage, but everything needs to begin some place. If we are to gain support for *brain-injury research* and *services for persons with brain injury,* we must come together to unite for a common purpose. Help IBIA end the silent epidemic, and make sure the Decade of the Brain is more than a paper promise.

A Databased Managed Care System of Catastrophic Neurological Injury Rehabilitation

D. Nathan Cope

This chapter introduces and discusses an organization (Paradigm Health Corporation, Concord, CA) that, over the past several years, has developed an innovative model of managed care for the treatment of severely brain-injured survivors. This model has integrated outcome-based service delivery with shared-risk reimbursement. There is increasingly widespread recognition that the clinical and technical ability to provide treatment for brain and other catastrophic injuries, as well as other health care problems, is inextricably linked with the organizational and economic structures through which such care is delivered. This "economic" influence on the dimensions of care delivery offers the rationale for a "systems" presentation.

This chapter derives much of its salience from the peculiar economic conditions and developments in the area of "health care reform" currently underway in the United States, and that may seem somewhat specific to this country. However, the economic aspects of the cost–benefit and quality assurance problems of brain-injury treatment addressed here are general and transcend any purely insular, American experience. These issues have relevance and application to the problems besetting the financing of health care services worldwide, and thus are of some general interest to this audience.

Developments in the cost of general health care have been dramatic. The statistics on the annual growth rate of all health care services in the United States continue to be depressingly familiar, despite that the growth rate appears to have moderated somewhat recently. Within this general context, brain injury is a subset of a general type of health problem generally encompassed under the term *catastrophic injuries.* I do

295

not mean to recapitulate the statistics in regard to the magnitude of
traumatic, accidental injury in the United States; they are well known
and are of immense magnitude. It is not unusual for the medical care
cost of one individual to approach $1 million, and it is possible for such
are to reach millions of dollars. When the cost of the long-term lifetime
care needs and support requirements are included, lifetime costs are
often as large as $5–$10 million per case. In response to this annual
growth in health care expenditures, those responsible for the payment
of health care services (i.e., insurance industries, various governmental
branches, etc.) have increasingly looked to managed care mechanisms to
bring this cost growth under control. Multiple managed care initiatives—including (a) development of preferred provider organizations
(PPOs) and discounted services, (b) utilization of review activities with
possible denial of payment of previously unsurveyed care, (c) institution
of diagnosis-related grouping (DRG) reimbursement system by the federal government in which a specific sum is paid for a treatment of
unique diagnosis, and (d) institution of external case management systems to monitor and influence the course of care—are all elements of
this payor response toward cost-containment. The combined effect of all
these managed care approaches has been the production of revenue
constriction on almost all health providers (e.g., hospitals, physicians,
clinics, allied health professionals, etc.). Increasing numbers of hospitals
in the United States are now finding that they are operating with an
increasingly large percentage of their beds vacant. Physicians are finding their freedom to manage patients as they see fit, and their ability
even to obtain referrals, increasingly defined by various managed care
organizations. Anxiety is pervasive for all health providers, as they
struggle to ensure an adequate volume of clinical work to survive as
economic entities.

   Rehabilitation has been a particularly unique component of the health
care industry. It has been exempted from DRGs by the federal government, in large part based on a formal study done by the Rand Corporation and the Medical College of Wisconsin. This study, which examined
many thousands of rehabilitation patient hospital records, concluded
that diagnosis alone was insufficient to explain resource consumption
for rehabilitation. Due to this complexity, rehabilitation care to this day
has continued to be reimbursed under traditional fee-for-service mechanisms. A consequence of this exemption has been that general health
care facilities (i.e., acute hospitals) have learned to perceive rehabilitation units as one means of off-setting the general revenue reduction
resulting from DRGs and other utilization review activities of payors.
General acute care hospitals have opened new rehabilitation facilities
over the last decade; these facilities serve as a new and supplemental

revenue source. The result has been the proliferation of many new, small, relatively unskilled rehabilitation programs that provide more or less inappropriate treatments to complex catastrophic cases. This occurs because of the economic need to fill the new rehabilitation beds and to generate revenue, rather than in response to balanced clinical judgment of clinicians. Along with this has come extended lengths of treatment, or hospitalization and treatment in less efficient settings (e.g., inpatient services are often provided where outpatient, postacute, or home care programs would be, according to current clinical thinking, not only more cost-efficient, but also more clinically efficacious). The general result of this trend has been that many brain-injured and other catastrophically injured patients achieve suboptimal and more costly outcomes. This is because for many of the psychosocial, behavioral, and functional problems of these patients, inpatient facilities are less effective and expert. In addition, in many cases, essentially all financial support for rehabilitation is consumed in these acute care settings, leaving no funds for later postacute community-integration goals.

A great deal of clinical experience and research has supported the concept that an optimal rehabilitation system would be organized to: (a) provide the rapid implementation of rehabilitation so that these services would be begun even within the acute trauma setting, in parallel and coincident with the care of the traumatologists and neurosurgeons; (b) provide that rehabilitation only for programs that have the volume of cases, expertise, and experience to understand the wide range of problems and multiple approaches relevant for this complex condition (the terms *centers of excellence* or *model systems* have been used to describe this concept of highly specialized expert treatment centers; and (c) facilitate the rapid movement of patients from one level of care to another, as rapidly as clinically appropriate. Patients would be transitioned smoothly and quickly from the trauma center to the acute inpatient rehabilitation center to the postacute behavioral, subacute, outpatient, and home-based rehabilitation levels of care.

However, as the economic dilemmas of acute hospital facilities have become more pressing, these traditional rehabilitation centers of excellence and downstream levels of care within the historical continuum have become increasingly removed from the referral process. Their traditional sources of referrals, the acute hospitals are now retaining, rather than referring, their brain-injured cases (and, in general, all possible other complex medical cases). The basic concept of the model systems or expert centers of excellence within a continuum of care has been seriously eroded.

A further problem involves the addition of managed care approaches to rehabilitation, which have increasingly relied on strict utilization review and rehabilitation benefit limitations to restrain what is seen by payors as uncontrollable hemorrhaging of treatment cost without clear, specific, objective returns. For example, much rehabilitation benefit by some health maintenance organizations (HMOs) in California is now provided by placing injured patients within nursing home settings, which provide some limited physical and other therapy, and treating this as equivalent to acute rehabilitation. Thus, this nursing home-based treatment has replaced traditional acute rehabilitation programs in many instances. HMOs typically offer 60 days of rehabilitation as a total rehabilitation benefit—a limit that has derived historically from original federal HMO enabling legislation, establishing a minimum benefit. Over time, HMOs have evolved this limit to a maximum rehabilitation benefit, and it has become a de facto clinical standard, irrespective of the patient's clinical needs.

The organization and founding of Paradigm Health Corporation occurred in 1991. It was derived from an awareness of these economic considerations, and the belief that an optional solution to the problems discussed would depend on a rational integration and balancing of both the payors' and providers' economic interests and the brain-injured survivors' clinical interests. This foundation was the result of several years of study and meetings involving multiple clinical providers and insurance or payor entities. The cofounders of Paradigm participated in multiple interviews, focus groups, and consensus gatherings around the country. Their goal was to understand the concerns of payors and providers, and subsequently design a delivery system that would respond to the needs and the concerns of all parties.

The organization has been in clinical operation for approximately 2.5 years. The structure of Paradigm includes: (a) the establishment of a provider network composed of expert providers, network managers, and physicians; (b) the establishment of an extensive prospective database of clinical and economic variables; (c) a shared-risk pricing mechanism; and (d) objectively defined outcomes. These components are discussed in turn.

It was felt that any solution to the problems discussed here required a network of expert providers that was both vertical and horizontal. The vertical dimension includes all levels in the continuum of care from acute rehabilitation through postacute, behavioral, subacute, community and home, and outpatient types of care. Comprehensive, yet efficient, rehabilitation for catastrophically injured patients requires the involvement of all these levels of service. Each of these levels has its own particular contribution and expertise to bring to the care of the brain-injured patient. In addition, the network needed to be horizontal (i.e., it needed to be geographically expansive) and national in coverage. Payors have obligations that generally are national in distribution. They may have a covered individual who acquires a brain injury anywhere in the United States, and the payors' desire and need was clearly for a uniform system through which their claimants could reliably obtain expert care at appropriate rates and cost. In addition, it is also clinically the case that patients often require movement of major distances from the site of their injury and acute care to the eventual site of their long-term reintegration into society. That is, a patient may be injured in one state and have his or her trauma care handled there. The patient may then be transferred to an acute rehab center of excellence for brain injury in a state of home residence, but that may nevertheless still be several hundred miles from his or her own community, where they finally receive community and vocational rehab. This could involve three, and sometimes four, geographically distinct and separate provider organizations. All providers in the network need to be expert (i.e., they need to have the experience and infrastructure necessary to provide optimal treatment for these complex cases). The purpose of this chapter is not to describe the parameters of these programs in more detail, except to acknowledge how a variety of clinical and administrative measures or dimensions of each program are characterized. These determinations go into the establishment of a program's "expertise." Many providers, although self-proclaimed "experts" in these areas, in fact lack many of the necessary features to efficiently and comprehensively manage severe traumatic brain injury (TBI) cases. In addition, the fact that a facility may be expert in the acute rehabilitation of brain injury does not necessarily indicate an expertise in the management of the behavioral or community reintegration aspects of these patients. Thus, expertise also implies a specific focus of capability. Further, the network providers need to demonstrate a commitment to a risk-sharing structure with the payor over the costs the individual patient's treatment, of which more is said later. Such elements as the structure of the program, the qualifications of individual clinical personnel, the quality assurance and program evaluation activity and efforts, the volume of the caseload of TBI and other relevant diagnoses, and each program's long-term experience, research, and leadership in the general field of head injury, including their general reputation (both locally and nationally), contributed to selection into the network. Finally, an on site review by Paradigm personnel was performed. Ongoing prospective review of performance by Paradigm, based on prospectively gathered data of patient care outcomes, and cost are continuing elements in the ongoing certification of network providers' expertise.

Paradigm utilizes network managers who function as the clinical on site representative of Paradigm. They are generally highly experienced nurse case managers whose role is to interface with providers, patients, and family in the clinical environment. They compose specific case plans of each patient in collaboration with the treating physicians and other expert provider clinicians. They also serve to monitor and coordinate the delivery of care detailed in these case plans. In particular, they ensure the efficient and seamless continuation of the thrust of the rehabilitation flow from one expert provider to another. They also attend to the details of environmental preparation, which geographically restricted providers are typically unable to deal with, such as communication with the patient's employer in preparation for return to work and other aspects of preparation in the community of ultimate residence. The network manager is also the individual who "certifies" the achievement of the specific outcomes of the care plan. Among the most important responsibilities of these individuals is the objective generation of data for Paradigm's prospective clinical database.

Paradigm provider physicians are chosen based on their expertise in the care of particular problems of brain injury and other catastrophic conditions. Physicians are felt to be the control point of the care-delivery process, and thus have primary responsibility for the construction of individual treatment plans and delivery of care. These physicians also share risk with Paradigm and the payor in regard to achievement of this plan's outcomes.

A further fundamental component of the Paradigm model is the specification of each patient of both general and specific treatment outcomes. A very important aspect of Paradigm's conceptualization of the rehabilitation process has to do with achievement of certain modular or nodal points in recovery. Paradigm structures these nodal points into five general outcome levels (I–V). The first is the achievement of a physiological stability, or Level I. Level II consists of appropriate rehabilitation sufficient to prepare the patient for safe discharge to a nonmedical environment (e.g., all long-term-care protocols, including routines for feeding, respiratory care, skin care, bowel and bladder management care, etc.). Level III encompasses all indicated rehabilitation to optimize function in the home or site of long-term care. Level IV involves all treatment and rehabilitation necessary to optimize function in the patient's community. Level V optimizes return to work or educational activity. At a more fundamental level, patient-specific outcomes address, in particular, the specific deficits and impairments of each patient, as well as the individual treatments and results necessary to achieve a chosen general outcome level for that patient.

The Paradigm prospective database also assesses and archives information regarding the significant clinical, demographic, and psychosocial variables of each individual patient. Thus, it establishes the overall complexity of that patient. As each patient's care proceeds, the site of care in which care is delivered and the resources consumed in achieving a specific outcome level are measured. With this data, Paradigm is able to statistically develop an equation, through multiple-regression techniques, that generates a "clinical index" in which the general resource requirements of the individual patient can be predicted with reliability.[1]Having the ability to predict resource consumption for specific outcome level change then allows the achievement of rational, empirically based, shared-risk pricing. This takes the form of a contract offering for a specific price, achievement of a specific defined outcome level, along with the associated patient-specific outcomes relevant to that outcome level. The consequence of this contractual risk sharing is profound. The economic incentive of all providers in this arrangement is immediately changed from the delivery of the maximum amount of care to delivery of the most effective and efficient care necessary to achieve the specified outcomes.

Thus, one would define a patient by the initially determined level of clinical complexity necessary to go from a Level 0 to a Level II outcome and attach a general resource requirement on that process. This complexity level then becomes the basis for a general pricing agreement between the provider and the payor. The provider would be responsible for achieving the specified outcomes under this contract. If the provider was expert, efficient, diligent, and able to produce these outcomes quickly, this payment would more than cover cost and provide for a positive reimbursement margin. If the provider was nondiligent or inexpert in the provision of this care, and the cost of such care exceeded the contract price, the provider would be responsible for continuing to provide care until the outcomes were achieved.

The effects of this pricing arrangement are similar to the effect of general capitation on a whole population (i.e., the incentive of the provider is changed from delivery of the maximum amount of care to the delivery of the most efficient necessary care). In this process, Paradigm serves as an auditor of the results, in which providers are accountable for the delivery of acceptably high-quality rehabilitation outcomes and cannot simply operate on the basis of maximizing cost savings. The intention of this prospective shared-risk pricing arrangement is not to transform providers into "mini" insurance entities. Therefore, the economic obligation of providers under this prospective pricing contract is

---

[1]For example, this equation might take the form of $y = k + x_1 (dbr) + X_2(a) + x_3(m) + x_4(h) + x_n(ipn)$, where y = the clinical index "score," dbr = diagnosis base rate, a = age cohort, m = clinical comorbidity measures, h = a general health index, n = other general independent predicators, and each x = the related weighting value derived from multiple regression.

not without limit. A stop loss is provided so that, should the cost of a case become truly excessive, the responsibility for payment would shift back to Paradigm and the parent insuring organization. However, this stop-loss mechanism does not reverse the primary objective of shared-risk pricing, which is to put the incentives structure of all participants in the catastrophic case process (i.e., the payor and provider) on the same side of the table—where all participants are motivated to provide a quality, durable outcome at the most reasonable and efficient price.

Another aspect of Paradigm's national prospective database is the ability to follow patients in a long-term manner (i.e., for years posttreatment) so that immediate as well as extended benefits of rehabilitation may be documented. Longer term outcomes, such as return to work, maintenance of independence in the community, and so on, are emerging as accepted measures of ultimate importance in general outcomes research in rehabilitation. Local individual providers are ill suited and have limited capability for providing such long-term documentation and study. With these comprehensive data, one may also begin looking at "critical pathway" analyses. For example, questions may be addressed: Is there a benefit to having an aggressive behavioral management program in the continuum of care for the general TBI patient? Do behavioral problems generally resolve "spontaneously" with general care? Another example might be the contribution a home-based rehabilitation component might make on either the durability of long-term, functional outcomes or on reducing the cost of care. Another benefit of this database's nature is that it is possible to recognize various providers that demonstrate unique patterns of competence, expertise, and efficiency, and one can also identify problem areas in the delivery system. For example, acute rehab providers who require excessive stays for the achievement of typical rehabilitation outcomes, or providers who perhaps show a pattern of poor family preparation or education, may be identified and corrective actions taken. These analyses then become the source of information in quality assurance and quality continuous improvement feedback loops.

Overall, the Paradigm methodology appears to integrate in the area of brain-injury rehabilitation the legitimate concerns of payors, the volume needs of centers of excellence and expert clinicians, an efficiency and cost-effectiveness in resource utilization, as well as optimum clinical and functional outcomes for the patients.

In reflecting on our progress to date, when we embarked on this process 4 years ago, we felt that we had an excellent theory of catastrophic injury management, but we were aware that we had little in the way of empirical data or experience in support of the theory. At present, based on several years of clinical experience and many hundreds of patients, I can report that this system seems to be working to a general or even high level of satisfaction of all parties. Insurance carriers have reported a great reduction in the administrative costs and complexities of managing these cases. They also feel that the incidence of disastrous outcomes and high-cost cases has been virtually eliminated. The satisfaction of the patients and families is routinely surveyed and is at a very high level. At the same time, providers are satisfied with their ability, within this system, to generate appropriate treatment plans free from the micromanagement and oversight of traditional utilization review systems and procedures. In addition, once a plan is established, providers can provide treatment essentially independently, free from multiple and frequent contact with payor organizations for justifications or authorizations of ordinary and quite straightforward expenditures. Providers find the reimbursement system both simple to administer and quite acceptable, given the information provided by the Paradigm database. Clinicians' initial anxiety over "guaranteeing a clinical outcome" has been managed quite successfully, both by the financial stop losses as well as various contingencies in the contract that address a new pathophysiological event, (i.e., a myocardial infarction occurring during the course of rehabilitation). In this event, reimbursement would be covered under a different, more traditional scheme.

I have provided a necessarily brief introduction/overview to my organization, which is a new and unique approach to the problem of managing both the quality and cost of TBI and other complex catastrophic conditions. I believe this model is proving to be a successful one. It has been sufficiently successful with our partners, major insurance carriers, and expert providers. Thus, we have been encouraged to move, and in fact have moved, into associated areas of complex difficulties, such as multiple trauma and severe burns. We are currently investigating the methodology's applicability for other complex medical conditions. It may be that the principles inherent in the Paradigm approach have a more general applicability to the management of medically complex and expensive conditions, and are not limited to neurological rehabilitation per se.

22

Neurolaw: Medicolegal Aspects of Traumatic Brain Injury

J. Sherrod Taylor

Neurolaw is the emerging field of medical jurisprudence that addresses the medicolegal aspects of neurological injuries. Supporters of this new discipline adhere to the fundamental belief that law—particularly the civil litigation process—may contribute to the achievement of better clinical outcomes for people who sustain such injuries. Although neurolaw embraces the legal ramifications of both traumatic brain injury (TBI) and spinal cord injury (Lemkuhl, 1993; Taylor, 1994a; Weed & Field, 1994), and also deals with the prevention of neurological injuries through legal means (e.g., helmet and seatbelt laws), this chapter focuses solely on law as it relates to recovery after brain injury.

TBI is a global public health concern. Millions of people worldwide acquire brain injury annually. Countless human lives are affected by the consequences of TBI. Brain injury is ubiquitous because it often results from events that are common in daily life. Although motor vehicle-related injuries are the most frequent cause of brain dysfunction, falls, assaults, injuries associated with sports or recreational activities, and pedestrian or bicycling injuries also produce deficits in brain function.

Many of the traumatic occurrences that cause TBI become the subject of legal investigation, inquiry, and action. For this reason, professionals who serve TBI survivors and their families require a unified multidisciplinary approach for dealing with neurotrauma from the legal perspective. By encouraging allied health and legal professionals to work together in a spirit of mutual cooperation, neurolaw provides a framework for collaborative action within the legal arena.

People with acquired brain injury often rely on the civil litigation process to obtain needed financial support. Proceeds derived from personal injury, workers' compensation, Social Security, and insurance-related cases are used by TBI survivors to: (a) fund programs of care and rehabilitation, (b) replace lost earnings, and, in appropriate cases, (c) compensate for physical pain and mental suffering. Although each of the several civil justice recovery systems named may be applicable to specific, individual TBI cases, this chapter focuses primarily on personal injury (tort) litigation.

INCREASING TBI POPULATION

Neurolaw emerged in direct response to the dramatic increase in the brain-injured population resulting from technological advances in medical care. Prior to the advent of modern shock trauma units and wide usage of neuroimaging procedures, many people with TBI died from their injuries. With new developments in patient care, most people who sustain brain injury now survive (Papastrat, 1992). Many of these survivors require treatment for a long period of time, but such care is costly. Indeed, Goodall, Lawyer, and Wehman (1994) observed that the greatest barrier to the development of long-term supports for people with TBI is lack of funding. Inadequate funding is most acute in severe TBI cases, where the National Head Injury Foundation (NHIF) estimates that the costs may exceed $9 million over the patient's lifetime. Neurolitigation may be employed to secure funding required for treatment.

This increase in the TBI survivor population created a profound shift of emphases within both the health care and legal communities. In former days, when brain injury often resulted in death, clinicians tended to focus on modalities of acute care designed principally to save the injured person's life. Because such efforts had high failure rates, many patients never moved from acute care into the rehabilitation setting. However, as more people began to survive brain injury, the health care community began establishing rehabilitation programs aligned along a comprehensive continuum of care.

The legal community also responded to increases in the TBI population. Where lawyers formerly based civil litigation on statutes pertaining to wrongful death, they may now institute legal actions predicated on laws dealing with personal injury. It is important for health care providers to appreciate the distinction between death and injury claims because the legal damages associated with death differ radically from those linked to personal injury. On the one hand, wrongful death damages are designed primarily to compensate living heirs for the loss of economic resources and intangible relationships previously provided by the deceased to the surviving family. On the other hand, personal injury damages are generally allocated for reimbursement of medical and rehabilitation treatment expenses and lost wages, while also, in proper cases, compensating the injured person for pain and suffering.

Because the elements of damages in these two types of cases are different in character, the legal proof required in each case is also different. When clinicians serve as expert witnesses in wrongful death cases, they are usually asked only to verify that death was caused by the traumatic event giving rise to the litigation. However, when they testify in personal injury actions, they are frequently asked to confirm not only the cause of the injury, but also the nature and extent of the injury. In many instances, the practitioner may also be questioned about the estimated costs of future health care. Because of these differences in proof requirements, lawyers representing clients in death actions commonly have only limited contact with health care professionals. But in personal injury cases, attorneys may have many contacts with care providers. When the size of the TBI population increased, conditions were ripe for establishment of a new approach to addressing medicolegal questions. Neurolaw emerged to provide an architecture for efficient interaction between clinicians and lawyers involved in legal cases brought on behalf of TBI survivors.

OUTCOMES IN TBI CASES

Legal and health care services share a common characteristic: Consumers determine the value of both services in terms of final outcome. Professional productivity is not measured by effort expended; rather, it is measured by results. Both law and rehabilitation medicine are outcome-driven systems. Practitioners in both fields have long recognized this fact. This is the reason that health care literature is replete with "outcome studies" (Brooks, 1982), and why marketers from for-profit TBI centers stress outcomes achieved by their facilities when they recruit patients. This is also the reason that trial lawyers proudly tell prospective clients about previous successful TBI cases during initial interviews.

Attorneys work diligently to obtain just and adequate compensation for their TBI clients, knowing well that the amount of money damages awarded in each case constitutes the measure of the legal outcome in neurolitigation. In a like manner, clinicians employ a vast array of treatment modalities designed to achieve optimal clinical outcomes for their patients. Although the recovery of money proceeds from a lawsuit will not necessarily result in favorable clinical outcomes in TBI patients, it does provide the financial support required to fund opportunities for maximum care and attention—thereby laying a foundation on which a favorable clinical outcome may be based.

To be sure, predicting the outcomes of TBI patients from the clinical perspective is difficult because they are determined by a host of complex factors, including: (a) premorbid circumstances (e.g., age, preexisting disease, preexisting psychosocial factors, alcohol/drug abuse, prior nutritional status), (b) specific mechanisms of injury (e.g., intracranial mass lesion and/or extracranial injury), (c) secondary brain injury (e.g., brain swelling, hypoxia, infection), and (d) success or failure of therapeutic interventions (Vollmer, 1993).

However, TBI survivors and their families tend to be chiefly concerned with outcome in a functional sense: They focus on a desire for the injured person to return, as closely as possible, to preinjury status. They want the brain-injured person to move in an orderly fashion through the continuum of care—toward regaining independence in the activities of daily life and reintegrating into the fabric of society. In pursuit of this stated goal, health care professionals generally accept the notion that early treatment after brain injury, followed by vigorous application of rehabilitative therapy, contributes to the injured person's reacquisition of at least some degree of prior function. Certainly these professionals acknowledge that it is the quest for a return to normalcy that motivates persons with brain injury and their families to embark on a course of treatment in the first place. If this were not the case, no real purpose for seeking health care would exist.

Fortunately, clinical studies (Levin, Benton, & Grossman, 1982) have demonstrated that there is a significant improvement in functional outcome after rehabilitative treatment. Mills, Nesbeda, Katz, and Alexander (1992) concluded that postacute TBI treatment aimed at retraining real-life functional abilities can lead to long-term improvements in independence. Spivak, Spettel, Ellis, and Ross (1992) demonstrated that both length of stay and intensity of treatment affect outcomes: Patients in the long-length stay group consistently made more progress across all outcome variables than patients in the short-length stay groups. Moreover, Malec, Smigielski, DePompolo, and Thompson (1993) determined that a group-oriented, comprehensive-integrated approach to postacute brain-injury rehabilitation is effective and cost-effective, and they recommended early intervention for optimal outcomes.

However, in today's health care environment, programs that provide substantial brain-injury rehabilitation cost large amounts of money. Thus, persons with acquired brain injury and their families confront many obstacles as they seek to assemble the multiple sources of funding required for therapeutic intervention. Even when TBI survivors are entitled to receive good benefits from health insurance, they may nonetheless require alternative sources of funding to obtain access to needed rehabilitative resources. For this reason, in appropriate cases, eligible survivors turn in increasing numbers to legal remedies—especially those grounded in personal injury (tort) litigation. It is a simple fact of modern life that economics influences the allocation of services. In the absence of adequate funding, rehabilitation efforts would be impossible. The need for substantial monies becomes acute, especially if, as it has been suggested, some rehabilitation providers set the length of stay in their facilities to coincide with the point at which funding becomes exhausted (Banja, 1992).

Although the goal of rehabilitation is to return individuals with brain injury to the status they enjoyed prior to injury, realism dictates that not all survivors regain that cherished position. Often the permanent sequelae of TBI prevent achievement of that admirable goal. Therefore, Evans and Ruff (1992) suggested that clinical outcome following brain injury may be measured in three areas: residential setting status, living assistance, and productive activity. The residential setting status varies between two extremes: return to the home environment and placement in long-term supported-living settings. Requirements for living assistance vary from a complete return to independence to the need for 24-hour supervision. Productive activity ranges from a return to competitive employment to no productivity at all. Of course, each of these measurable outcomes has intermediary points located between the best and worst possible extremes.

From the legal perspective, clinical outcomes that result in less than a full return to preinjury status present needs for greater amounts of compensatory damages for TBI survivors. In such cases, awards secured through the legal system may be the sole avenue for long-term funding needed to care for these injured people. Yet the precise amount of money required to sustain TBI survivors is difficult to estimate. In the present health care environment, it may be argued that TBI survivors simply cannot have too much money if they wish to participate in rehabilitation therapy. In the final analysis, Malec et al. (1993) were probably correct when they wrote: "When the benefit of a post-acute rehabilitation programme is the salvage of a human life, it follows that any degree of cost that does not jeopardize human life in another sector of society is offset by the benefit" (p. 28).

With these considerations firmly in mind, it is readily apparent that lawyers and allied health professionals have significant roles to play in assisting TBI survivors in the procurement of funds through neurolitigation. Thus, from the outset of every TBI lawsuit, health care providers should recognize the capability of the legal system to contribute to favorable clinical outcomes in their patients. Concomitantly, attorneys must recognize that, without the dedicated assistance of clinicians who serve as expert witnesses, successful prosecution of neurolegal cases will not occur. Thus, providers and lawyers must develop a dynamic, synergistic relationship during the course of neurolitigation to promote their patients' and clients' overall interests. Recognizing the desirability of forming such a relationship led attorneys and clinicians to join in developing the field of neurolaw.

ORIGINS OF NEUROLAW

Neurolaw is a recent development in the history of medical jurisprudence. In his seminal study, Mohr (1993) observed that medical jurisprudence is a separate professional field focusing on interaction between those who possess medical knowledge and those who exercise legal authority. Thus, this area of study became a sort of facilitating or mediating field between medicine and law. Although it may seem curious to modern practitioners, Mohr noted that, in the first half of the 19th century, medical schools endorsed with unanimity and tenacity the notion that medical jurisprudence should be an essential aspect of professional training for future physicians. At that time, it was believed that, with knowledge of medical jurisprudence, physicians could work with attorneys, judges, and legislators to enhance both the public contribution and the social role of professionals in the new nation. Lamentably, interest in the field of medical jurisprudence waned during the late 1800s. By the beginning of the 20th century, courses on this subject almost totally disappeared from medical school curricula.

Brain injury has been the subject of civil litigation for over 100 years, yet many health practitioners and attorneys remain ignorant of how best to work in concert during such cases. In 1987, recognizing that the medicolegal aspects of TBI were not being addressed adequately by concerned professionals, the NHIF initiated an annual seminar entitled "The Head Injury Case: What the Trial Lawyer Needs to Know." During this conference, health and legal specialists came together to share current information pertaining to brain disorders and the legal environment. American attorneys were reintroduced to the nuances of brain injury. Health care providers who attended this meeting became reacquainted with how law could be employed for the benefit of their patients. Later, other professional groups began to hold similar meetings worldwide, encouraging health practitioners to participate in legal actions designed to promote favorable clinical outcomes for their TBI patients. Neurolaw was beginning.

The term *neurolaw* was coined during the early part of the "Decade of the Brain" (Taylor, Harp, & Elliott, 1991a, 1991b). Neurolawyers became recognized as those attorneys who, through interest, education, and training, possess special expertise in representing clients with brain injury. Soon articles in professional journals described the new field (Taylor, 1991, 1993a, 1993b; Taylor, Harp, & Elliott, 1992). From the outset, Charles W. Haynes, a former NHIF president, supported this emerging specialty by publishing *The Neurolaw Letter,* a monthly newsletter for health care and legal practitioners. Also, Professor D. Neil Brooks, a past president of the International Neuropsychological Society (INS), championed its development. The *Martindale–Hubbell© Law Directory*—the world's definitive source of information for and about the legal community—stimulated further interest among attorneys when it began accepting listings for this field (Martindale-Hubbell, 1994).

Neurolaw has come before the international community of TBI professionals in a variety of other ways. Commentators have disseminated information about this topic in respected periodicals (Braithwaite, 1992; Bush, 1993; Litvak, Amin, & Senf, 1993). Books authored or edited by physicians (Roberts, 1991; Rothenberg, 1994) and lawyers (Simkins, 1994) have emphasized the importance of neurolegal inquiry. Other organizations (e.g., European Brain Injury Society [EBIS], International Association for the Study of Traumatic Brain Injury [IASTBI], Commonwealth Association for Mental Handicap and Developmental Disabilities [CAMHADD], and World Health Organization [WHO]) have followed the lead of the NHIF by including programs devoted to neurolaw in their professional seminars. Today neurolaw stands as a field that unites concerned professionals from myriad disciplines who serve people with TBI.

MEDICOLEGAL ALLIANCE

Health care practitioners and neurolawyers generally know that the interests of persons with acquired neurological injuries are best served through employment of a multidisciplinary TBI team (Howard, 1988; Taylor, 1994b). The team usually involved in neurolegal cases includes: neurosurgeons, neurologists, physiatrists, psychiatrists, psychologists, neuropsychologists, physical and occupational therapists, speech/language/hearing pathologists, life care planners, vocational experts, nurses, and neurolawyers. Members of the TBI team recognize the value of mutual cooperation among all concerned professionals, and commonly acknowledge that such cooperation may be the key to favorable clinical outcomes in survivors of brain injury. Indeed, a cardinal principle of neurolaw provides: the success of neurolitigation is largely dependent on the quality and quantity of expert evidence.

Each member of the TBI team plays a significant part in the successful resolution of any neurolegal matter. The concept of "team" necessarily implies "teamwork" (collective, rather than individual, action). Of all areas of personal injury practice, neurolaw is the most "expert intensive" because proving the cause, nature, and extent of brain injury in court is sometimes a formidable endeavor requiring input from many specialists. For this reason, neurolaw cuts across traditional professional boundaries by including experts from disparate fields.

To participate successfully in neurolitigation, health professionals must acquire at least a modicum of *litigation literacy*. That term may be defined as basic awareness of the intricacies of the justice system (Taylor, 1992). Appreciation of legal procedures, as well as trial tactics and strategies, is embodied in this concept. By understanding the complex, multidimensional legal process, care providers may effectively contribute their expertise in any legal proceeding. Similarly, neurolawyers must have insight into matters involving neuroscience, medicine, and rehabilitation. Apprehending the work of disciplines other than their own allows concerned professionals to develop the relationships necessary to provide full service to patients and clients involved in litigation.

All health specialities recognize the need for their members to provide expert testimony in litigated cases. A provision found in the *Code of Medical Ethics* (American Medical Association, 1994) underscores this requirement:

> 9.07 Medical Testimony. As a citizen and as a professional with special training and experience, the physician has an ethical obligation to assist in the administration of justice. If a patient who has a legal claim requests a physician's assistance, the physician should furnish medical evidence, with the patient's consent, in order to secure the patient's legal rights. (p. 138)

Virtually all other TBI professionals are required by the ethical codes of their own specialties to provide similar services. From the legal perspective, both statutory and appellate case law uniformly recognizes the desirability and admissibility of evidence from expert witnesses in all personal injury cases.

Although adherence by concerned professionals to the principle of mutual cooperation promotes the interests of TBI survivors and their families, achieving a high level of cooperation has proved to be a difficult undertaking in many instances. One physician (Omenn, 1993) went so far as to pose this question: Can lawyers and scientists get along? This nagging question has permeated the attorney–health professional relationship for generations. As previously shown, lawyers, judges, and juries have long believed that health experts are needed to address disputes over the cause, nature, and extent of personal injuries. However, in the recent past, health care providers have sometimes been loathe to participate in legal inquiries for which they clearly have relevant expertise. Omenn suggested five possible reasons for this reluctance:

1. There is widespread suspicion for those experts who do regularly appear in court as expert witnesses—they are often called "hired guns" by their colleagues, as well as the lawyers who recruit or oppose them.
2. There is a clash of cultures. Litigation emphasizes differences, whereas science seeks consensus based on empirically demonstrable "facts." The legal construct of *most likely* is far less certain than scientists usually apply [in their own work]. Courtroom jargon is unfamiliar to scientists.
3. Scientists and physicians lack training for this work—they are unprepared for personal attack on their credentials and motives, for questions about their compensation, for questions designed to reveal deficiencies in their knowledge.
4. The expert witness may even be confused about her role with the lawyer who hired her. There are often conflicts between the role of consultant/advisor and the role of "expert" testifier.
5. There are serious logistical problems. Lawyers may line up experts whom they have no intention of using, partly to block the opposition from recruiting the same persons and partly to intimidate the opposition. Seldom can the date [or] times of required testimony be predicted.

Omenn's concerns constitute many valid criticisms of the legal system, generally, and the way lawyers work, specifically. They may be addressed with the following observations.

First, although it is certainly true that some health professionals express suspicion or even disdain for experts who often appear in TBI cases, such expressions should be confined to comments about well-known, incompetent "experts." To make such observations about competent, well-credentialed health experts is to do them a grave injustice at a time when they are endeavoring to provide valuable services for TBI survivors. Although some experts may be referred to as *hired guns,* this derogatory term is inappropriate in most instances. The previously cited portion of the *Code of Medical Ethics* (American Medical Association, 1994) is as follows:

> The medical witness must not become an advocate or a partisan in the legal proceeding. The medical witness should be adequately prepared and should testify honestly and truthfully. The attorney for the party who calls the physician as a witness should be informed of all favorable and unfavorable information developed by the physician's evaluation of the case. (p. 138)

This admonishment fully recognizes the distinction that trial lawyers often make during pretestimony conferences with their experts: It is one thing to be an advocate for a particular litigant and quite another to be an advocate for one's own professional opinions while giving testimony. Competent and ethical attorneys only want their experts to testify honestly when they present or defend their own professional opinions.

Second, the "clash of cultures" mentioned by Omenn becomes manifest when we consider the burden of proof that TBI plaintiffs have in civil cases. Under this burden, litigants are required to show the cause, nature, and extent of their injuries by a "preponderance of the evidence" (i.e., by what Omenn referred to as the legal construct of *most likely*). Simply stated, *preponderance* means "probability" or a "greater weight of evidence." Clinicians who object to using this legal standard do so, they say, because the notion of "preponderance" embodies a lesser degree of proof than that commonly used to establish a scientific "fact." Thus, those experts maintain that the concept of "probability" does not satisfy the exacting criteria of science to be considered "true" (Malec, 1993).

However, the failure of health experts to employ the notion of "preponderance" when testifying presents TBI litigants with many problems in court. Clinicians become especially vulnerable on cross-examination when defense attorneys seek to suggest "possible," rather than "probable," causes for the plaintiff's brain dysfunction. To avoid this potential trap, clinicians are well advised to acknowledge that courts do not require testimony to be based on 100% certainty in civil cases. Recognition of this fact demonstrates that the expert witness possesses litigation literacy.

Frequently, the issue of brain-injury causation is hotly contested during neurolitigation. Therefore, this issue demands further attention here. Regarding the question of causation, Kolpan (1989) observed that TBI experts must only state that the plaintiff's current condition was likely (i.e., probably, more likely than not, with 51% probability) caused by the traumatic event that is the subject of the neurolitigation. This should not be difficult to do in the majority of cases. As Jennett (1982) pointed out in his discussion of behavioral outcome: "Unless reliable data are available about the pre-morbid state, it may be assumed that such behavior after head injury is the result of brain damage" (p. 42). Thus, to comply with the legal rules pertaining to "preponderance of the evidence," practitioners only have to use the scientific principle of parsimony (i.e., William of Occam's Razor), which provides that no more causes should be assumed than are necessary to account for the facts (i.e., in science, the simplest theory that fits the facts of a problem is the one that should be chosen).

Regardless of how uncomfortable the notion of "preponderance" may make some health witnesses, it is nonetheless essential that they accept this concept. To participate successfully in litigation, brain-injury professionals must enter the domain of law and use applicable legal rules to govern their testimony. Besides, when medical practitioners are sued for malpractice, they frequently urge that "medicine is an inexact science" (*Branch v. Anderson*, 1933). Similarly, in its guidelines for expert witnesses, at least one medical specialty organization reminds members of "the innate uncertainty inherent in all of medicine" (American Academy of Pediatrics, 1989). Thus, in reality, health professionals already apply the concept of "probability" to their own practices. Therefore, predicating expert testimony on "probability" should impose no significant burden on testifying clinicians.

Third, Omenn was also correct when he observed that health care providers may lack training in being an expert witness. Supporting Omenn's position, Goodall, Dedrick, Zasler, Kreutzer, and Riddick (1993) reported that a majority of experienced case managers they surveyed expressed a desire to receive more training in the medicolegal aspects of TBI. Thus, if providers desire to assist their patients in acquiring funds required to pay for treatment and rehabilitation, they must develop proficiency in this area. (Recognizing the need for such training, the Department of Rehabilitation Medicine at the Emory University School of Medicine has added three neurolawyers to its adjunct faculty.) Again, the concept of "litigation literacy" provides assistance. By working closely with attorneys who intend to call providers as expert witnesses, TBI professionals can prepare for the onslaught of cross-examination questions designed to promote the thorough and sifting inquiry to which opposing counsel is legally entitled.

Fourth, in the real world of neurolitigation, health experts seldom become confused about their roles. It is unlikely that practitioners will ever be retained for purposes other than to present evidence in some form (e.g., reports, depositions, or in court). Usually TBI experts testify by deposition or in person.

Fifth, the first part of Omenn's final criticism is valid. Expert TBI clinicians, as well as neurolawyers, confront serious logistical problems. Today's busy court dockets require all participants in neurolitigation to be patient because dates and times of testimony are somewhat unpredictable. But in complex TBI cases, judges often set aside specific dates for trials. However, knowing the precise time of an expert's testimony is almost never possible because judges and counsel cannot predict how the presentation of evidence will "flow" on any given day. As a final comment, it must be pointed out that TBI experts are not generally retained by lawyers who have no intention of using them during the course of the proceedings. Thus, Omenn's concern over that issue is generally without merit.

There may be at least one additional reason for the reluctance of some health care providers to cooperate with lawyers during TBI litigation. At the very time medical treatment innovations produced a sizable increase in the TBI survivor population, a rift developed between clinicians and attorneys due to the so-called "medical malpractice crisis." It is indeed fortunate for people with brain injury that this perceived crisis has ended because now, more than ever, the services of cooperating specialists from both the health and legal professions are required to prosecute cases fully. Recently, the Utah Supreme Court placed the "crisis" into the proper perspective when it observed in *Lee v. Gaufin* (1993) as follows:

> [a]lthough it was well-established that malpractice insurance premiums had substantially increased [during the 1970s and 1980s], the evidence for the asserted causes was largely anecdotal.
>
> Initially, little effort was made to investigate empirically the real causes of the malpractice insurance crisis. The medical profession and the insurance industry blamed malpractice lawsuits, and as a result, "tort reform" legislation was enacted in a number of states. . . .
>
> In time, however, the presumed causes of the "malpractice crisis" were challenged, as was the efficacy of the legislative responses. (p. 584)

Later in the same appellate decision, the justices observed:

> the dramatic increases in medical malpractice insurance premiums and the increased costs of health care were not caused by significant increases in malpractice lawsuits or claims . . . or by significant increases in the size of jury verdicts. (p. 588)

However, the hostile environment created by the "crisis" was inhospitable to mutual cooperation among cognate TBI disciplines. Clearly it had a deleterious effect on the health–law relationship. It encouraged professionals in both fields to revert to a "we–they" viewpoint. But even children who read Dr. Seuss know that, by dividing ourselves into "we" and "they," we lose our ability to grasp our fundamental interdependence (Geisel, 1961). In the world of neurolaw, there must be no we–they dichotomy—only the "us" mentality should prevail. Lingering effects of the "malpractice crisis," like a ghost from the not too distant past, may still make some clinicians reluctant to cooperate with neurolawyers, and may remain in some quarters as a potential source of future conflicts. But the number of brain-injury practitioners who harbor those feelings is steadily declining. The medicolegal alliance grows stronger day by day under encouragement given by neurolaw supporters.

OTHER PRACTICAL APPLICATIONS

The emergence of neurolaw has had other profound effects on the medicolegal paradigm. For example, in an effort to integrate health concepts pertaining to brain injury into the fabric of law, neurolegal advocates have urged state legislatures to enact statutory definitions of TBI into their codes. Although law has been influenced by descriptions of brain injury appearing in health literature, law has tended to lag behind and has been slow to incorporate those health ideas into legal principles. But this is changing. Legislators are moving toward placing concrete definitions of TBI, which mirror those found in health literature, into state codes. Presently, at least 11 states (i.e., Arizona, Georgia, Kentucky, Michigan, Minnesota, Montana, Nevada, New York, North Dakota, Rhode Island, and Tennessee) have passed such legislation. Although the specific wording of these various laws differs slightly from state to state, the Minnesota law (Minn. Stat. § 256B.093) is typical:

> 'Traumatic brain injury' means a sudden insult or damage to the brain or its coverings, not of a degenerative or congenital nature. The insult or damage may produce an altered state of consciousness and may result in a decrease in cognitive, behavioral, emotional or physical functioning resulting in partial or total disability.

By using the term *TBI* in their records, reports, and litigation testimony, health experts practicing in states that have enacted such definitions into their statutory laws will be using a term with a recognized legal meaning. Such use will reduce the opportunity for confusion regarding a patient's condition if the professional's opinions are later scrutinized by an appellate court. Employment of the term *TBI* may also result in care providers being reimbursed maximum amounts for their charges by health insurers, who pay full benefits for organic injuries but lesser amounts for charges associated with mental illness. Moreover, by using the legal definition of TBI, clinicians and neurolawyers may avoid confusion arising from professional jargon, which is commonly wrapped in mysterious obscurity. Utilization of the legal definition of TBI will result in concerned professionals "speaking the same language" to some degree.

The development of neurolaw has also encouraged health care practitioners to develop refined protocols for the forensic evaluation of TBI patients. Whether they are called to testify as plaintiff's or defense expert witnesses, clinicians know that, at some time during the neurolitigation process, they will probably be asked to render professional opinions regarding the cause, nature, and extent of the patient's brain injury. A proper forensic evaluation requires the provider to conduct a thorough review of the injured individual's pre- and postinjury status. By reviewing pertinent health, school, military, employment, and criminal records, and conducting the appropriate examination, the expert is well positioned to provide forensic testimony.

Plaintiff's attorneys use these forensic evaluations to: estimate damages, prepare settlement demands, identify strengths and weaknesses of their cases, and gain insights into treatment interventions that may increase their client's daily functioning. Defense lawyers use these evaluations to: identify strengths and weaknesses of their own positions, evaluate claims, set insurance reserves, and identify malingering or symptom magnification.

Finally, the advent of neurolaw has made health care providers more aware of the roles that lawyers play in TBI cases. Now health care providers tend to become more personally involved in the legal aspects of TBI. Indeed, it is common for these providers to be called on by TBI survivors and their families to recommend specific attorneys to work on the legal problems faced by their patients. However, O'Hara and Harrell (1991) observed that choosing an appropriate attorney may be a difficult task under the best of circumstances, and is certainly not made easier when patients are in the midst of recovering from their injuries. For this reason, those authors suggested that a patient's case manager aid in the selection process by providing names of people who are familiar with the legal ramifications of brain dysfunction. Noting the need for survivors, families, and care providers to have ready access to lawyers who handle brain-injury litigation, in 1992 the NHIF published *The Directory of Legal Resources in Brain Injury and Disability*, which contained biographical information about specific neurolawyers (National Head Injury Foundation, 1992). In 1993, NHIF recognized that attorneys were becoming full-fledged members of the multidisciplinary TBI team, and for the first time included information about attorneys in its *National Directory of Head Injury Rehabilitation Services* (National Head Injury Foundation, 1993). Likewise, the Rehabilitation Research and Training Center on Severe Traumatic Brain Injury (1993) established a listing of attorneys in its *National Directory of Lecturers and Resources in Traumatic Brain Injury*. Using the information presented in these directories, providers can assist TBI survivors in locating competent neurolawyers. Additionally, Taylor (1993c) provided survivors, families, and health practitioners with criteria for use in selecting attorneys experienced in conducting neurolitigation. Armed with this valuable information about neurolawyers, TBI patients become better equipped to prosecute their claims before appropriate tribunals.

CONCLUSION

As shown herein, the emerging field of neurolaw engenders a spirit of mutual cooperation among professionals who deal with TBI. Although the notion of "cooperation" is beguilingly simple to understand in theory, it may be difficult to implement in practice. Members of individual disciplines concerned with TBI sometime tend myopically to pursue their own areas of interest until a reason arises to seek collaboration. Brain-injury litigation affords an opportunity for multidisciplinary, collective action by TBI professionals.

A neurolegal perspective encourages concerned professionals to develop and maintain constructive relationships and interactions. Such relationships and interactions are clearly beneficial to brain-injured people who are involved with the legal process because they lead to favorable outcomes in neurolitigation. Favorable legal outcomes result in increased availability of funding for programs of treatment and rehabilitation. Early application of medical and rehabilitation care enhances the probability of favorable clinical outcomes for TBI patients. In these ways, neurolaw represents a synthesis of medicine, rehabilitation, and law that can contribute to improving the quality of the lives of TBI survivors and their families (Taylor, 1995).

REFERENCES

American Academy of Pediatrics. (1989). Guidelines for expert witness testimony. *Pediatrics, 83*(2), 312.

American Medical Association. (1994). *Code of medical ethics: Current opinions with annotations,* § 9.07 (p. 138).

Banja, J. D. (1992). Ethics, fraud, and the misallocation of rehabilitation resources. *Journal of Head Trauma Rehabilitation, 7*(3), 114–116.

Braithwaite, B. (1992). Head injury litigation. *New Law Journal,* 942–943.

Branch v. Anderson, 171 S.E. 771 (Ga. App. 1933).

Brooks, N. (1982). Head injury and the family. In N. Brooks (Ed.), *Closed head injury: Psychological, social, and family consequences* (pp. 123–147). New York: Oxford University Press.

Bush, D. S. (1993). Malingered claims of brain damage and neuropsychological evidence. *Defense Counsel Journal, 60*(1), 122–126.

Evans, R. W., & Ruff, R. M. (1992). Outcome and value: A perspective on rehabilitation outcome achieved in acquired brain injury. *Journal of Head Trauma Rehabilitation, 7*(4), 24–36.

Geisel, T. S. (1961). *The sneetches, and other stories.* New York: Random House.

Goodall, P., Dedrick, D., Zasler, N. D., Kreutzer, J. S., & Riddick, S. (1993). Survey of case manager training needs in traumatic brain injury. *Brain Injury, 7*(5), 455–468.

Goodall, P., Lawyer, H. L., & Wehman, P. (1994). Vocational rehabilitation and traumatic brain injury: A legislative and public policy perspective. *Journal of Head Trauma Rehabilitation, 9*(2), 61–81.

Howard, M. E. (1988). Behavior management in the acute care rehabilitation setting. *Journal of Head Trauma Rehabilitation, 3*(3), 14–22.

Jennett, B. (1982). The measurement of outcome. In N. Brooks (Ed.), *Closed head injury: Psychological, social, and family consequences* (pp. 37–43). New York: Oxford University Press.

Kolpan, K. I. (1989). Expert courtroom testimony. *Journal of Head Trauma Rehabilitation, 4*(1), 95–96.

Lee v. Gaufin, 867 P.2d 572 (Utah 1993).

Lemkuhl, L. D. (1993). *Brain injury glossary.* Houston, TX: HDI Publishers.

Levin, H. S., Benton, A. L., & Grossman, R. G. (1982). *Neurobehavioral consequences of closed head injury.* New York: Oxford University Press.

Litvak, S. R., Amin, K., & Senf, G. M. (1993, Dec.). Neurolaw: Update on traumatic head injury. *Arizona Trial Lawyers Association Advocate,* pp. 1–10.

Malec, J. F. (1993). Ethics in brain injury rehabilitation: Existential choices among Western cultural beliefs. *Brain Injury, 7*(5), 383–400.

Malec, J. F., Smigielski, J. S., DePompolo, R. W., & Thompson, J. M. (1993). Outcome evaluation and prediction in a comprehensive-integrated post-acute outpatient brain injury rehabilitation programme. *Brain Injury, 7*(1), 15–29.

Martindale-Hubbell. (1994). *Martindale-Hubbell® Law Directory.* New Providence, NJ: Author.

Mills, V. M., Nesbeda, T., Katz, D. I., & Alexander, M. P. (1992). Outcomes for traumatically brain-injured patients following post-acute rehabilitation programmes. *Brain Injury, 6*(3), 219–228.

Minnesota Statutes § 256 B.093.

Mohr, J. C. (1993). *Doctors and the law: Medical jurisprudence in nineteenth-century America.* New York: Oxford University Press.

National Head Injury Foundation. (1992). *The directory of legal resources in brain injury and disability.* Washington, DC: Author.

National Head Injury Foundation. (1993). *National directory of head injury rehabilitation services.* Washington, DC: Author.

O'Hara, C. C., & Harrell, M. (1991). *Rehabilitation with brain injury survivors: An empowerment approach.* Gaithersburg, MD: Aspen Publishers.

Omenn, G. S. (1993, June 16). Can lawyers and scientists get along? *Daily Journal of Commerce,* p. 2.

Papastrat, L. A. (1992). Outcome and value following brain injury: A financial provider's perspective. *Journal of Head Trauma Rehabilitation, 7*(4), 11–23.

Rehabilitation Research and Training Center on Severe Traumatic Brain Injury. (1993). *National directory of lecturers and resources in traumatic brain injury.* Richmond, VA: Author.

Roberts, A. C. (1991). *Litigating head trauma cases.* New York: Wiley.

Rothenberg, M. A. (1994). *Emergency medicine malpractice* (2nd ed.). New York: Wiley.

Simkins, C. N. (Ed.). (1994). *Analysis, understanding, and presentation of cases involving traumatic brain injury.* Washington, DC: National Head Injury Foundation.

Spivak, G., Spettel, C. M., Ellis, D. W., & Ross, S. E. (1992). Effects of intensity of treatment and length of stay on rehabilitation outcomes. *Brain Injury, 6*(5), 419–434.

Taylor, J. S. (1991). Proving long-term soft tissue damage. *Insurance Settlements Journal, 3*(1), 21–26.

Taylor, J. S. (1992). Litigation literacy. *The Neurolaw Letter, 1*(10), 4.

Taylor, J. S. (1993a). La compensation due prejudice [Obtaining compensation for brain injury]. *Revue Francaise du Dommage Corporel, 19*(2), 149–151.

Taylor, J. S. (1993b). Neuropsychological evidence in Georgia: New law. *Verdict, 18*(4), 46–48.

Taylor, J. S. (1993c). Traumatic brain injury cases: Selecting a neurolawyer. *Journal of Head Injury, 3*(2), 54–56.

Taylor, J. S. (1994a). Head and spinal injuries: Legal aspects. In M. A. Rothenberg (Ed.), *Emergency medicine malpractice* (2nd ed., pp. 465–486). New York: Wiley.

Taylor, J. S. (1994b). Lawyers as part of the TBI team. *Viewpoints, 28,* 2.

Taylor, J. S. (1995). Neurolaw: Towards a new medical jurisprudence. *Brain Injury, 9*(7), 745–751.

Taylor, J. S., Harp, J. A., & Elliott, T. (1991a). Meeting the legal challenge. *The Neurolaw Letter, 1*(1), 1.

Taylor, J. S., Harp, J. A., & Elliott, T. (1991b). Neuropsychologists and neurolawyers. *Neuropsychology, 5*(4), 293–305.

Taylor, J. S., Harp, J. A., & Elliott, T. (1992). Preparing the plaintiff in the mild brain injury case. *Trial Diplomacy Journal, 15*(2), 65–72.

Vollmer, D. G. (1993). Prognosis and outcome of severe head injury. In P. R. Cooper (Ed.), *Head injury* (pp. 553–581). Baltimore, MD: Williams & Wilkins.

Weed, R. O., & Field, T. F. (1994). *Rehabilitation consultant's handbook* (rev. ed.). Athens, GA: Elliott & Fitzpatrick.

23

Final Thoughts: Speculations for the Future

B. P. Uzzell
Henry H. Stonnington

Head injuries have been around since the beginning of life on this planet and, contrary to what people want to believe, are not 20th-century phenomena. Ancient forebearers knew devastation and functional changes after head injury. Some of the oldest known writings dealing with surgical topics in the 17th century B.C. describe treatment for head injuries (Wilkins, 1985). Throughout the centuries, lay and professional observations and treatment of head injuries have occurred, accelerating during wartime.

ACUTE CARE

The onset of a head injury is abrupt, causing changes throughout the nervous system and subsequent behaviors. Throughout time, it has been known that age is an important factor. The older the head-injured victim, the more likely an injury will be severe and chance of survival will be less. But not all those 40-, 50-, 60-year-olds or older die. Many of them survive. Regardless of age, the abruptness of the injury produces physical, social, and psychological harm. The neuronal events set in motion by the head injury and their ensuing consequences are measured from the time of the abrupt onset, and continue throughout the individual's life. For that reason, investigations and treatment tend to follow a similar timeline. Generally, information and writings near the event of head injury are labeled acute, and treatments and research related to that time period have been separated from those more distant from the time of injury in the chronic stage. However, this book does not address only one of those areas, but contains chapters written by well-known authors working on separate, but equally important, acute and chronic aspects of head injury. This blending of two separate, but equally important, sides of head injury was deliberate. It allows the reader, scientist, and professional to gain a more complete view of the status of head-injury treatment, research, and outcome, and to "cross-fertilize" across acute and chronic areas. We believe the future requires some knowledge about both areas.

Within the past 20 years, acute care medicine has been exploding with interest in researching and treating head injury. As a result, more individuals than ever before are surviving after head injuries. This interest was facilitated by the introduction of the Glasgow Coma Scale in the 1970s. The scale was used in emergency rooms and intensive care units, allowing comparability of clinical states of head-injured cases throughout the world (Teasdale & Jennett, 1974). This led to international comparisons of morbidity and treatments to prevent secondary insults acutely, such as hypothermia, mannitol, hyperventilation, and barbituate coma. Many of these treatments have strong advocates and opponents, although these difficult-to-obtain data are still being collected.

For one thing, it is difficult to randomly assign a patient to one treatment and not to another, or to withhold treatment in emergency rooms and intensive care units, because this raises ethical questions. Second, there is a timing factor that is so important to head injury. It may be that a given treatment will be effective at a specific time, but not at another in the recovery from head injury. It appears that, within minutes after a head injury, a process is initiated; either the outpouring of excitatory amino acids, neutrophils giving off toxins after crossing the blood-brain barrier to extracellular space, or other neural or metabolic activities. If not reversed, these processes will have deleterious effects. Certain aspects of the patient's clinical condition after head injury may or may not indicate the most effective treatment at that time. If appropriate treatment is not applied, secondary effects may develop. This raises the need for further acute care research of ionic events at the cellular level, inflammatory processes, and cerebral metabolism. We need to disclose why certain patients develop secondary insults from intracranial hypertension, ischemia, hyperemia, and vasospasm and other patients do not. Recent findings suggest that cerebrovascular and metabolic changes associated with traumatic brain injury (TBI) are due to pathological alterations in endogenous neurochemical systems, including those involved with normal neurotransmission, neuroprotection, autodestruction, regional inflammation, or growth factors (McIntosh, 1994). Future acute care management will undoubtedly include selective treatments based on further acquired knowledge.

NEUROIMAGING

High technology has played a tremendous role in both acute and chronic domains. With the advent of the computed tomography (CT) techniques in the 1970s, primary lesions to the brain resulting from injury, as well as some secondary insults, could be visualized and studied. Treating physicians were no longer dealing with the brain as a "black box," but were actually able to see the brain structures initially after the injury, and as many days later as clinically required. These images had a tremendous influence on treatment and care, particularly in cases of prolonged coma.

During the 1980s, the magnetic resonance imaging (MRI) technique appeared with better resolution of lesions (Gentry, 1994). For instance, areas of the brain near the skull that had been obscured on a CT scan could be visualized on an MRI. Both CT and MRI produce static, nonfunctional images of neural structures. Dynamic techniques such as positron emission tomography (PET) and single photon emission computed tomography (SPECT) appeared, providing information about brain metabolism after head injury. Later, combinations of functional and structural techniques emerged (e.g., stable Xenon CT or magnetoencephalography [MEG] and MRI data). Some of these have become useful not only with other illness, such as neoplasms and cerebrovascular disease, but with the identification of abnormalities after minor head injuries, which were not revealed by either technique alone. It is anticipated that refinements and combined techniques will develop in the future concurrently with each improvement in various functional and structural techniques.

Presently in most emergency rooms, CT images are used prior to MRI to detect bleeding because the MRI technique does not detect the presence of blood as well as CT in the early hours after head injury. However, the MRI, or combined MEG and MRI, seem to be the techniques of choice for detecting lesions and their disappearance (or lack of disappearance) in the later chronic phase postinjury. But knowing only the location and/or volume of lesions is not the whole story in the chronic phase, where other nonphysiological factors influence survivors' outcomes. Neuropsychological examinations can be useful here, correlating with high-technology findings, and elucidating functional strengths and weaknesses to provide guidance for rehabilitation treatment in the chronic phase. Neuropsychology in rehabilitation is distinctive. Just as other techniques (including high-technology techniques) are fallible, so are neuropsychological measures. Refinement is needed in the future. Just because a functional weakness may not be observed, it does not mean it does not exist. Possibly, insensitive instruments or other factors are masking true findings.

CHRONIC CARE

In the chronic phase, rehabilitation is based on principles of plasticity of the nervous system, which presumably facilitates the rehabilitation process. Recovery depends on posttraumatic ionic or neurotransmitter environment and neurotrophic substances. However, not all aspects regrowth are good; some are maladaptive. The consequences of an insult on a developing brain vary with the developmental stage, but the timing for rehabilitation procedures in that developing brain and the adult brain are unknown. Timing of rehabilitation treatment has been less explored than timing of acute treatment. We do know that the earlier the rehabilitation after an injury, the better the recovery. In the future, we may discover that maladaptive functioning may be prevented if rehabilitation is rendered at a specific postinjury time.

The timing application to brain-injured children has a very interesting consequence, suggesting that they "grow into" a deficit. A cyclic cortical reorganization occurs during childhood, involving the development of connections between the frontal lobes to all other parts of the brain during the first 20 years of life (Thatcher, 1992). If this is disrupted by a head injury, damage in childhood may not become apparent for many years (Case, 1992). Thatcher's method of "EEG coherence" may be a way to detect whether such damage has occurred, and the future may bring ways to counteract this delayed damage onset.

Delayed appearance of cortical events has occurred in brain-injured adults as well. Some 20 or 30 years after head injury, vascular deterioration and even Alzheimer's disease may emerge (Rasmusson, Brandt, Martin, & Folstein, 1995). This type of central nervous system deterioration is consistent with delayed events occurring in postpolio syndrome and spinal cord injuries.

Age factors influence acute management as well as rehabilitation. Although survival after severe injuries is reduced in older individuals, many people over 40 years of age survive moderate and minor injuries. Rehabilitation programs require pacing that is different for older individuals, whose nervous systems are not as resilient as children or young adults. Other aspects associated with age-appropriate rehabilitation will no doubt be uncovered and utilized in the future.

New neuropharmacological agents are being developed and used in the early stages of treatment to prevent secondary damage, as well as during the rehabilitation phase. Neuropharmacology is becoming one of the most important ways of improving the management and outcome of rehabilitation. Much work is being done in manipulating neurotransmitters in a way that will help and not harm. Many pharmacological agents are actually harmful, whereas others promote recovery. Thus, the use of neuropharmacological agents in rehabilitation has changed, and will change further in the future, the way we rehabilitate patients. More and more agents will be developed to counteract agitation, improve cognition and communication, and affect behavior. As in the acute stage of recovery, there may be a critical time period to receive a specific treatment. Once this window of opportunity is passed, it will lose neuropharmacological effectiveness.

Entering the chronic phase, with primary and secondary injuries, as well as residual effects of acute treatment, head-injured survivors and their families must deal with reactions to their circumstances. Rehabilitation specialists deal with the whole individual, and must tailor or individualize their programs to meet their individual patients' needs. Head-injured survivors live in an environment with family and friends, not in a vacuum. Some families' attitudes and beliefs facilitate recovery, whereas others do not. Both families and caregivers need to know how and why. Patients have unique personalities prior to the injury, which are modified posttraumatically, but are there any common personality trends that are conducive to rehabilitation? A number of variables affect rehabilitation. In fact, unpredictable influences are overwhelming to patients, families, caregivers, friends, and other individuals in the community. No person or group can deal with it alone. The family, no matter how loving, cannot be expected to bear the brunt after formalized treatment has stopped. Most countries have family advocacy groups seeking help and services so this does not occur. For those who say chronicity is forever, something must be done. A return to productivity or employment of the head-injured person requires support from employers, families, or individuals in the community.

We expect rehabilitation techniques to continue changing. This change will be brought about partly by the impact of new health care standards. Rehabilitation has been an extremely expensive modality. In the future, less and less rehabilitation will occur within hospital or residential walls. In the acute phase of rehabilitation, much of the treatment will be performed at home or in intensive day rehabilitation outpatient programs. The so-called "rehabilitation without walls" may replace some outpatient programs.

Health care professionals may be curtailed due to need and cost reductions. Outcomes may or may not be improved with new treatment methods requiring fewer rehabilitation personnel. It is possible that in the future, we will have rehabilitation technicians trained by professionals to provide a brain-injured person with one-on-one therapies. These will include physical, occupational, speech, and cognitive therapy, and will maintain behavioral-modification type of attitude with the patient and family. Possibly a rehabilitation therapist, who is qualified to perform all therapies, will supervise the rehabilitation technician. As required for today's rehabilitation programs, quality control needs to be determined to see if future rehabilitation programs meet the standards of that time and make a difference in the lives of head-injured survivors. More sensitive instruments to measure rehabilitation outcomes and an array of individuals not involved in rehabilitation today will be involved in assessing the quality of rehabilitation programs.

Throughout the rehabilitation process, the patient and family will be key members of the team that is in charge of setting goals and making a variety of choices, particularly at the time when the community-reintegration process begins. Interdependence among health care professionals, the patient, the family, the workplace, and the school system will be taken for granted. As the client and family become active in setting goals and selecting choices, they will assume the responsibility arising from those privileges and may require legal counseling. Having acute rehabilitation at home, as well as transitional living programs, qualifies the family for the assistance of a home health aide. More respite care may become available to families. This will relieve family members and enable their continued employment, lessening complete financial and psychological collapse, which is frequent at the present time.

PREVENTION

Although many unanswered questions remain, many positive things are happening that bode well for the future. Much is being done in the area of prevention. A lot of development is occurring to minimize bodily damage in motor vehicles and other forms of transportation. Safety features continue to be added to motor vehicles. Prevention programs will be part of the curriculums of schools in the future, teaching children about the consequences of risk factors such as alcohol, drug consumption, and firearms. Head injury will not be eliminated. Undoubtedly, TBI will remain a catastrophe in some cases. However, hope and optimism prevail in the future for survivors in improved management of both acute and chronic stages of their recovery.

REFERENCES

Case, R. (1992). The role of the frontal lobes in the regulation of cognitive development. *Brain and Cognition, 20,* 51–73.

Gentry, L. R. (1994). Imaging of closed head injury. *Radiology, 191,* 1–17.

McIntosh, T. K. (1994). Neurochemical sequelae of traumatic brain injury: Therapeutic implications. *Cerebrovascular and Brain Metabolism Reviews, 9,* 109–162.

Rasmusson, D. X., Brandt, J., Martin, D. B., & Folstein, M. F. (1995). Head injury as a risk factor in Alzheimer's disease. *Brain Injury, 9,* 213–219.

Teasdale, G., & Jennett, B. (1974). Assessment of coma and impaired consciousness. A practical scale. *Lancet, 2,* 81–84.

Thatcher, R. W. (1992). Cyclic cortical reorganization during early childhood. *Brain and Cognition, 20,* 24–30.

Wilkins, R. H. (1985). History of neurosurgery. In R. H. Wilkins & S. S. Rengachary (Eds.), *Neurosurgery* (Vol. 1, pp. 3–15). New York: McGraw-Hill.

Author Index

Grip, J. C., 105, *111*
Groah, C., 262, 263, *271*
Grossman, R. I., 9, *28*, 129, 130, *138,*
    257, *271*, 308, *320*
Grosswasser, Z., 8, *28*, 85, *96*, 227, *233*
Gualtieri, C. T., 101, 102, 105, 106, *110,*
    111
Guinto, F. C., Jr., 30, *37*
Guitar, B., 173, *183*
Gulenchlyn, K. Y., 9, *28*
Gurney, J. G., 140, *147*
Guyot, J. F., 68, *79*

H

Haas, J. F., 107, *111*
Haas, L. J., 106, *111*
Habib, A. H. A., 57, *62*
Hadley, D. M., 9, *28*, 29, *37*
Haggerty, R., 283, *288*
Haig, A. J., 103, *111*
Haining, J. L., 43, *48*
Haley, E. C., 42, 45, *49*
Halgren, E., 156, *160*
Hall, E. D., 45, *50*
Hall, K. M., 229, *233*
Halley, M., 68, 69, 70, 71, 76, 78, *79*
Halliday, A., *28*
Halstead, W. C., 119, 126, *127*
Hamm, R. J., 52, *62*, 68, 70, *79*
Hansen, A. J., 51, 53, 54, 55, *62*
Hanson, D. G., 168, *183*
Hardy, J. C., 164, *183*
Harlow, H. F., 201, *216*
Harp, J. A., 310, 311, *321*
Harrell, M., 318, *320*
Harris, B. S. H., 257, *271*
Harris, J. A., 116, 122, *127*, 142, 143,
    147, 148
Harris, R. J., 57, *65*
Hart, B. L., *28*
Hartman, D. E., 116, *127*
Hasan, D., 47, *48*
Hausen, J., 42, *50*
Haut, A. E., 277, *286*
Haut, M. W., 124, *127*
Haut, W., 277, *286*
Hawkins, J. D., 283, 284, *286*
Hayashi, N., 68, *72*
Hayes, R. L., 51, 52, 57, 59, *62*, 68, 70,
    71, 72, *79*, 101, *111*
Heaton, R. K., 119, 126, *127*
Hebb, D. O., 200, *216*
Hegedus, K., 189, *194*

Heinrichs, W. R., 122, *127*
Heiskanen, O., 42, 46, *49*
Heitzer, M. L., 67, *79*
Heller, D., 129, *138*
Hepworth, J., 275, *287*
Hernandez-Caceres, J., 55, *62*
Hieshima, G. B., 8, *27*
High, W. M., Jr., 30, *37*, 105, *111*
Hijdra, A., 47, *50*
Hillered, L., 51, *64*
Hinton, V. A., 169, *183*
Hirayam, T., 68, *72*
Hirayama, T., 94, *97*
Hixon, T. J., 164, *184*
Hof-Van Duin Van, J., 191, *194*
Holloway, K. L., 76, *78*
Holness, R. D., 45, *49*
Hopkins, K., 229, *233*
Hoppe, D., 60, *64*
Horii, Y., 168, *183*
Horn, L. J., 191, 192, *194*
Hovda, D., 51, 52, 53, 54, 57, 58, *63*, *65*
Howse, D. C., 57, *62*
Huber, P., 44, *49*
Humphrey, M., 277, *287*
Humphrey, P. R., 45, *49*
Hundley, M. B., 45, *49*
Hunt, W. E., 40, *48*
Hunter, K. M., 45, *49*
Huttenlocher, P., 201, *216*
Hwang, P., *28*
Hyatt, M. S., 9, *27*

I

Ichise, M., 157, *160*
Iengo, M., 168, *183*
Ikezaki, K., 55, 56, *64*
Illingworth, R., 45, *49*
Ingram, C. R., 45, *48*
Ingram, J. C. L., 166, 173, *183*
Isaacs, M. L., 141, *147*
Ishige, N., 67, *79*
Ishikawa, K., 58, *63*
Isseroff, A., 201, *216*
Iwai, A., 72, *80*

J

Jackson, R. D., 106, *111*
Jackson, W., 130, *138*
Jacobs, H., 226, *233*
Jaffe, K. M., 275, 282, 283, *287*
Jampala, V. C., 156, *160*

Subject Index

S

Sepsis, 67
Seritonergic tricyclic, 106
Serotonin, 109
Spinal cord injury, 95
Single photon emission computed tomography (SPECT), 8–9, 18, 116, 150–151, 155, 157, 252, 325
Skull fracture, 8, 153
Speech, 104, 165, 172–176, 178, 182, 221, 242
Spinothalamic, 94
Stroke, 27
Substance abuse, 139–144, 146
Sulcus, 15–16
Superconducting quantum interference device (SQUID), 10

T

Tachycardia, 187
Tactual Performance Test, 126
Tardive dyskinesia, 101
Temporal lobe disease, 150, 155
Temporoalis muscle, 69
Tetraethylammonium, 55
Tetraethyltris-methylammonium, 55
Thalamotomy, 90, 93
Thalamus, 71–72
Therapy, 47, 172–174, 176, 179, 240, 309

Transcranial Doppler ultrasound, 44
Traumatic Brain Injury (TBI), 7–9, 39, 51–53, 55, 59–61, 67–73, 76, 78, 83–85, 96, 99, 101, 103–110, 115–123, 129–130, 139–147, 150, 157, 185, 190–192, 219–221, 223–224, 226–229, 231–232, 247–248, 251–252, 254, 257, 259–260, 262–265, 269–270, 275–286, 289, 292–294, 299, 302–319, 324, 328
Tremor, 93–94
Tumors, 236

V

Valproate, 108
Vascular endothelium, 45
Vasospasm, 39, 42, 44–47, 324
Vegetative state (VS), 185–193
Velopharyngeal function, 168, 171–172
Videostroboscopy, 168

W

Wechsler Adult Intelligence Scale (WAIS), 32, 123, 260
Wechsler Intelligence Scale for Children (WISC), 210
Wechsler Memory Scale (WMS), 32
Wide Range Achievement Test-revised (WRAT-R), 260
World Health Organization, 250, 255

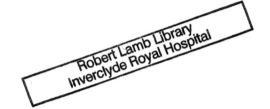